THE Blue Zones
American Kitchen

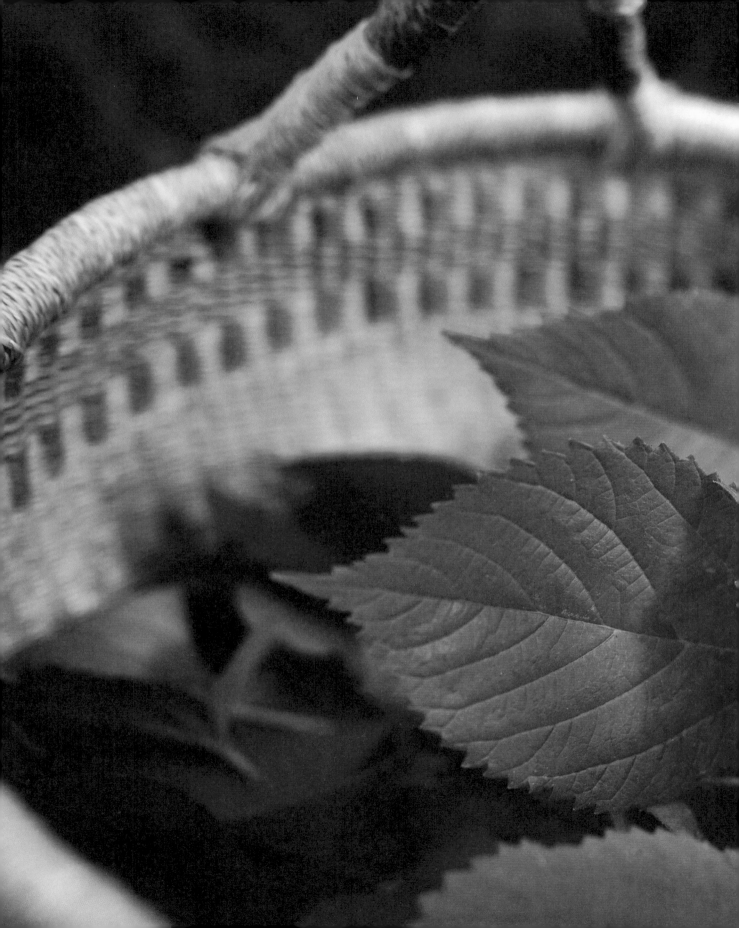

THE
Blue Zones
American Kitchen

100 RECIPES TO LIVE TO 100

DAN BUETTNER

WITH PHOTOGRAPHS BY DAVID McLAIN

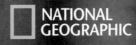

NATIONAL
GEOGRAPHIC

WASHINGTON, DC

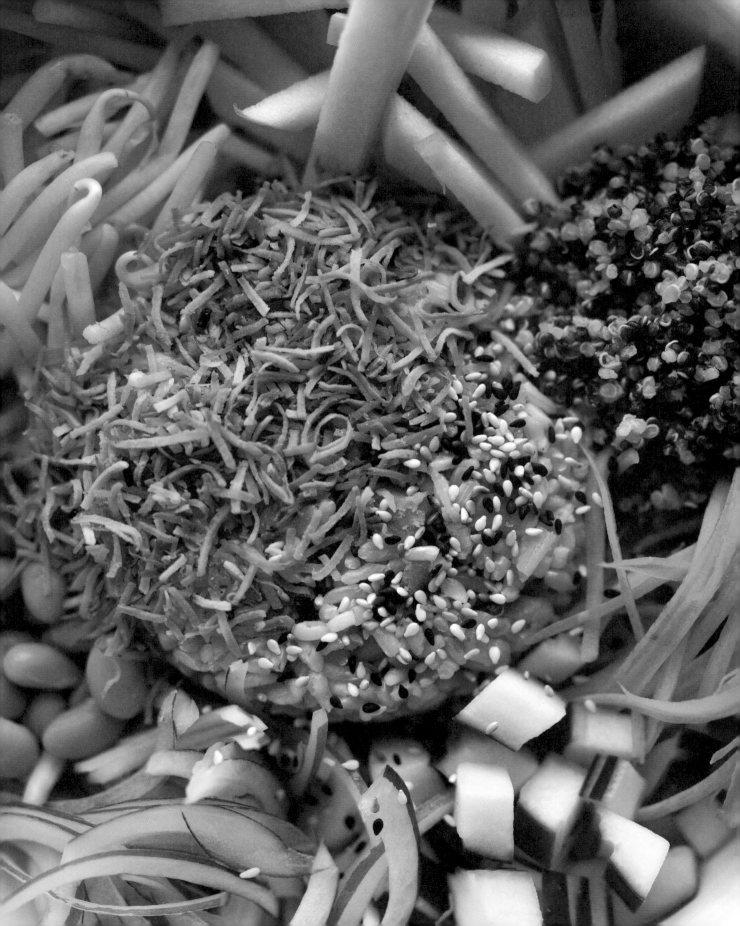

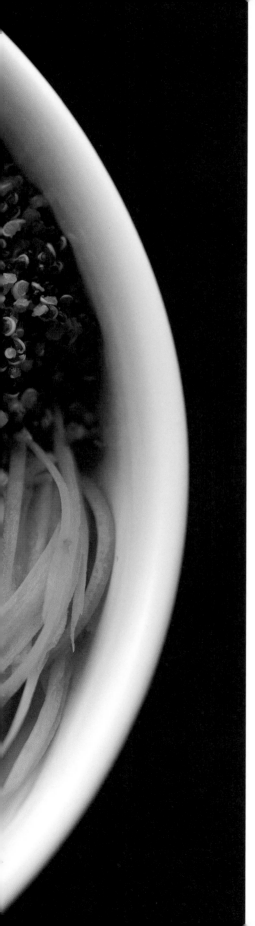

CONTENTS

Opposite: Thai chef Nat Ruengsamutr prepared Khao Yum (Rainbow Rice Salad, page 183). Pages 2–3: On a visit to Minneapolis, we foraged for wild greens with chef Alan Bergo (page 243).

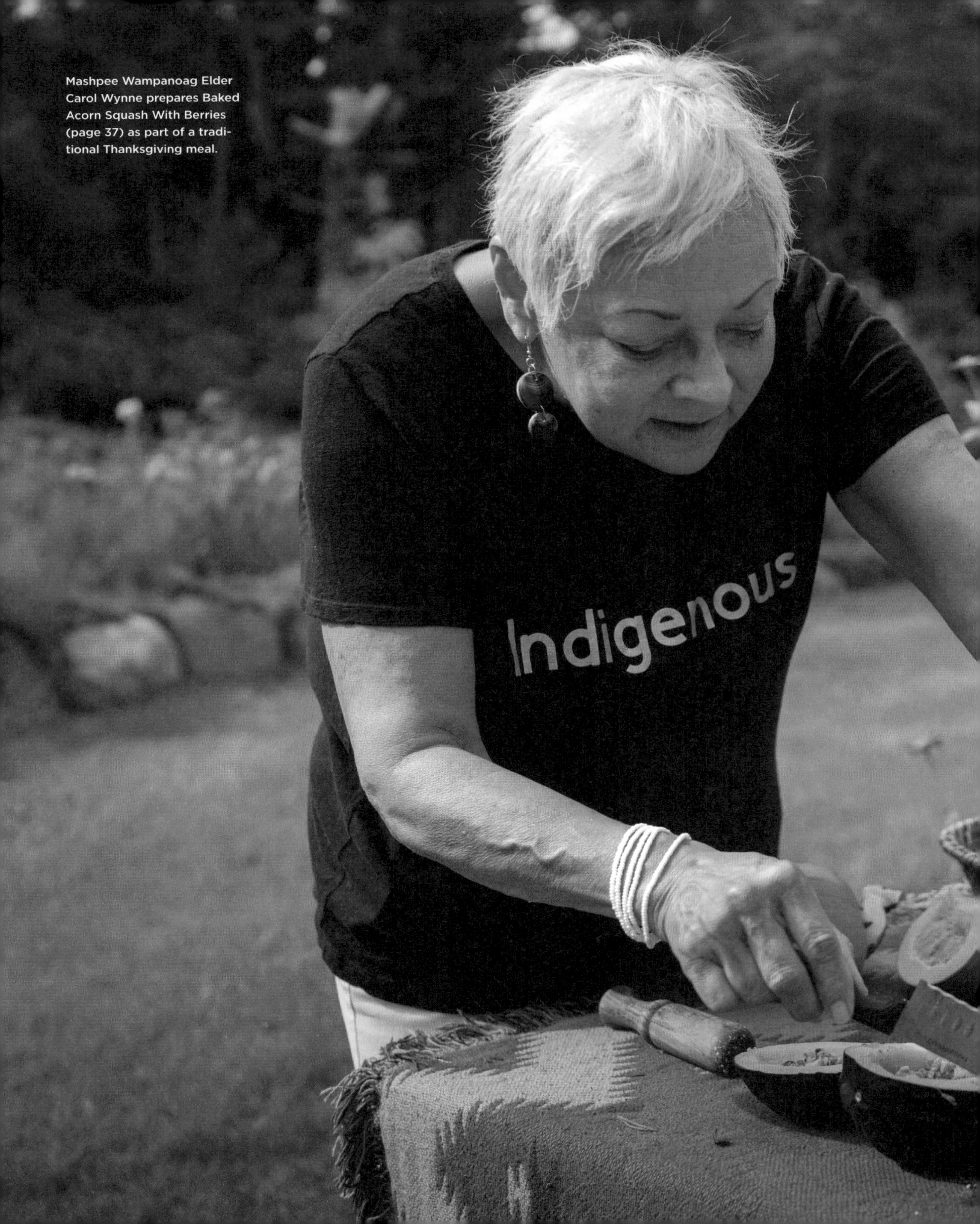

Mashpee Wampanoag Elder Carol Wynne prepares Baked Acorn Squash With Berries (page 37) as part of a traditional Thanksgiving meal.

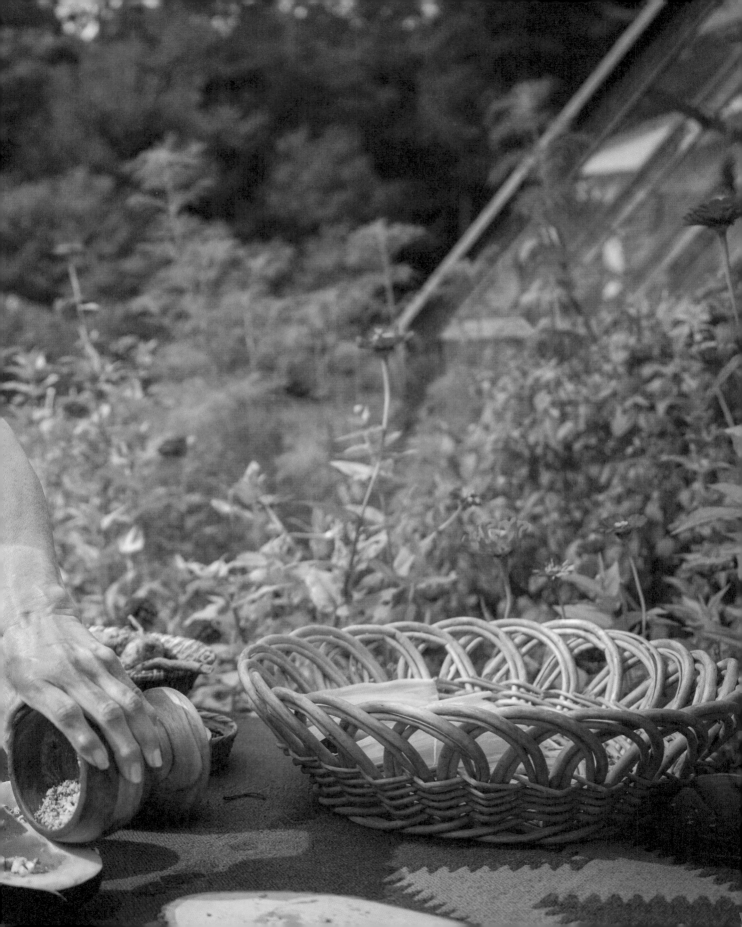

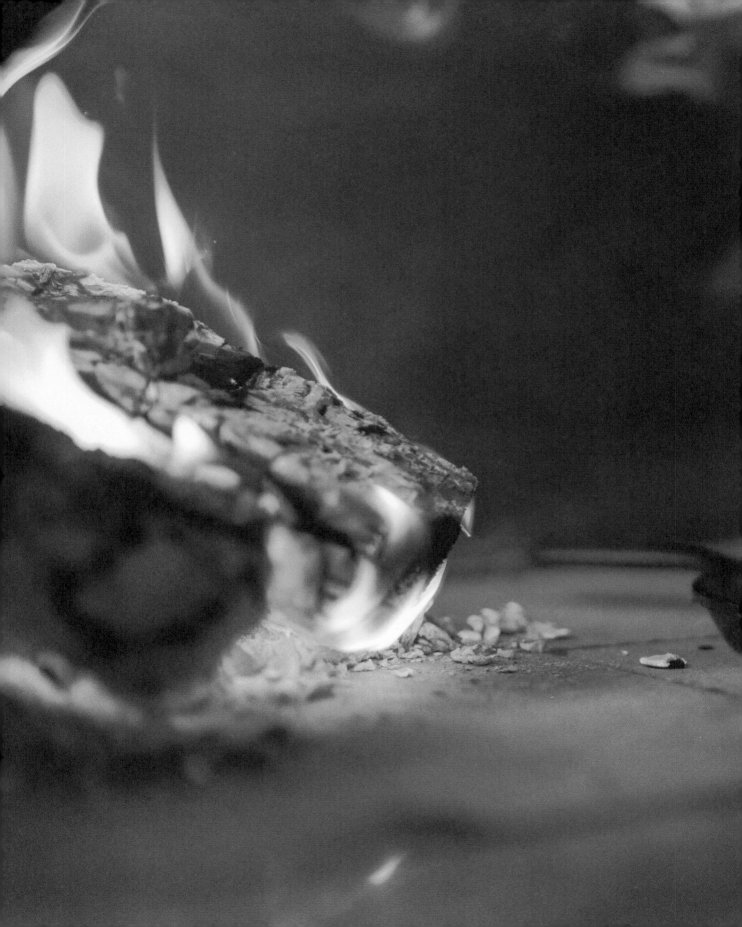

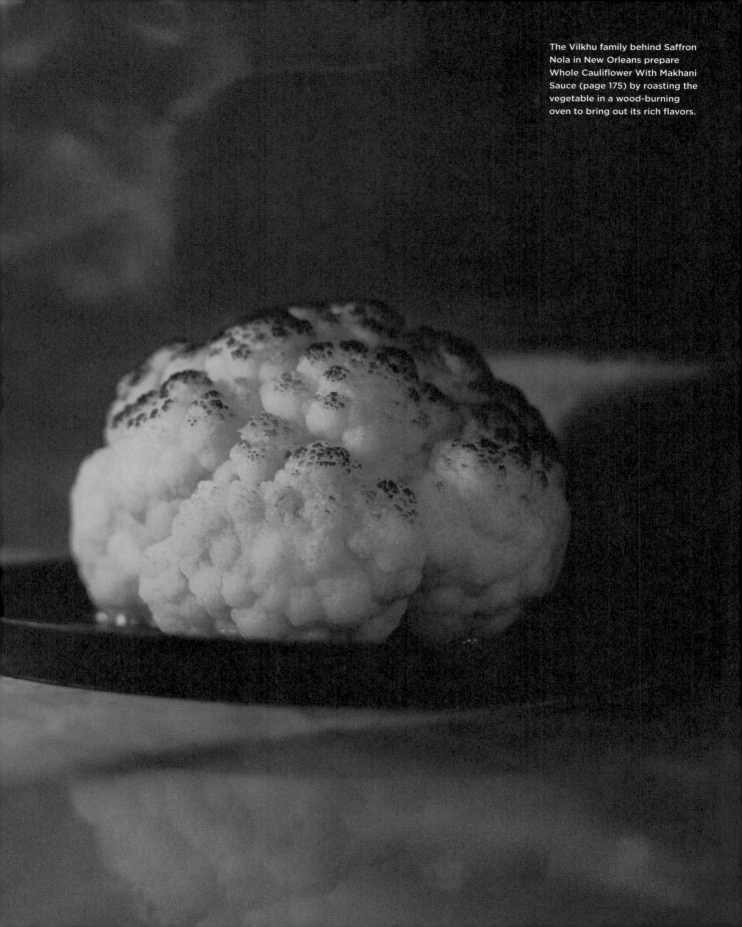

The Vilkhu family behind Saffron Nola in New Orleans prepare Whole Cauliflower With Makhani Sauce (page 175) by roasting the vegetable in a wood-burning oven to bring out its rich flavors.

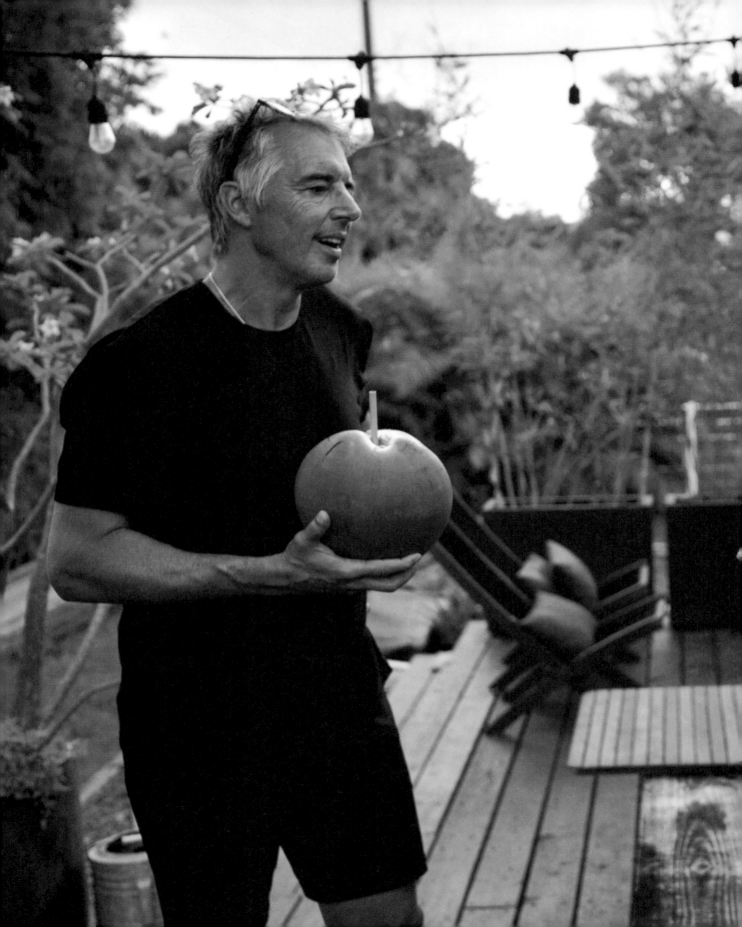

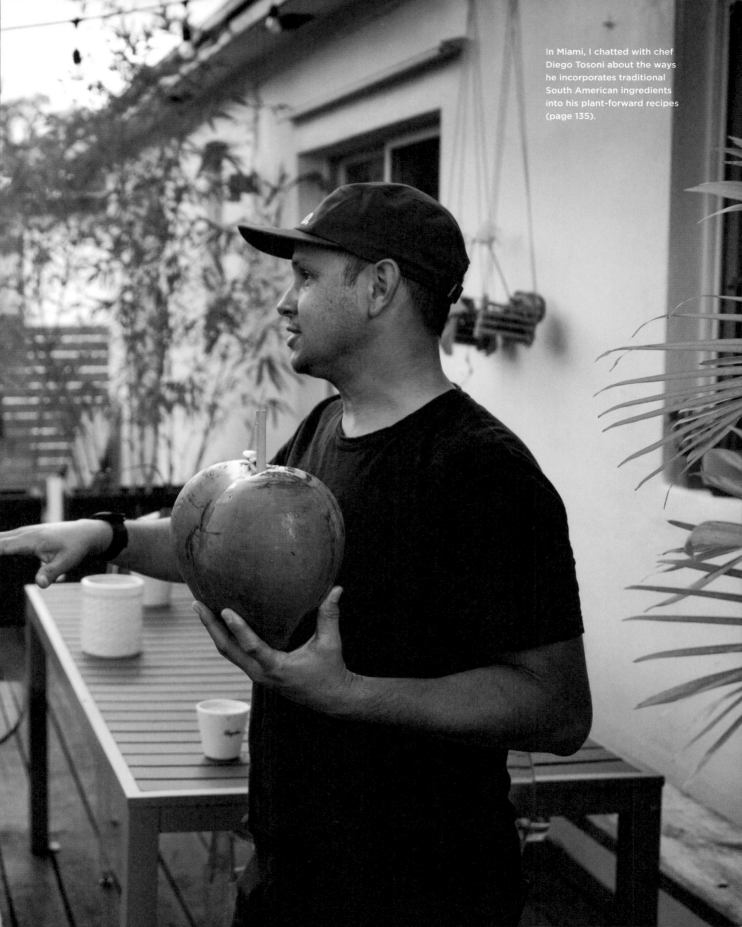

In Miami, I chatted with chef Diego Tosoni about the ways he incorporates traditional South American ingredients into his plant-forward recipes (page 135).

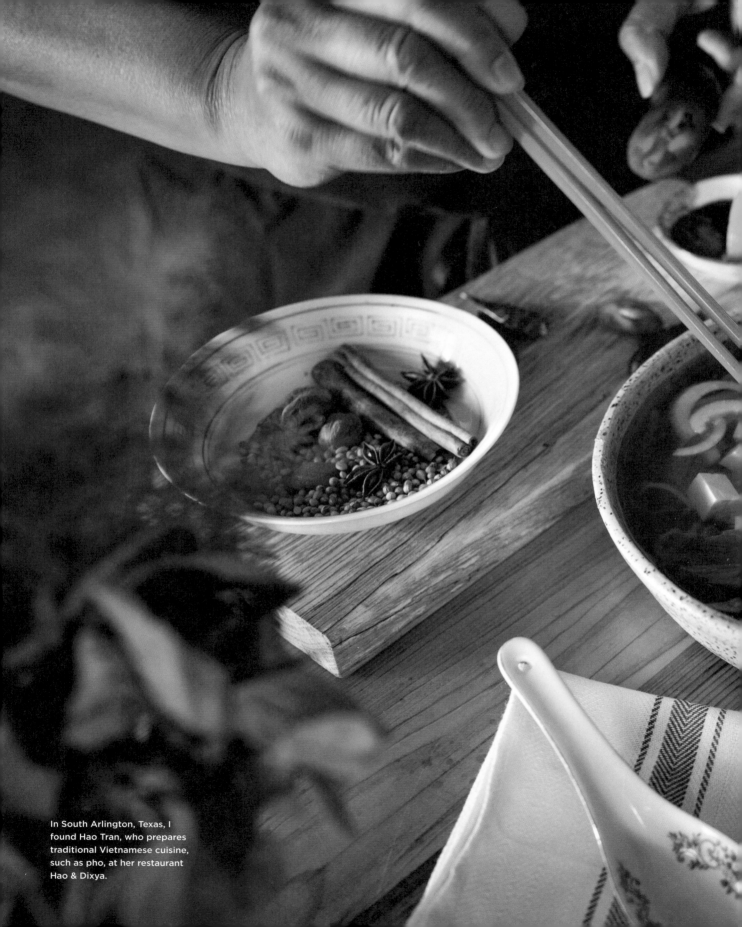

In South Arlington, Texas, I found Hao Tran, who prepares traditional Vietnamese cuisine, such as pho, at her restaurant Hao & Dixya.

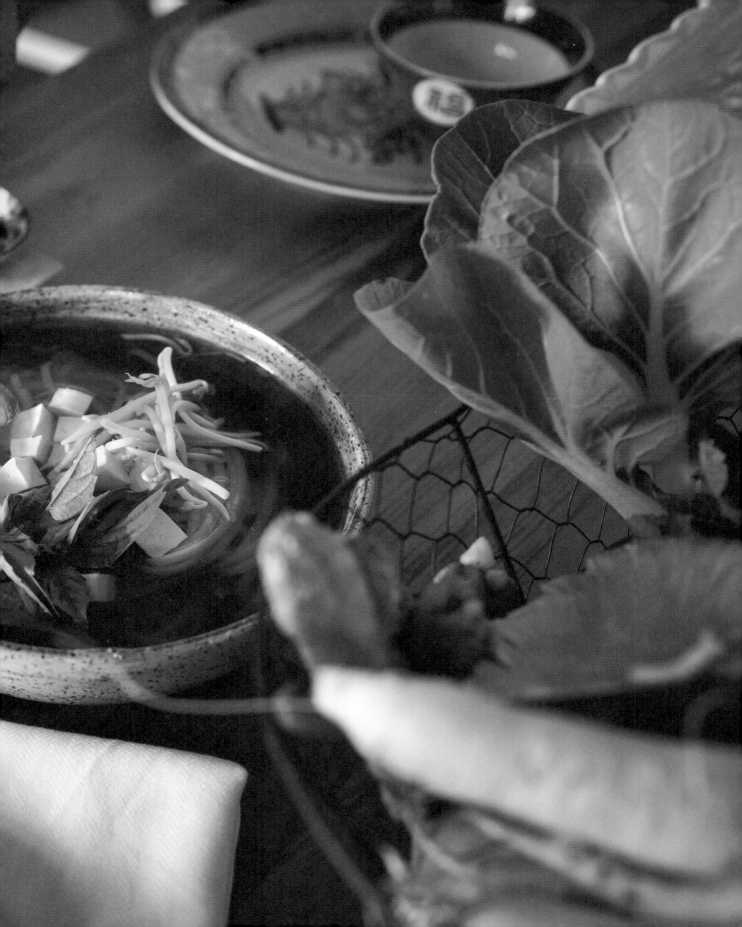

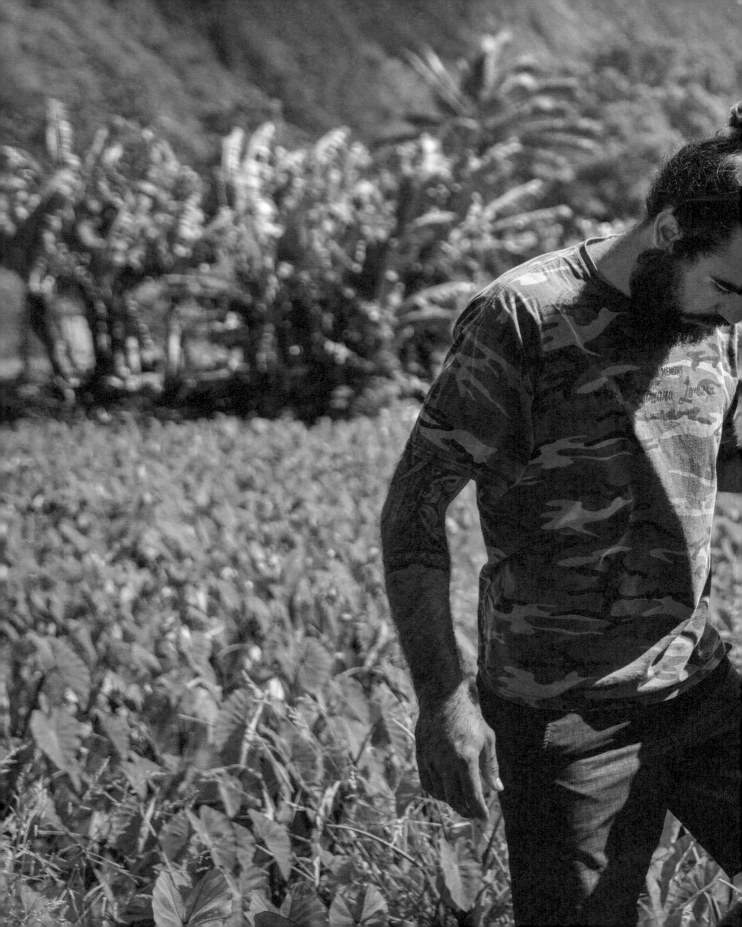

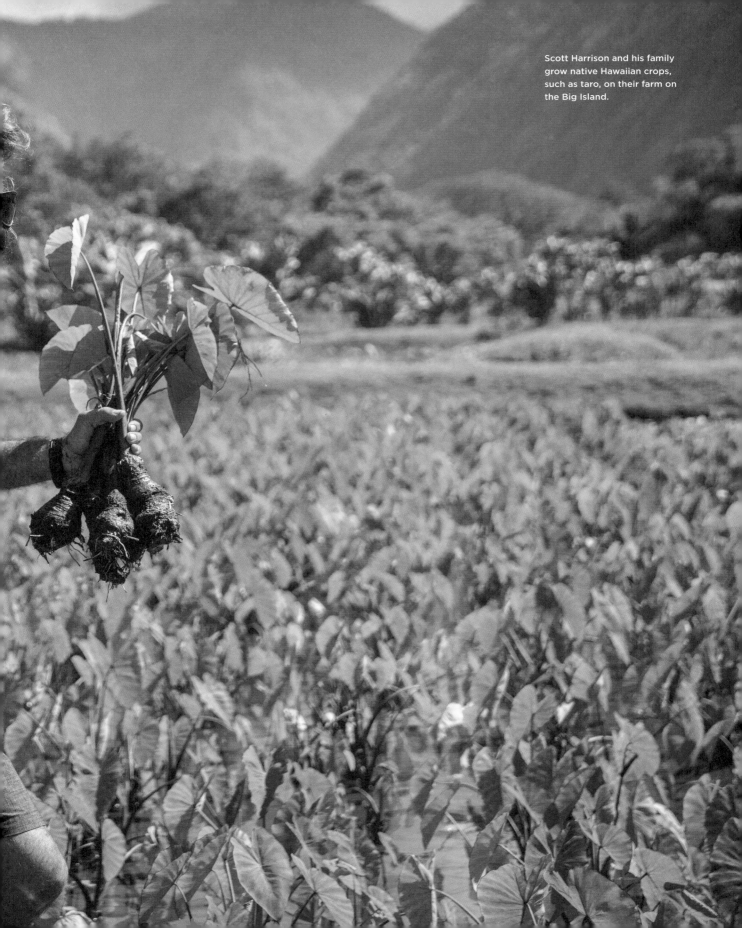

Scott Harrison and his family grow native Hawaiian crops, such as taro, on their farm on the Big Island.

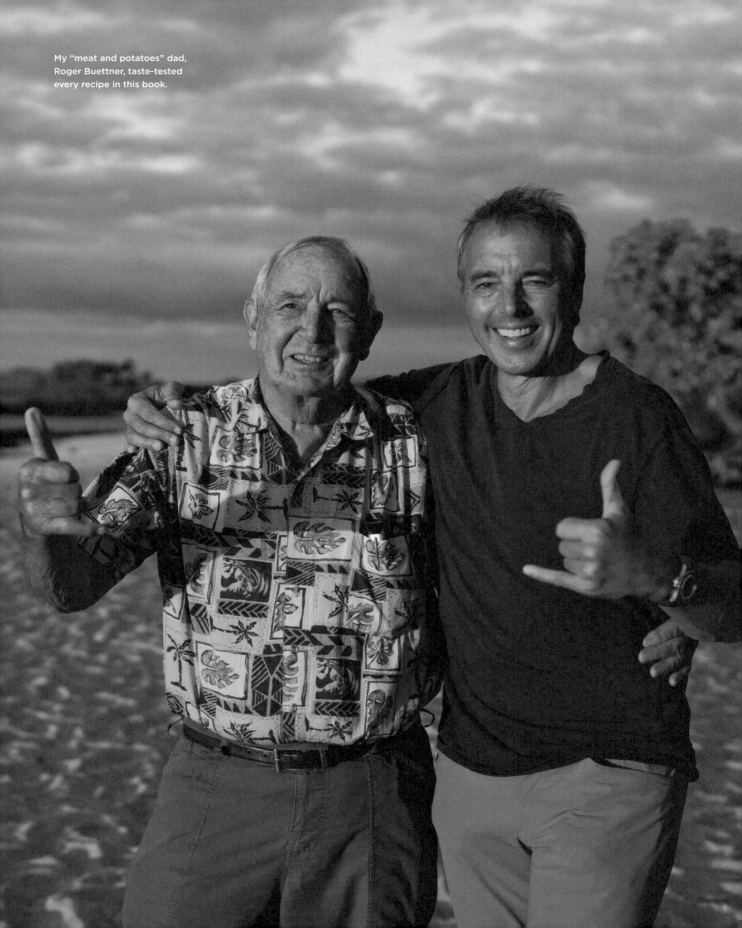

My "meat and potatoes" dad, Roger Buettner, taste-tested every recipe in this book.

Introduction

This book could help you live an extra 10 good years.

In 2022, 750,000 people in the United States will die from eating the standard American diet. Among those deaths, nearly 443,000 will die from high blood pressure, 213,000 from high blood sugar, and 158,000 from high cholesterol. Meanwhile, in 2022, Americans will spend approximately $3.7 trillion on health care, 85 percent of it on treating preventable diseases largely driven by what we eat.

This may not come as a shock when you consider that each year the average American consumes about 144 pounds of meat (the equivalent of 856 hamburgers), 130 pounds of sugar (including some 39 gallons of soda pop), 17 gallons of milk, and 35 pounds of cheese—some of which tops our annual 46 slices of pizza. Seventy percent of our calories come from processed foods, which collectively contain about 2,700 artificial food additives, many of them known to cause cancer.

There is strong evidence that eating less meat, especially processed meat, reduces the risk of heart disease, and moderate evidence that it reduces the risk of obesity and cancers of the colon, liver, lung, and pancreas. The World Health Organization classifies processed meats (lunch meats, hot dogs, bacon, etc.) in the same category as cigarettes, a known carcinogen. "Replacing one serving per day of red meat with a serving of nuts would reduce total mortality by approximately 20 percent," says Dr. Walter Willett, professor of epidemiology and nutrition at the Harvard T.H. Chan School of Public Health and professor of medicine at Harvard Medical School.

According to the Centers for Disease Control and Prevention, Americans consume more sugar than people in any other country in the world. Added sugars contribute to obesity, type 2 diabetes, hypertension, stroke, gout, and Alzheimer's disease, and they fuel the growth of many cancers.

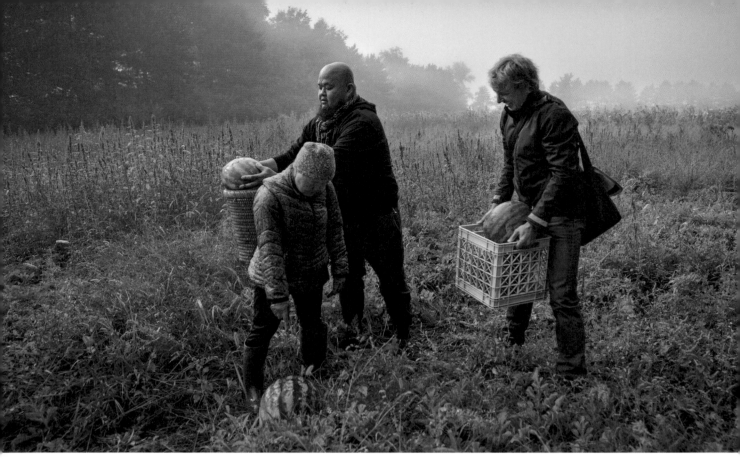

Yia Vang and I help his mother, Pang Vang, harvest traditional Hmong crops from her robust back-yard garden in a suburban area outside Minneapolis, Minnesota.

But what if I told you there is another American diet, one that could actually increase your life expectancy by up to 10 years and in some cases reverse disease? This is not a fad diet invented by a South Beach doctor, paleo pseudoscientist, or social media influencer. This diet was developed by common Americans. It is affordable for almost everyone and sustainable, and it has a minuscule carbon footprint. Most important, it is hearty and delicious, developed over centuries by fusing flavors from the Old World and the New World in ingenious and uniquely American ways.

For the past 20 years writing for National Geographic, I have identified the world's longest-lived areas (blue zones) and studied the patterns and lifestyles that seem to explain their populations' longevity. These places—Okinawa, Japan; Sardinia, Italy; Ikaria, Greece; Nicoya, Costa Rica; and the Seventh Day Adventist community in Loma Linda, California—produce populations with the highest centenarian rate and the highest middle-age life expectancy. People in these places suffer, in some cases, a fifth the rate of heart disease, a sixth the rate of dementia, and a sixth the rate of certain cancers compared with Americans. Until very recently, the obesity and diabetes rates in each were under 5 percent. The people in the blue zones live up to a decade longer than average Americans and spend a fraction of what most the rest of us do on health care.

How do they achieve this extraordinary longevity? It's never one thing but rather a cluster of mutually supporting factors that keep people doing the right things and avoiding the wrong things for long enough not to develop chronic diseases.

Essentially, they live in environments that make healthy choices unavoidable. As a result, they're not developing heart disease, type 2 diabetes, obesity, dementia, certain cancers, and other diseases that would otherwise shorten their lives. They live in places where every time they go to work, to a friend's house, or out to eat, getting there involves a walk. Their lives are underpinned with purpose, so they're not experiencing existential stress or waking up wondering what the day holds. Loneliness—a life-shortening condition (as bad as smoking 10 cigarettes daily) that affects some 25 percent of Americans—isn't an option in blue zones: Streets are full of walking neighbors, village festivals are regularly attended, and religious services are full. They also eat a special diet.

In my book *The Blue Zones Solution,* I explored a legitimate diet of longevity. Working under the guidance of Dr. Walter Willett, I aggregated more than 150 dietary surveys capturing the daily eating habits of people in the blue zones over the past 80 years. When we "averaged" those diets over time, we discovered that long-lived people eat remarkably similarly all over the world.

What are they eating? Ninety to 100 percent of their calories come from whole-food, plant-based sources. In a word, they eat a high-carbohydrate diet. The term *carbohydrate* is probably the worst dietary term ever coined, as it encompasses everything from jelly beans to lentil beans. Simple carbohydrates like chips, white flour, and sweets are probably the most toxic foods in our diet, while complex carbohydrates like whole grains, tubers, and beans are probably the healthiest foods we eat. In blue zones, 65 percent of the dietary intake comes from those healthy complex carbs; in fact, whole grains, greens, tubers, nuts, and beans are the five pillars of a longevity diet on four continents.

In the blue zones, long-lived people eat very little fish and eggs. Meat is a celebratory food, consumed only five times a month. And though they enjoy small amounts of sheep and goat cheese, dairy from cows is almost completely absent from the diet.

Sugar doesn't figure much into their diets either, except as honey for drinks or desserts and occasionally in baked goods for festivals. In all, people of the blue zones consume about seven teaspoons of sugar a day, about a third of the 22 or so teaspoons the average American consumes daily. They drink water, teas of all kinds, black coffee, and wine, including a garnet-red Cannonau in Sardinia that is rich in heart-healthy antioxidants like resveratrol and flavonoids like procyanidins. Soda pop was unknown to most of the 350 centenarians I interviewed.

How much longer can you live if you eat a Blue Zones diet? Up to 10.7 years for women and 13 for men in the United States, according to a recent study. A team of

Norwegian researchers developed a methodology to examine the impact of food choices as indicated by recent meta-analyses of the Global Burden of Disease study, which includes data on 286 causes of death in 204 countries and territories. They calculated that sustaining changes made by moving from a typical Western diet to an optimized intake could add years to almost anyone's life span. "The largest gains would be made by eating more legumes, whole grains and nuts, and less red and processed meat," the study concluded. They estimated that for the U.S. population to improve their diet in this way, a 20-year-old could add up to 13 years to their life, a 60-year-old could add up to 8.8 years, and even an 80-year-old could add 3.5 years. The kicker: Eating a Blue Zones diet would likely add even more good years.

In 2019, as the COVID-19 pandemic set in, National Geographic photographer David McLain and I hatched an idea to search for an American Blue Zones diet. Sensing that our great-grandparents may have eaten similarly to the way people eat in the original blue zones, we began by looking into dietary surveys conducted in the early 1900s. To our dismay, we found that some of our ancestors (immigrants from northern and central Europe) brought their cows, pigs, and pickles with them. The average family in 1900 was made up of 4.6 persons and on average consumed 855 pounds of dressed weight meat, which equals 680 pounds of edible meat.

That amount is comparable to what we eat in the United States today—147.8 pounds per person versus 144 pounds per person every year.

Sugar consumption, which has been described today as food enemy number one, was somewhat less prevalent in the 1900s, when the average American ate about 90 pounds per year, compared with the 130 pounds eaten today.

Processed foods are a different story. One might argue that processed foods have been around ever since early humans used salt to preserve meat and fish. In ancient China, paraffin was burned to ripen fruit. Egyptians colored food with saffron; Romans added alum (potassium aluminum sulfate) to bread to make it whiter. In 1869, chemist Hippolyte Mège-Mouriès invented margarine, and a decade later a chemist isolated saccharin (the main ingredient of artificial sweeteners) after noticing a sweet taste on his hands as he experimented with a coal tar derivative. But other than these junk food vanguards, people were eating mostly real food.

America's food environment progressively deteriorated as the 20th century unfolded. Before World War II, food processing was relatively simple and mechanical—for example, breaking down wheat kernels into still identifiable flour, germ, and chaff, and vacuum-sealing vegetables in tin cans. But after the war, food technologists began to go much further, breaking raw grains down to their basic molecular structure and reassembling them into foods that bore no resemblance to the raw materials out of which they were fabricated.

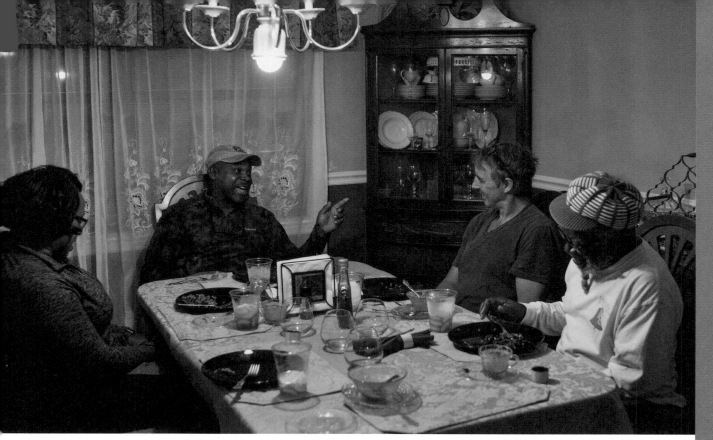

Over a meal of Hoppin' John (page 90), Rollen Chalmers (head of the table) shares stories of his family's food lineage and his experience cultivating heritage crops like Carolina Gold rice.

In 1957, the process for high fructose corn syrup (HFCS) was developed, and within a decade it was being rapidly introduced into foods. Derived from corn, which was (and still is) subsidized by the U.S. government, HFCS quickly became a cheaper sweetener for soft drinks and the preferred sweetener for food and beverage manufacturers. HFCS is metabolically very different from sugar because it tells the body to store calories and is linked to obesity, hypertension, and diabetes. By 2008, the average American was consuming about 38 pounds of HFCS annually.

The 1970s seems to have been the worst decade for the food environment. Factory farms became the preferred business model for meat production, subjecting animals to enclosed, unclean, dark, poorly ventilated, and horribly overcrowded indoor industrial settings. Disease and infections ran rampant. The use of bovine growth hormone and antibiotics, and the addition of vitamin supplements to corn and soy feed, created fast-growing and fatter but less nutritious livestock.

Meanwhile, the food industry revolutionized. Artificial sweeteners like aspartame and saccharin were approved by the Food and Drug Administration. Earl Butz, secretary of agriculture under President Richard Nixon—responding to pressure from his boss to increase the food supply—built the infrastructure to favor corn, wheat, soybeans, and sugar beets: inexpensive, government-subsidized inputs for the meat and junk food industries. He also encouraged large-scale importation of palm oil, a cheap but unhealthy fat. These policies resulted directly in the larger and larger portions offered by fast-food outlets and soft-drink producers.

The fat-free craze drove the development of citrus fiber, maltodextrin, sucralose, gums, and carrageenan to mimic the mouthfeel and flavor-enhancing characteristic of fat. As Mark Schatzker argues in his book *The End of Craving,* these artificial ingredients conspire to confuse the brain into craving more calories while leaving our bodies nutritionally wanting. And that nutritional mismatch disrupts metabolism on an elemental level, harming the human body.

As unhealthy calories got cheaper, they also got harder to escape. The number of fast-food establishments grew significantly—from 58,000 in 1970 to more than 253,000 in 2015. More than 50 percent of all retail outlets, including tire repair shops, car washes, and pharmacies (which sell diabetes medicine) force us to shop through a gauntlet of sugar-sweetened beverages, snacks, and candies. We are hardwired to crave sugar, fat, and salt from our evolution in an environment of hardship and scarcity. Now we live in an environment of overabundance and ease. We're told to muster discipline and self-control all day every day. But discipline is like a muscle, and muscles fatigue. Our food supply today provides about 4,000 calories daily per person, twice the average need. In 1980, 15 percent of Americans were obese. Now 45 percent of us are. Between 1979 and 2008, the weight of the average American woman increased by more than 20 pounds; the weight of the average American man increased by about 23 pounds.

Still, I was hell-bent on searching for a Blue Zones diet in America. I called my friend Jeff Gordinier, former food writer for the *New York Times.* He told me about a vegan movement in the African American community that is bringing back pre-1920s traditions. He also introduced me to the James Beard Award–winning chef Sean Sherman (founder of the Sioux Chef), who is popularizing cuisines of Indigenous peoples, and chef-historian Adán Medrano, who is bringing back true Texas-Mexican cuisine. As I spoke with each chef and explored their cuisines, I noticed the ingredients of these food traditions closely resembled what people were eating in blue zones.

To confirm the hunch, James Edward Malin, a food studies researcher and an engineering and science librarian at the Cooper Union in New York, and I exhumed more than 60 oral histories, scientific reports, and academic papers to reconstruct several traditional American diets. The mother lode, however, came from the work of an agricultural chemist named Wilbur Olin Atwater. In 1887, he and his colleagues at the U.S. Department of Agriculture's Office of Experimental Stations launched the first "dietaries" in various communities. For this project, field researchers went directly into households and recorded every bit of food the families ate over a period of several weeks. The resulting reports provide a remarkably data-driven representation of exactly what people were eating more than a century ago.

Fortunately, Atwater wasn't interested only in white people, as many scientists of

AVG % ANIMAL-BASED CALORIES PER DAY

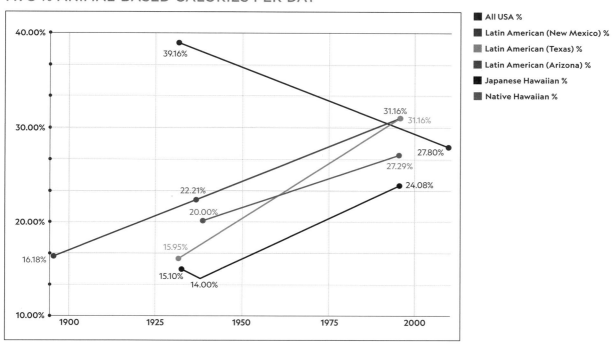

Legend:
- All USA %
- Latin American (New Mexico) %
- Latin American (Texas) %
- Latin American (Arizona) %
- Japanese Hawaiian %
- Native Hawaiian %

AVG TOTAL CALORIES PER DAY

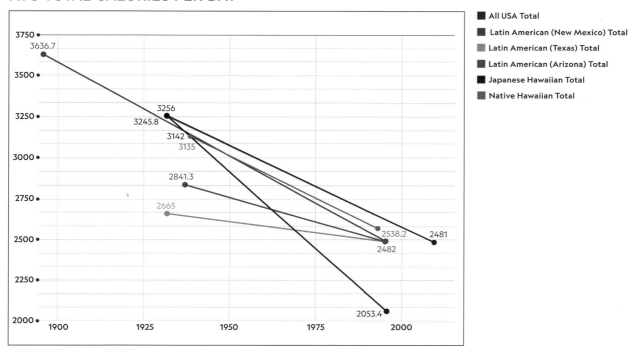

Legend:
- All USA Total
- Latin American (New Mexico) Total
- Latin American (Texas) Total
- Latin American (Arizona) Total
- Japanese Hawaiian Total
- Native Hawaiian Total

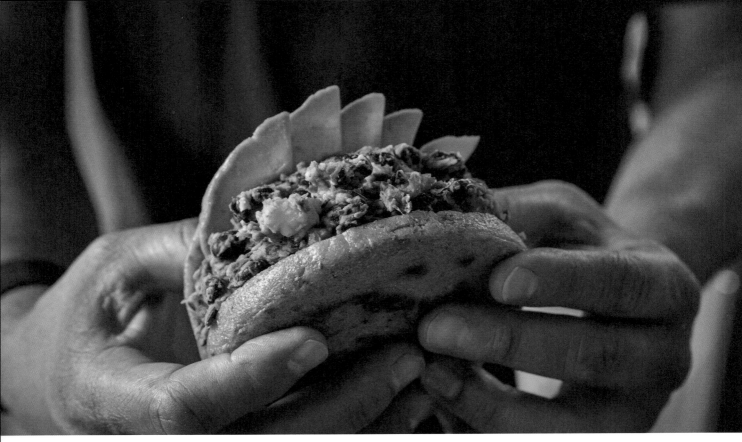

Diego Tosoni, chef of Love Life Café in Miami, prepared a Plant-Powered Arepa (page 135) that is as delicious as it is versatile for meals.

the day were. The scope of his work was ethnically and racially diverse, precisely capturing the diets of Mexican, Asian, and African Americans. His data from the late 1880s to the early 1930s shows that Mexican American and Asian American diets were 84 percent and 88 percent plant-based, respectively.

African Americans living in the Deep South also have a long tradition of eating blue-zones-type foods. A West African plant-based diet, passed along through centuries of enslavement, persecution, and oppression, amalgamated into a vivid and delicious food culture focused on local and nutritious ingredients. Dietary surveys dating back to the 1890s indicate that the vast majority of foods eaten by Southern African Americans were vegetables and grains. Aside from salt pork—mostly added for flavor—animal products played a minor role in the African American diet of the late 19th and early 20th centuries. One 1928 study from Mississippi observed lean meat intake was as low as 3.5 percent. Furthermore, Southern African Americans living in 1897 consumed about a third as much sugar as we do today.

Latin Americans had similar Blue Zones diets. Dietaries from before WWII indicate that the Indigenous communities in New Mexico and Texas ate only about 16 percent animal calories—likely the lowest recorded at the time. Early records show native Latin American sugar consumption was close to 10 teaspoons a day. This food culture contrasted sharply with that of non-Hispanic white Americans around 100 years ago, who ate a diet with almost 40 percent animal products and double the amount of sugar.

Asian Americans one century ago had the bluest Blue Zones diet of all. Combining information from different communities around the country, one report indicated that Asian Americans got about 5.5 percent of their calories from sugar and about 19 percent from animal products.

Armed with these dietary surveys—and with the help of producer Karen Foshay, my amazing editor, Naomi Imatome-Yun, and chief of staff, Sam Skemp—David and I hit the road to search for chefs and food historians who could re-create these cuisines from 100 years ago. On six separate trips, often traveling in a Sprinter van, David and I canvassed the United States. I recorded the ingredients, cooking techniques, and oral histories of how these chefs are preserving their cultural traditions. Meanwhile, David captured the setting, portraits, and creations of these culinary historians. Then I commissioned my dad, Roger Buettner, to taste-test and approve the recipes. Dad grew up on a meat-and-potatoes farm in the Midwest. We reasoned that if he didn't like the food, the average American wouldn't either.

We traveled from New England (where a Wampanoag chef prepared a true "Thanksgiving dinner"), to Pennsylvania (where abolitionists and vegetarians grew out of the same compassionate impulse), to Appalachia (where we discovered how coal-mining stores corrupted a very healthy cuisine), and to Miami, with its budding Latin-vegan scene. On we went to New Orleans (where a first-generation Senegalese chef demonstrated a $100-a-plate re-creation of the "last meal" once fed to his enslaved ancestors), to Oklahoma (where a Native American chef made tortillas from 1,000-year-old corn varieties she's preserved), and to Hawaii (where we captured the diverse and healthy pre-WWII fusion of Hawaiian, Chinese, Japanese, Portuguese, and Filipino cuisine that Spam nearly destroyed). Finally, we ended our journey in the Midwest, where a Wisconsin chef-forager showed us how to fine-dine off the land and where we met the most amazing 80-year-old Hmong chef in her garden, 200 feet from a Target parking lot.

Ultimately, this book is a celebration of a uniquely American but largely overlooked American diet. Its more than 100 recipes showcase the ingenuity of our Indigenous people and our immigrants who brought their time-honored cooking techniques from the Old World and blended New World ingredients to produce ingenious food that just may help you live to 100.

AUTHOR'S NOTE

I've chosen only plant-based recipes for this book. First and foremost, because the daily meals eaten in these communities a century ago were overwhelmingly vegetarian. Second, because if you're eating healthy, plant-based food, you're much more likely to live to 100 than if you're eating like an average American. Whether you're cooking for yourself, your family, or your friends, the recipes here will be delicious and will put you on a path to live to 100. Enjoy!

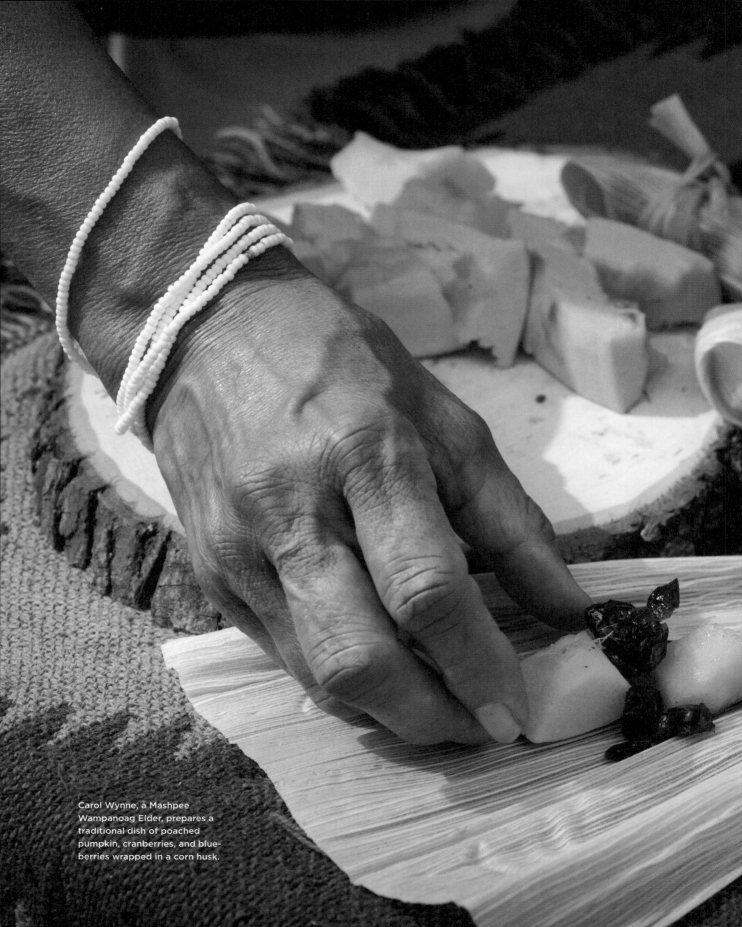

Carol Wynne, a Mashpee Wampanoag Elder, prepares a traditional dish of poached pumpkin, cranberries, and blueberries wrapped in a corn husk.

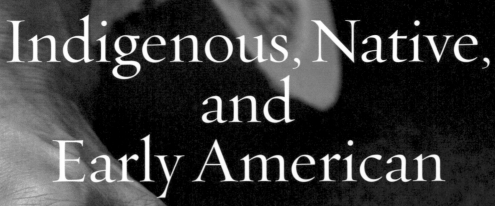

Indigenous, Native, and Early American

Mashpee Wampanoag, Mohawk, Cherokee, Oglala Lakota Sioux, Hawaiian, and Pilgrim Cuisines

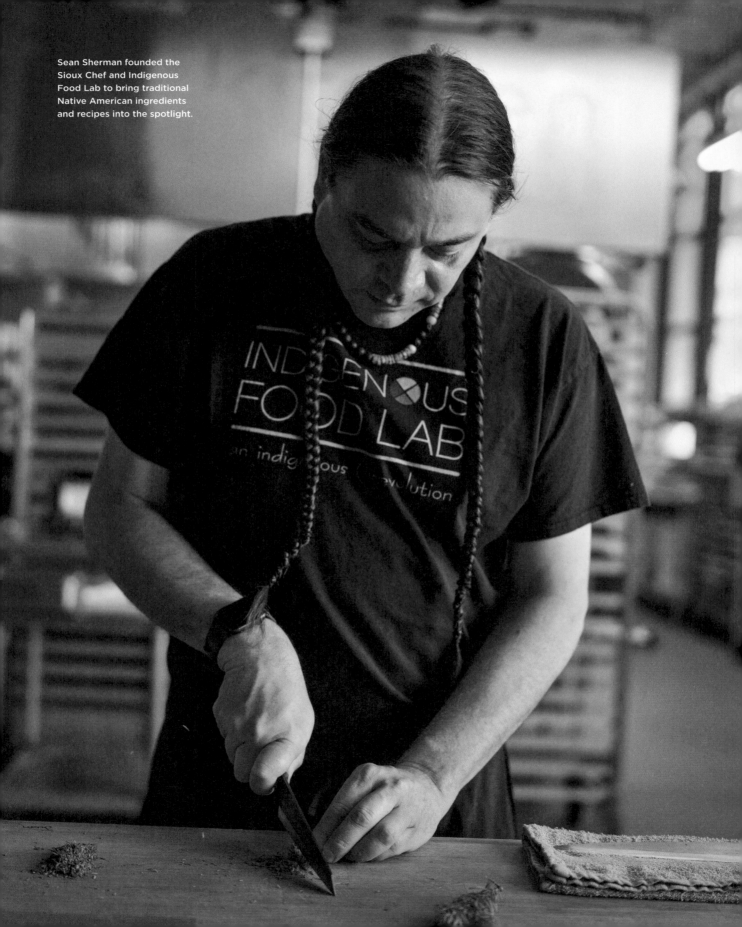

Sean Sherman founded the Sioux Chef and Indigenous Food Lab to bring traditional Native American ingredients and recipes into the spotlight.

"There's a huge world of food that is overlooked, misunderstood, and ignored..."

~PAULA MARCOUX

In late fall 1620, 102 sea-weary Pilgrims arrived at Plymouth Rock, mostly sick and suffering from malnutrition. After 55 days surviving on rations of dried meat, hard biscuits, and beer, they reached a cold, strange world where they had little knowledge of local food sources. Almost half the new arrivals died that winter—probably from scurvy and pneumonia. If not for the generosity of the Indigenous Wampanoag people, who observed the floundering immigrants, the rest might have perished too. But they took pity and taught the Pilgrims how to tap maple trees for syrup and where to find blueberries and cranberries, which likely cleared up their scurvy. Most important, the Wampanoag showed them how to cultivate local corn, squash, and beans—staples that had sustained their tribe for generations and would fuel the Pilgrim descendants' survival for centuries to come.

A year later, probably in October 1621, the two peoples came together for a harvest celebration that two centuries later European descendants called "Thanksgiving." But that occasion was nothing like the Thanksgiving we celebrate today. It was "less about celebration and more about exchanging knowledge and a show of force," Carol Wynne, a Mashpee Wampanoag culture keeper and clan mother tells me. "Most of what we think of as Thanksgiving is a myth."

That includes the food.

Little is known of what was on the menu at that original Thanksgiving harvest meal except a reference to fowl and deer in a letter from colonist Edward Winslow. Though the Wampanoag did hunt wild game and collect scallops and oysters, those made up less 20 percent of their diet. More than 70 to 80 percent of their diet came from plant-based sources, both farmed and gathered. That's why I asked Carol and her friend the food anthropologist Paula Marcoux, author of *Cooking With*

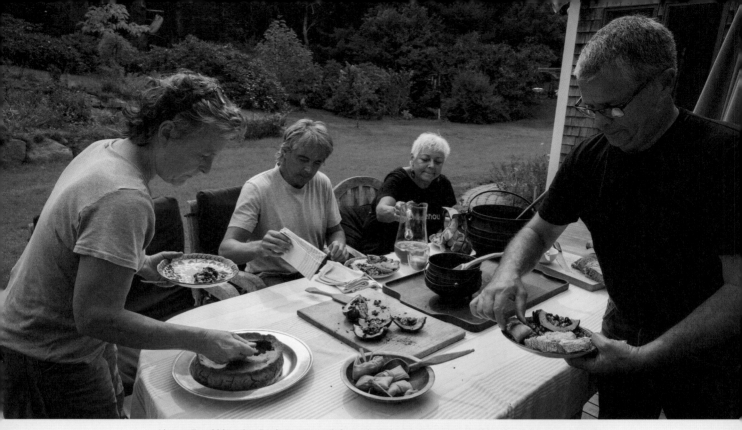

Above: Food historian Paula Marcoux (left) and Mashpee Wampanoag Elder Carol Wynne (seated on my left) prepare a true Thanksgiving dinner. Opposite: Ingredients for Sean Sherman's Lion's Mane and Nettle Tamales With Plum Sauce (page 51)

Fire, if they would put their heads together to re-create an early 17th-century meal.

In the courtyard of Paula's home, Carol looks serene and seemingly impervious to the summer heat. Wearing a lilac blouse, a necklace of small white shells, and Nike running shoes, she prepares dishes from traditional Wampanoag ingredients. Over an open fire, she roasts squash stuffed with hazelnuts, dried blueberries, and maple syrup. In a pot off to the side, she boils samp, a cornmeal of sorts. In a third pot filled with sassafras tea, she poaches slices of pumpkin wrapped in corn husks.

Over another fire Paula, wearing an olive green tank top and matching fatigues, shuttles between three black pots hanging from a wooden cooking tripod. In one pot, she boils pumpkin and apples for a pie filling. In another bubbles a 1620s Plymouth Succotash (page 60) made from a recipe dating to the early 17th century. Paula has adapted this Wampanoag *msiquatash* stew of hominy, beans, and squash by gussying it up with green beans, onions, and herbs. The Wampanoag were also known to add Jerusalem artichokes, peanuts, acorns, chestnuts, and walnuts, the latter ingredients sometimes powdered to serve as a thickener.

"My particular obsession with history affords me the fun of networking with long-dead cooks in their long-gone kitchens through archival and archaeological sources," Paula says while stirring a pot. "It's a thrilling privilege to conjure their wisdom through fire."

Paula tells me of the incredible culinary wealth that Native Americans gave us, including sunflowers, wild rice, sweet potatoes, tomatoes, peppers, peanuts, avocados, papayas, potatoes, vanilla, and cacao. Without the ingenuity of Indigenous people, we'd know nothing of vanilla ice cream, Hershey bars, or french fries. Then again, perhaps that would be a good thing . . .

On the northern tip of Hawaii's Big Island, we see another version of Native ingenuity. Three miles back from a black-sand beach, through a forest of giant trees reminiscent of those seen in *Jurassic Park,* and hemmed in by a 2,000-foot-high escarpment of rioting vegetation, we find the farm of 25-year-old Scott Harrison.

Here, Scott and his family have been cultivating native plants for three generations. Scott wears a camouflage shirt, flip-flops, Oakley glasses, and a man bun—and his yard abounds with native plants that Hawaiians have eaten for more than 1,000 years: sweet potatoes, bananas, pineapples, papayas, mangos, and breadfruit. In a neatly tended paddy field, Scott reaches into inches of water and extracts a taro plant. "You can eat the leaves like spinach and boil the stalks like asparagus," he says, holding it up like a trophy. "Mostly we survived off of the root, which we mash into a paste that we eat every day."

The traditional Hawaiian diet, which included seafood and wild game, was very healthy. Sadly, the onslaught of processed and fast food has spoiled the health of Native Hawaiians. Currently, they are the least healthy ethnicity in Hawaii.

Back in the continental United States, David and I meet extraordinary chefs practicing a sort of neo-Indigenous cooking. On the White Hills Lavender farm near

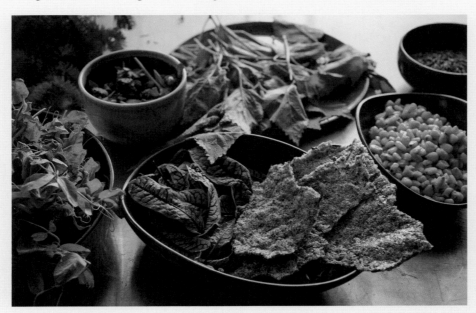

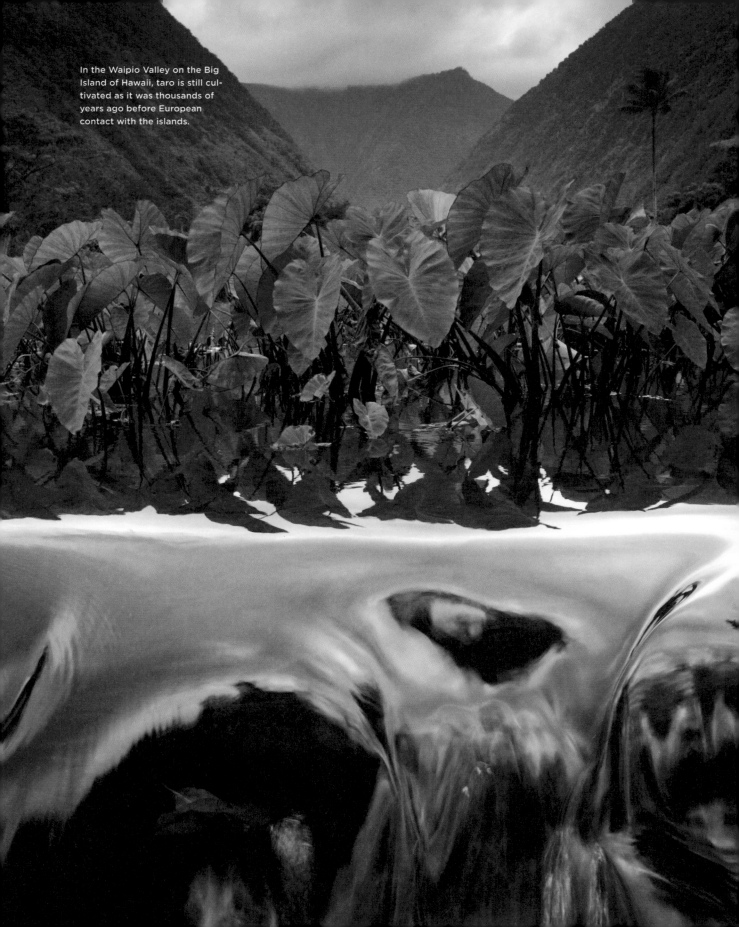

In the Waipio Valley on the Big Island of Hawaii, taro is still cultivated as it was thousands of years ago before European contact with the islands.

Dearing, Georgia, Dave Smoke McCluskey, an ebullient chef of Irish Mohawk ancestry, prepares three of his creations over a fire pit. His Mohawk Baked Beans (page 38) add mustard and tomato paste to the traditional bean-and-maple-syrup staple.

In my hometown of Minneapolis, I catch up with Sean Sherman, founder of the Sioux Chef. Born to the Oglala Lakota Sioux tribe in South Dakota's Pine Ridge Reservation, he moved to Minneapolis as a young adult with a zeal for innovative food and social justice. Sean's nonprofit, North American Traditional Indigenous Food Systems, works to bring back Indigenous foods and disseminate them throughout the community. Meanwhile, his restaurant, Owamni, takes a "decolonized approach to dining" avoiding dairy, wheat flour, cane sugar, beef, chicken, and pork—colonial foods not originally from this land. Instead, the restaurant serves Indigenous-inspired dishes like stuffed squash pasta with mushrooms, nasturtium, black tepary beans, and sweet corn.

This innovative food, all rooted in a disappearing tradition, reminds me of something Paula has told me. "There's a huge world of food that is overlooked, misunderstood, and ignored because of our preoccupation with the familiar present," she says. "A world of cooking has opened up for us, as many people have become less jingoistic about our food choices."

She must be right. A few years ago, Owamni would have been hopelessly arcane. In 2021, *Esquire* named it one of the "best new restaurants in America" and Sean as Chef of the Year.

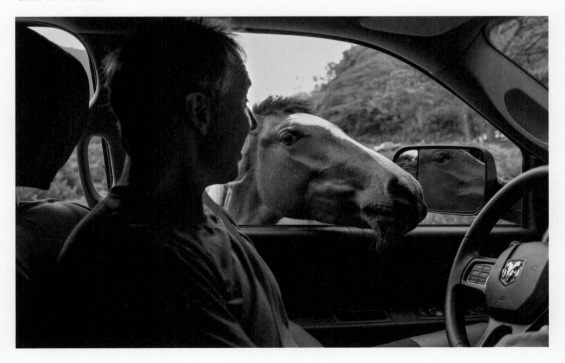

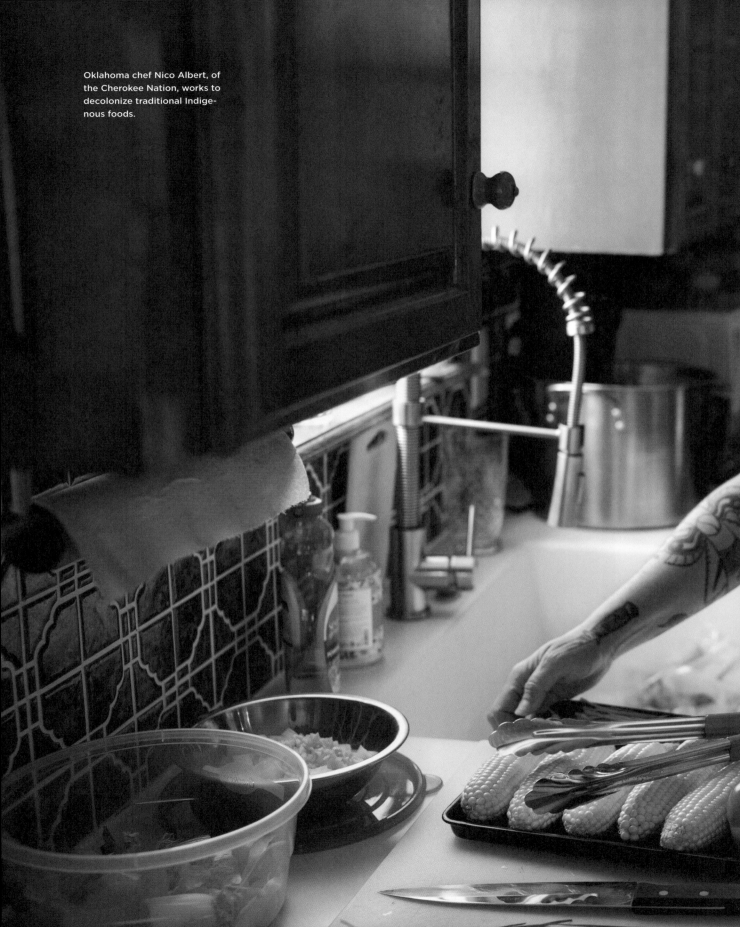

Oklahoma chef Nico Albert, of the Cherokee Nation, works to decolonize traditional Indigenous foods.

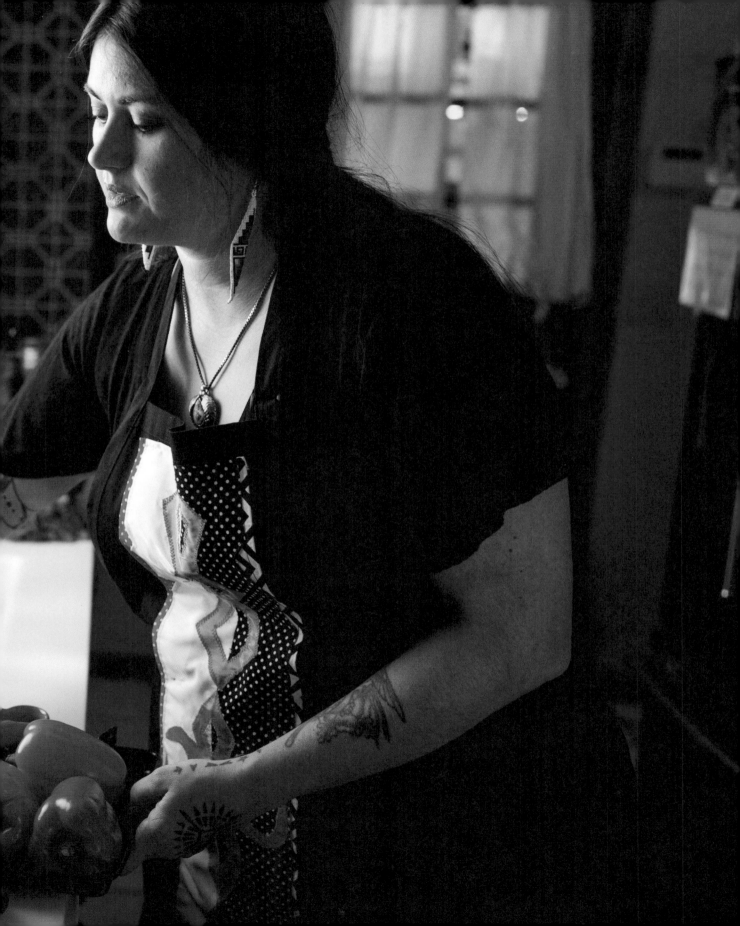

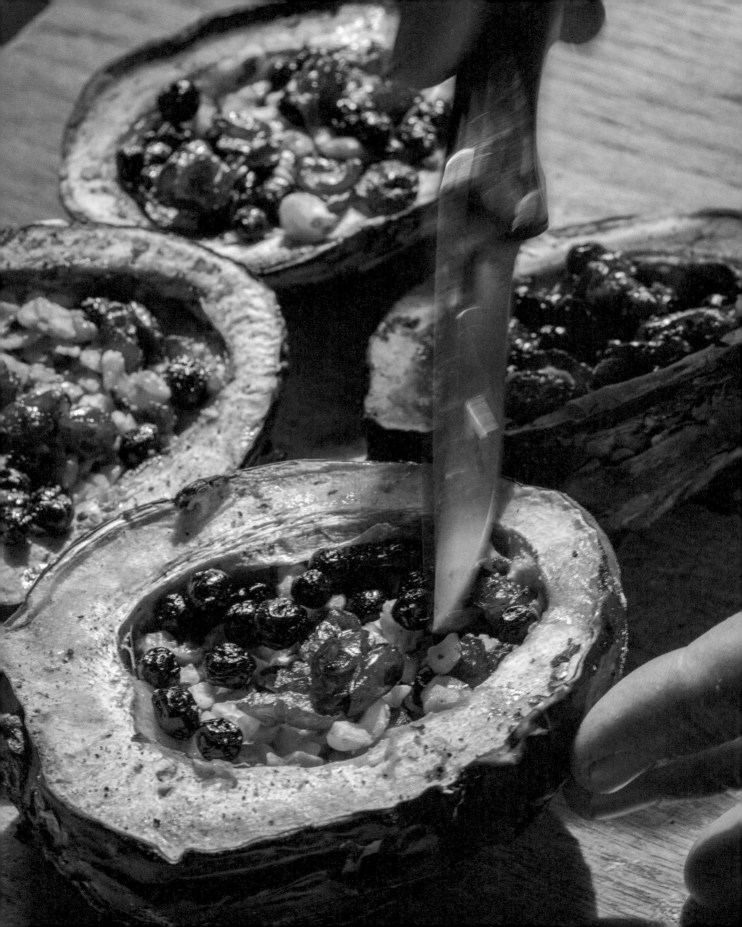

Baked Acorn Squash With Berries

TOTAL COOK TIME: 45 MINUTES • SERVES 6

Corn, beans, and squash have been staple foods in the diet of Native American tribes for more than 2,000 years. Acorn squash is abundant, and lasts for weeks in the refrigerator and months in a cool, dark place. You can cook the squash on a grill wrapped halfway in foil or in an open fire pit close to the flames and red-hot coals, rotating them a few times so that they don't catch on fire. This recipe is adapted from one of the many ways Wampanoag ancestors cooked acorn squash over an open fire.

3 acorn squash, halved lengthwise and seeded

½ cup coarsely ground roasted hazelnuts

½ cup dried blueberries

½ cup dried or fresh cranberries

½ cup brewed sassafras tea or berry tea

½ cup maple syrup

Preheat the oven to 400°F.

Make a bed of crumpled foil on a baking sheet and arrange the squash halves on top, flesh side up (the foil keeps the squash from sliding).

Spoon the hazelnuts into the center of each squash half, dividing them evenly; do the same with the blueberries and cranberries. Drizzle the tea over the top.

Bake for about 45 minutes, checking halfway through and reducing the heat to 350°F if the squash is browning too quickly; if you reduce the oven temperature, you may need to cook the squash for a few minutes longer. When finished cooking, the squash should be soft enough to eat with a spoon.

Serve hot and with maple syrup on the side for drizzling.

VARIATIONS
You can make your own toppings, or simply top the acorn squash with olive oil and seasoned salt or plain maple syrup. Carol likes to include a crunchy ingredient when experimenting. Here are a few of her favorite ideas for alternative toppings: raspberries, pecans, and brown sugar; or diced apples, crumbled walnuts, honey, and nutmeg.

Mohawk Baked Beans

TOTAL COOK TIME: 2 DAYS • SERVES 6 TO 8

2 pounds dried cranberry beans

1 large onion, diced

¼ cup darkest maple syrup

2 teaspoons tomato paste

2 tablespoons yellow mustard

Salt

Freshly ground black pepper

Place the beans in a large pot and cover them with cold water. Soak them overnight. Drain.

Put the beans in a Dutch oven or oven-safe pot and cover them with water. Bring them to a boil over medium-high heat, then reduce the heat to low and simmer for 1 to 1½ hours, until the beans are al dente.

Once the beans are al dente, add the onion, maple syrup, tomato paste, and mustard. Put them in the oven and set the oven to 225°F. Let the beans cook 8 hours or overnight, checking occasionally and adding water if needed. Season with salt and pepper to taste.

Serve hot.

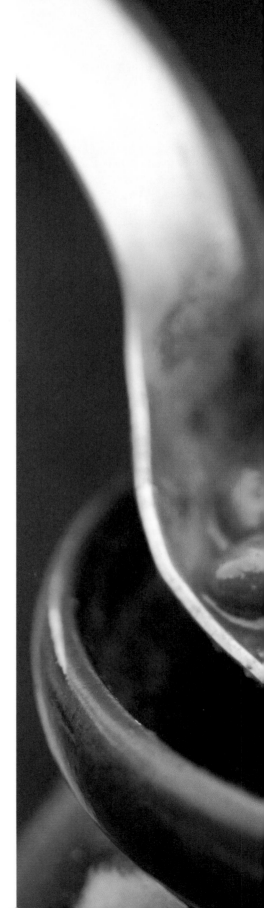

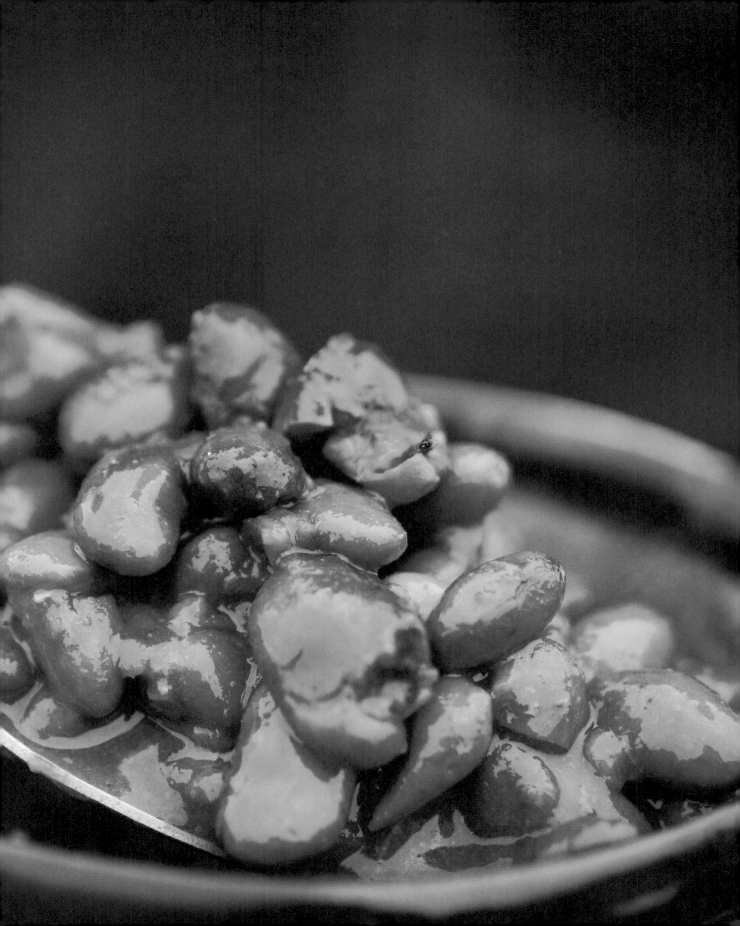

Warriors of the Rainbow Cranberry Mush

TOTAL COOK TIME: 1 HOUR • SERVES 6

Chef Dave Smoke McCluskey cooks what he calls "neo-Indigenous" cuisine. He's a trained chef in classical European techniques who cooks farm-to-table food that draws heavily on his Mohawk heritage and the foods of the Cape Cod community where he was born and raised. Here he uses hominy grits—corn that has been nixtamalized, or boiled in alkaline water. Nixtamalization is a 3,500-year-old process first used by Mesoamerican peoples to make the corn they grew more digestible and nutritious. Traditionally, this recipe would have been made with hickory milk, but we use almond milk.

4 cups water

4 cups almond milk

1 pound fresh cranberries or ½ pound dried cranberries

3 cups hominy grits

1 cup maple syrup, or to taste

Optional toppings: pumpkin seeds, pecans, dried cherries, or maple sugar

In a large pot, combine the water, almond milk, and cranberries and bring to a boil over high heat.

Reduce the heat to medium low, stir in the grits, and let simmer for 45 to 60 minutes, stirring occasionally, until the grits have absorbed the liquid and are very tender.

Stir in the maple syrup and serve hot with desired toppings, if using.

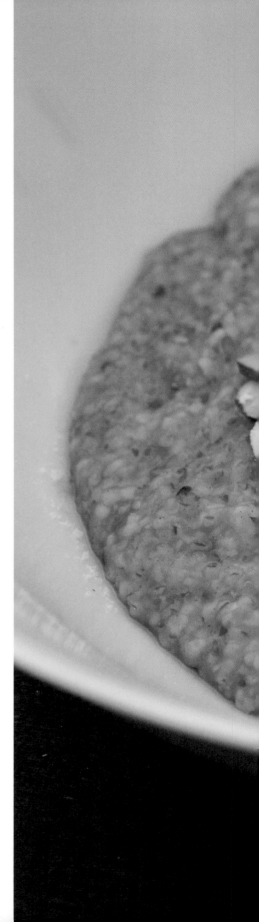

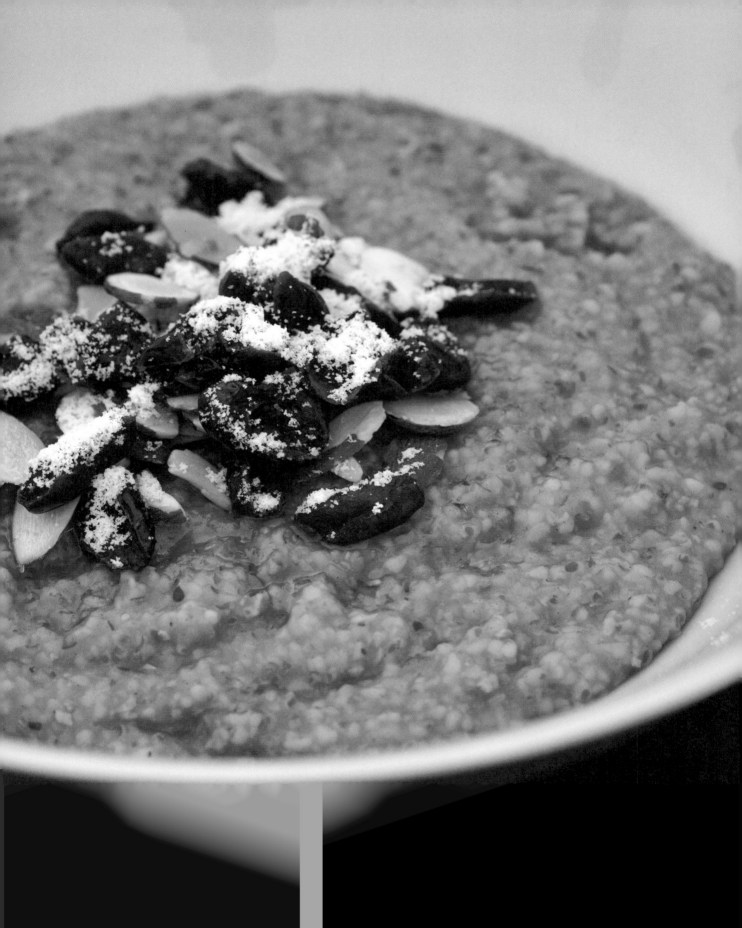

Fire-Roasted Cabbage With Roasted Chili-Chestnut Sauce

TOTAL COOK TIME: 6 HOURS • SERVES 4

This cabbage dish is a good one to make ahead—the cabbage is even better when it has a few hours or even overnight to chill before you grill! Nico Albert makes this dish using a sous vide for maximum flavor and melt-in-your-mouth texture, but it's just as delicious slow roasted in the oven. You can finish this dish on a grill over a wood fire or bed of charcoal, but it can be prepared on the stovetop as well.

FOR THE FIRE-ROASTED CABBAGE:

1 head green cabbage, cut into four wedges (with the core left intact)

2 tablespoons sunflower oil

2 tablespoons ground sumac

2 tablespoons chopped fresh sage

Salt

Freshly ground black pepper

2 scallions, thinly sliced (optional)

FOR THE ROASTED CHILI-CHESTNUT SAUCE:

1 red bell pepper

1 dried guajillo chili, split lengthwise and seeded

1 dried ancho chili, split lengthwise and seeded

7 whole roasted chestnuts

2 tablespoons pure maple syrup

1 tablespoon salt

To make the fire-roasted cabbage, drizzle the cabbage wedges with the sunflower oil. Use your hands to spread the oil all over to coat the outside. Season with the sumac, sage, salt, and pepper, making sure all sides get seasoning.

If you have a sous vide machine, place the wedges in a vacuum bag (depending on the size of the bags, one to two wedges will fit in each), and seal according to directions. Place the cabbage wedges in an immersion bath set at 180°F and cook for 4 hours.

If you don't have a sous vide, roast the cabbage wedges in the oven with low heat to achieve a similar effect. Preheat the oven to 325°F. Place the prepared cabbage wedges on a rimmed baking sheet or in a baking dish that fits them snugly. Add ¼ cup of water to the baking sheet and cover it with foil. Bake for 1 hour, then turn the cabbage wedges over. If needed to prevent burning, add a splash or two more of water. Bake for another hour.

Once cooked, chill the cabbage in the refrigerator while you prepare the sauce.

To make the roasted chili-chestnut sauce, roast the bell pepper. You can do this over a wood or charcoal grill, on the stovetop, or in the oven. If using a grill, place the pepper directly on the grill before the initial flames die down and cook, turning occasionally, until it is blackened on all sides.

On a gas stovetop, roast the bell pepper directly in the flames of the burner. In an oven, use the highest setting of the broiler. Cook until it's blackened on all sides.

Place the charred pepper in a resealable plastic bag or wrap it in foil to allow it to steam as it cools.

While the bell pepper cools, bring ⅔ cup of water to boil. Then, toast the dried chilis over the fire. Place the chilis directly on the grill and toast them briefly—you want the color to darken and the chilis to puff slightly—but remove them before they blacken. You can also toast the chilis in a hot, dry skillet on the stovetop. Once the chilis are cooked, place them in a small bowl and cover them with the boiling water, weighing them down with a small plate, if necessary, to keep them submerged.

When the bell pepper has cooled enough to handle, remove the charred skin by gently wiping it away with your fingers. Remove the stem and seeds, and place the roasted pepper in a blender.

When the water for soaking the dried chilis has cooled enough to touch, the chilis will have softened enough. Remove them, reserving the soaking liquid, and place the chilis in the blender with the roasted bell pepper. Add the roasted chestnuts, maple syrup, and salt. Add about ½ cup of the chili-soaking liquid to the blender. Blend the mixture starting on low speed, then increase the speed to high until a smooth sauce forms. Add additional chili-soaking liquid if the mixture is too thick; it should have a smooth consistency that coats the back of a spoon.

Take the precooked cabbage out of the fridge and allow it to come to room temperature. Start your grill: When the cooking fire has burned enough to have a good bed of hot coals, or the charcoal has burned to the point that it's completely gray, your grill is ready for the cabbage. Cook the cabbage until it has caramelized and has been charred on all sides and heated through. If preparing the dish on a stovetop, you can sear the outside of the cabbage in a skillet over high heat to caramelize the outside and heat it through.

To serve, pour a generous amount of the roasted chili-chestnut sauce on each plate, and place each roasted cabbage directly in the pool of sauce. Garnish with sliced scallions, if desired.

Creamy Squash Soup
With Corn Salsa and Wild Onion Chimichurri

TOTAL COOK TIME: 45 MINUTES • SERVES 5

Chef Nico Albert celebrates Native foodways and believes they are the key to connection for Indigenous peoples. Native cooking is naturally nutrient-dense and sustaining, and Nico believes food is essential for restoring the well-being of Native people. Her winter squash soup blends traditional Indigenous cooking with some global inspiration. Feel free to use any type of winter squash for this soup: Georgia candy roaster, butternut, or any type of pumpkin will work well.

FOR THE CHIMICHURRI:

12 wild onions or 4 to 5 green
  onions, trimmed
¼ cup chopped parsley leaves
  (stems removed)
¼ cup apple cider vinegar
1 tablespoon pure maple syrup
2 teaspoons salt
¼ cup sunflower oil

FOR THE SOUP AND SALSA:

6 ears sweet corn, shucked
2 tablespoons sunflower oil
1 large yellow onion, diced
4 large garlic cloves, minced
6 cups water
2 pounds winter squash, peeled,
  seeded, and cut into 2-inch cubes
Salt
Freshly ground black pepper
2 small jalapeño peppers, seeded
  and very finely diced

To make the chimichurri, on a grill or in a very hot, dry cast-iron skillet over high heat, cook the wild onions until nicely charred in some spots but not totally blackened.

Coarsely chop the charred onions and add them to a blender or food processor with the parsley, vinegar, maple syrup, salt, and oil. Puree the mixture until it reaches a slightly chunky, pesto-like consistency.

To make the soup, cook the ears of corn on a grill, turning occasionally, until they are lightly charred on all sides. Remove the corn from the heat and set it aside to cool.

Add the oil to a large (5- to 7-quart) Dutch oven or stockpot and heat over medium heat.

Add the yellow onion and garlic. Cook, stirring frequently, until the onion and garlic have caramelized and turned a light golden brown.

Cut the corn from the cobs, reserving the cobs for the soup and the kernels for the salsa.

Put the cobs in the pot with the sautéed onion and garlic. Add the water to the pot, place it over high heat, and bring it to a boil. Reduce the heat to a simmer (if cooking over a fire, move the pot to a cooler spot on the grill to maintain a simmer). Allow the mixture to simmer for 15 to 20 minutes, until the broth becomes fragrant with the aroma of sweet corn and the liquid has reduced to about 4 cups.

Add the cubed squash, bring the liquid back to a simmer, and cook until the squash is very tender.

Working in batches, use an immersion blender or a countertop blender (allow to cool slightly before putting into blender) to puree the soup until smooth. Season with salt and black pepper to taste.

To make the salsa, combine the reserved corn kernels with the jalapeño and stir to mix well. Season with salt and pepper to taste.

To serve, ladle the soup into bowls, garnish with a generous scoop of the roasted corn salsa, and drizzle with the wild onion chimichurri.

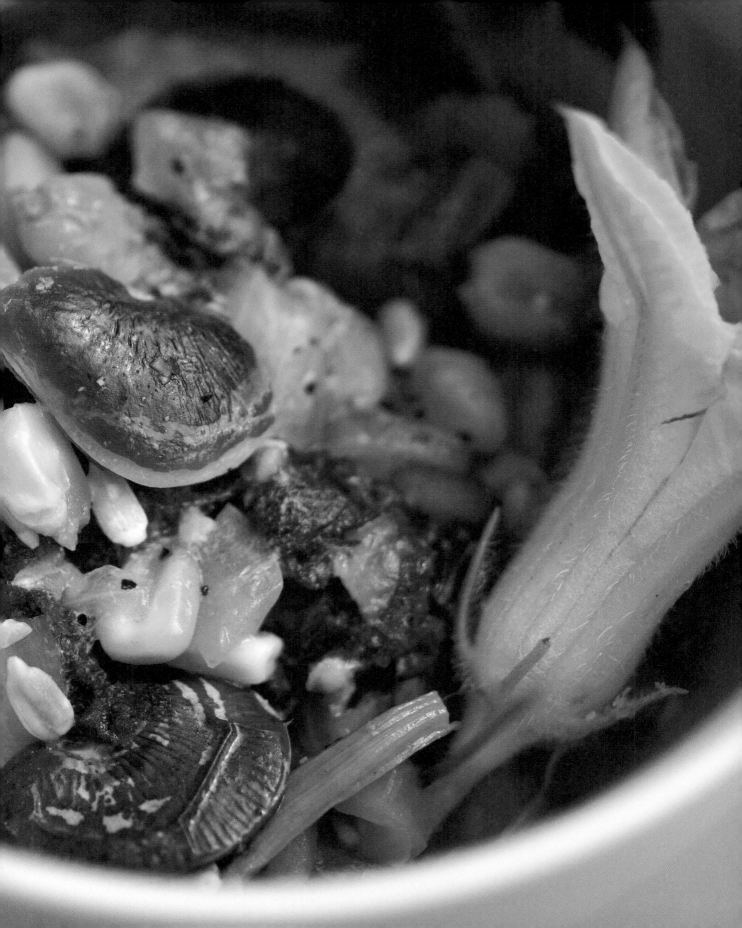

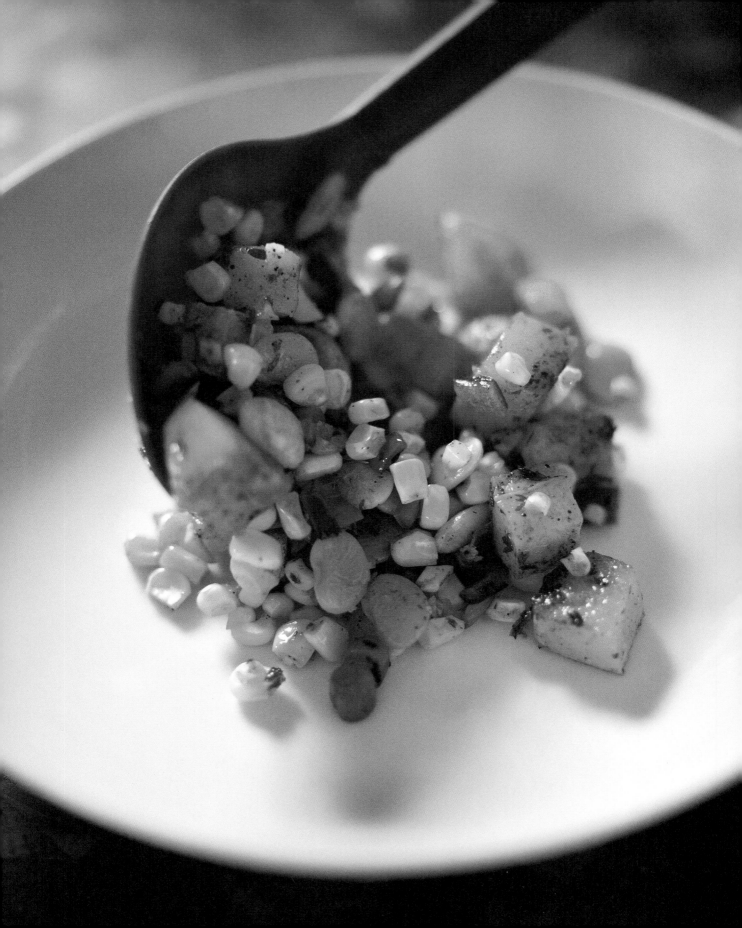

Three Sisters Cherokee Succotash (left)

TOTAL COOK TIME: 30 MINUTES • SERVES 4

Throughout the Smoky and Blue Ridge Mountains, the Cherokee people traditionally grew squash, corn, and beans—the "three sisters." This succotash combines the three sisters with fresh herbs and aromatics.

2 cups peeled and diced butternut squash

2 tablespoons plus 1 teaspoon olive oil

1 teaspoon paprika

1 teaspoon salt

1 teaspoon freshly ground black pepper

1 teaspoon minced fresh garlic

½ cup finely diced red onion (about 1½ medium onions)

½ cup finely diced red pepper (about 1 medium pepper)

½ cup chopped green beans (such as haricots verts)

1 cup fresh corn kernels (cut from 1 to 2 ears of corn)

1 cup fresh or frozen lima beans

2 tablespoons chopped parsley

½ cup finely chopped spring onions

Preheat the oven to 375°F.

Place the squash on a small baking sheet and sprinkle with 1 teaspoon of the olive oil, the paprika, salt, and pepper.

Roast the squash in the oven until soft and caramelized, about 20 minutes.

Heat the remaining 2 tablespoons of olive oil in a sauté pan. Add the garlic and cook, stirring, for about 1 minute to release the oils.

Add the red onion, red pepper, and green beans and cook, stirring occasionally, for about 2 minutes. Add the corn kernels and cook for 2 more minutes.

Add the lima beans and cook for another minute. Season with additional salt, pepper, and paprika. Sprinkle with the parsley.

Add the spring onions last so that they don't overcook. Taste and adjust the seasoning as needed.

Add the roasted squash, toss, and serve immediately.

Salagi (Grape Dessert Dumplings)

TOTAL COOK TIME: 50 MINUTES • MAKES 12 DUMPLINGS

1 gallon grape juice

1½ cups all-purpose flour

1½ teaspoons baking powder

2 teaspoons granulated sugar

¼ teaspoon salt

1 teaspoon vegetable shortening

Reserve ½ cup of the grape juice, then pour the remainder of the gallon into a large stockpot and bring it to a boil.

In a large bowl, combine the flour, baking powder, sugar, and salt. Add the shortening and mix the dough until it is the consistency of a coarse meal.

Add the reserved grape juice and knead the dough just until it comes together. Be careful not to overwork the dough.

On a floured surface, use a floured rolling pin to roll it out into a ¼-inch-thick sheet. Use a sharp knife to cut the dough into 1-inch-wide strips, and then cut the strips into 2-inch lengths.

Reduce the heat so that the juice is at a rolling simmer. Add the pieces of dough to the pot, about seven or eight pieces at a time. Cook for about 5 minutes, until they are cooked through and double in size. Use a slotted spoon to remove them.

Serve the dumplings hot with vanilla ice cream or sorbet.

Stuffed Squash Halves With Blueberry Wojapi

TOTAL COOK TIME: 45 MINUTES • SERVES 2

Wojapi is a thick berry dish that has the consistency of a chunky sauce or pudding. It's traditionally made and enjoyed by different tribal nations. If your berries are very sweet and ripe, you may not need any additional sweeteners.

FOR THE WOJAPI:

6 ounces fresh blueberries, plus additional for garnish

1 tablespoon cedar leaf or thyme

¼ cup maple syrup, more or less to taste

FOR THE SQUASH:

1 delicata squash, halved lengthwise and seeded

2 tablespoons sunflower oil

Salt

FOR THE FILLING:

Sunflower oil

½ cup hominy

½ cup cooked white beans

½ cup sprouted beans

1 teaspoon bergamot juice

1 teaspoon sage

1 teaspoon cedar leaf or thyme

1 tablespoon maple syrup

Salt

To make the wojapi, in a medium saucepan, combine the blueberries, cedar leaf, and maple syrup. Cook over medium-low heat until the blueberries begin to break down and the sauce thickens. Use a fork to mash the berries if needed; the mixture should be chunky. Transfer it to a bowl and chill it in the refrigerator.

To make the squash, preheat the oven to 350°F.

Drizzle the squash halves with the oil and season generously with salt. Place the squash halves, cut sides down, on a baking sheet. Bake the squash for 15 to 20 minutes, until it is tender.

To make the filling, heat a skillet over medium heat and drizzle with enough sunflower oil to coat the bottom. Add the hominy, white beans, and sprouted beans. Cook, stirring occasionally, for 4 minutes. Add the bergamot juice, sage, cedar leaf, maple syrup, and salt to taste, and cook for about 4 minutes more, until the hominy and beans are golden brown.

To serve, spoon some of the wojapi onto two plates. Place one half of a squash off-center on each plate, skin side down. Spoon the filling into the squash halves. Finish with a sprinkling of salt and some fresh berries.

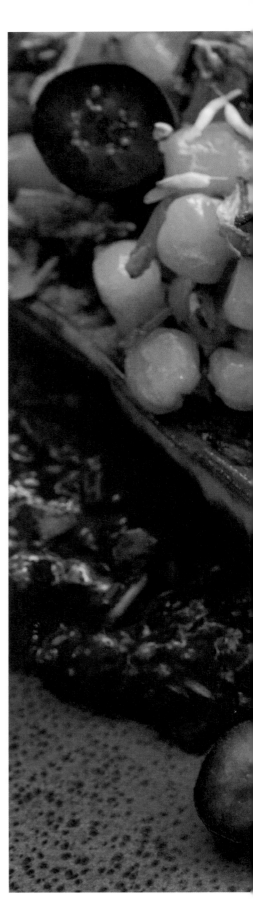

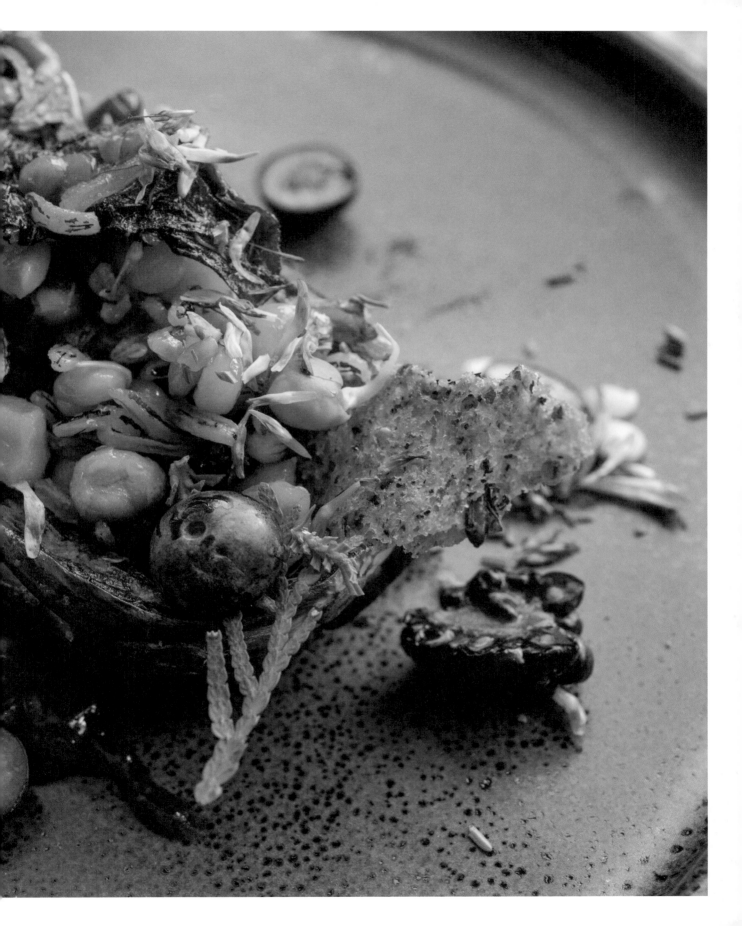

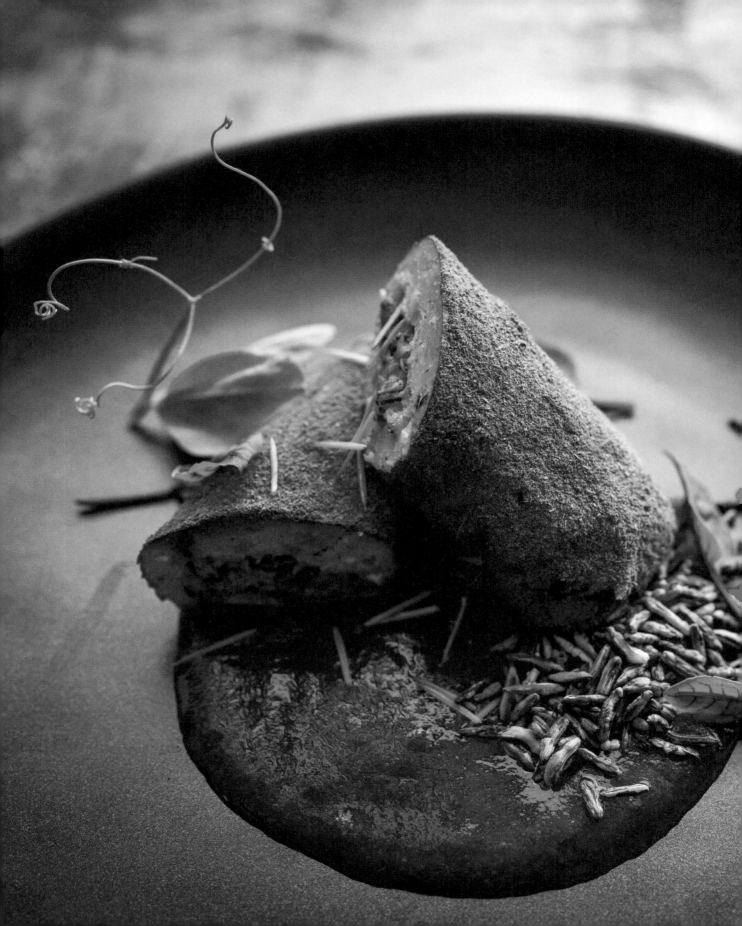

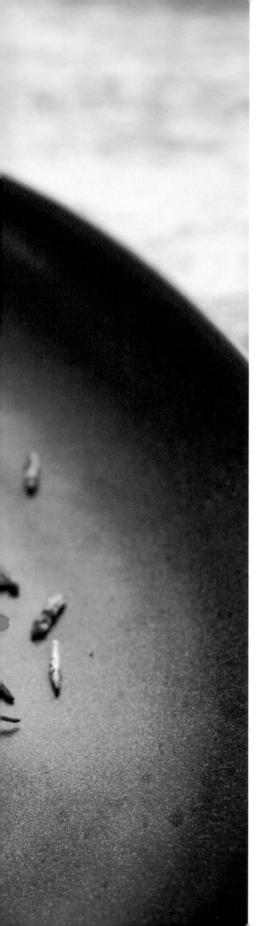

Lion's Mane and Nettle Tamales With Plum Sauce

TOTAL COOK TIME: 45 MINUTES • MAKES 4 TAMALES

FOR THE FILLING:

2 tablespoons sunflower oil

2 ounces fresh lion's mane mushrooms or any wild mushroom, chopped into 2-inch pieces

1 teaspoon bergamot (or Mexican oregano)

Salt

¼ cup cooked wild rice

FOR THE TAMALES:

2 cups fresh masa or masa harina (masa flour)

2 tablespoons sunflower oil (if using fresh masa)

4 large nettle leaves

3 tablespoons nettle powder

FOR THE SAUCE:

2 fermented or fresh plums, pitted

3 tablespoons maple syrup

Coarse salt, for garnish

To make the filling, set a skillet over high heat. Add the oil. When the oil begins to smoke, add the mushrooms and bergamot and a pinch or two of salt. Cook, stirring occasionally, until the mushrooms are golden brown. Remove from the heat and stir in the rice. Let cool.

To make the tamales, in a large bowl, combine the masa with the oil and mix well. If you are using masa harina, follow the package directions for 2 cups.

Wearing gloves to work with the nettle, soak the nettle leaves for about 30 seconds in room-temperature water. Lay two leaves on a cutting board, overlapping them by about ½ inch. Spread a quarter of the masa onto the leaves, leaving the edges of the leaves clear. Spoon the mushroom filling down the center of the masa. Wrap the masa leaves to enclose the filling, like a burrito. Repeat with the remaining ingredients.

Place the tamales in a steamer basket and steam for 12 minutes. Remove them from the steamer and place on a cutting board. Sprinkle the nettle powder over the tamales, covering them thoroughly, and then let them rest.

To make the sauce, put the plums and maple syrup in a blender and blend on high speed, adding 1 tablespoon of water at a time, until the mixture is a smooth puree.

Pour the plum sauce onto four serving plates. Place one tamale on top of each pool of sauce and garnish with salt. Serve immediately.

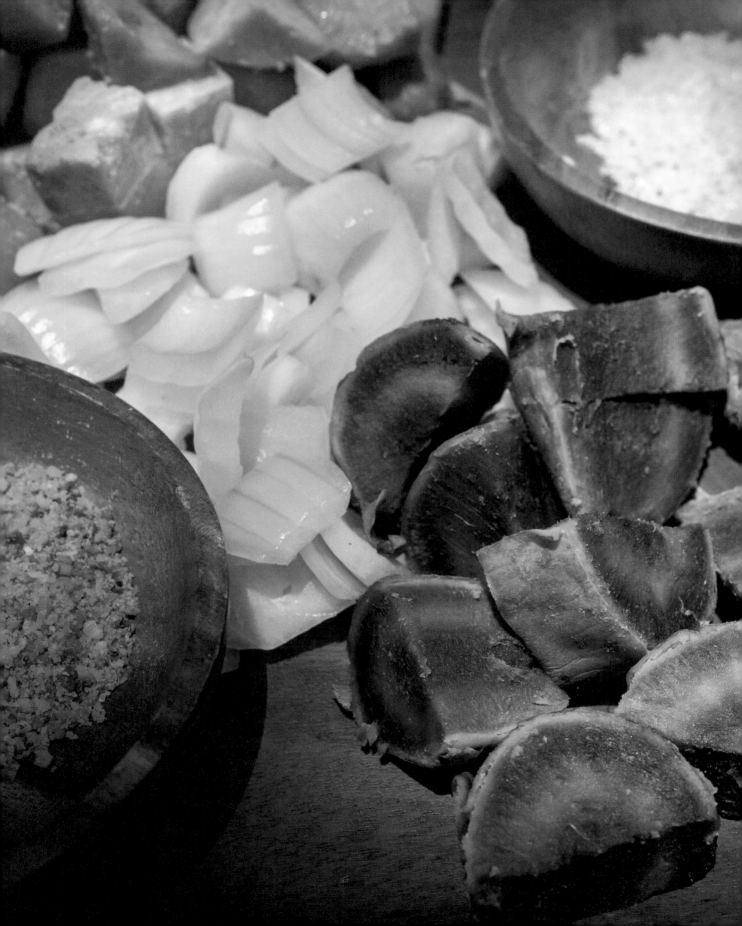

Uala Laulau
(Taro Leaves Stuffed With Sweet Potato and Breadfruit) (left)

TOTAL COOK TIME: 30 MINUTES • MAKES 6 LEAVES

"Aunty" Tammy Mahealani Smith can trace her lineage back 10 generations, and her family has been feeding people for many decades. She is passionate about sharing the knowledge and techniques of *ulu* and other traditional Hawaiian foods.

Laulau is a traditional Hawaiian and Polynesian dish of stuffed taro or ti leaves that are filled and steamed. This version is filled with *uala* (Hawaiian sweet potato), uala leaves, *kalo* (taro), and ulu (breadfruit).

Handful fresh sweet potato leaves

1 cup cooked uala (Hawaiian sweet potato), cubed

1 cup cooked kalo (taro), cubed

1 cup cooked ulu (breadfruit), cubed

1 whole sweet onion, diced

Hawaiian salt

Inamona (kukui nut), roasted and finely chopped

1 pound ti leaves, center vein removed

Lay a handful of sweet potato leaves flat on a clean work surface.

Add about 4 cubes each of the uala, kalo, and ulu, and a quarter of the onion on top of the leaves, down the center. Season with salt and inamona.

Wrap everything in a bundle like a burrito, folding in the sides, and then place the bundle on a ti leaf and wrap it up. Wrap the ti leaf bundle in a second ti leaf.

Repeat with the remaining ingredients.

Place the bundles in a steamer over simmering water for 30 minutes.

Serve hot, removing the ti leaves and eating everything inside.

Aina Momona Stew With Taro, Breadfruit, and Sweet Potato

TOTAL COOK TIME: 2 HOURS • SERVES 6

Kalo (or taro) is considered sacred to the people of Hawaii and is a nutritious root vegetable that sustained Hawaiian society for centuries. Kalo leaves need to be cooked in boiling, salted water before being added to the stew. The older the leaves are, the tougher they will be, and the longer they'll need to cook.

4 cups kalo (taro) leaves, chopped

4 cups water

2 tablespoons vegetable broth seasoning (such as bouillon powder)

2 cups kalo (taro root), cut into bite-size pieces

2 cups ulu (breadfruit), cut into bite-size pieces

2 cups uala (Hawaiian sweet potato), cut into bite-size pieces

Salt

Freshly ground black pepper

Bring a pot of water to boil, then add the kalo leaves and let boil until softened, 45 minutes to 2 hours, depending on the age of the leaves. Remove them from the water and drain.

Add the leaves, 4 cups of water, vegetable broth seasoning, kalo, ulu, and uala to a soup pot. Bring to a boil, then lower the heat to a simmer.

Cover and simmer for 20 to 30 minutes, until the vegetables are soft, stirring occasionally.

Add salt and pepper to taste before serving. Enjoy with poi (mashed kalo).

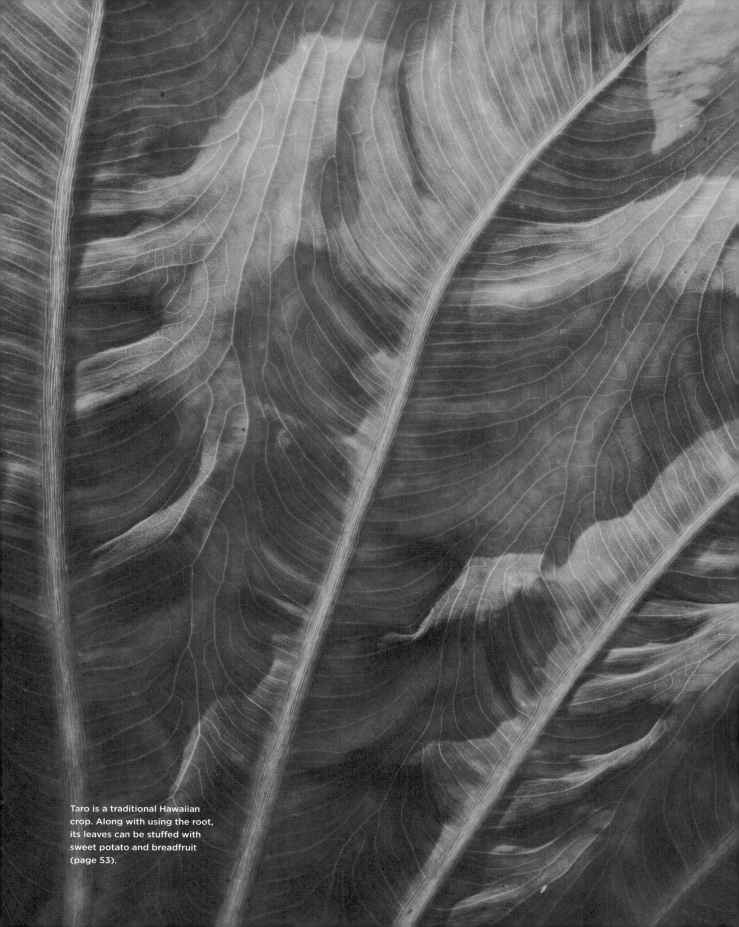

Taro is a traditional Hawaiian crop. Along with using the root, its leaves can be stuffed with sweet potato and breadfruit (page 53).

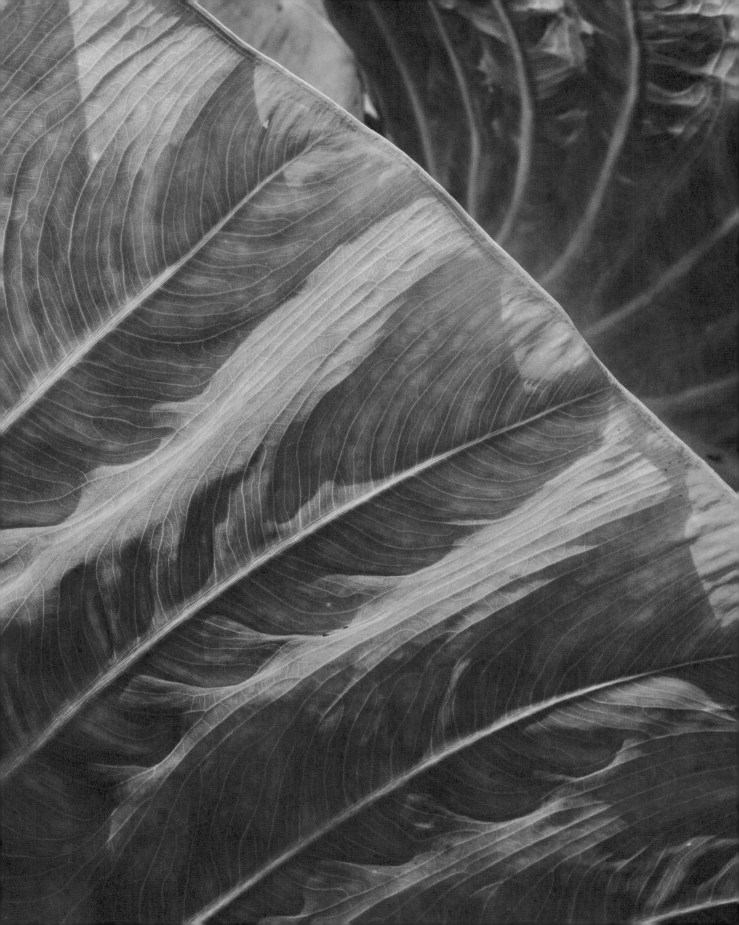

Ulu (Breadfruit) Poke

TOTAL COOK TIME: 1 HOUR 15 MINUTES • SERVES 4

Jasmine Silverstein is a whole-food chef in Hawaii who is passionate about the power of food and medicine and about helping Hawaii build its independence and break free from its reliance on the global food system.

Ogo, called *limu* in Hawaiian, is a reddish-colored seaweed that is harvested in Hawaii. In the blue zones region of Okinawa, Japan, seaweeds and sea vegetables are a core part of the traditional diet. Besides being umami-rich and low in calories, they are also nutrient-dense with carotenoids, folate, magnesium, iron, calcium, and iodine, and they have compounds found only in sea plants that seem to serve as effective antioxidants at the cellular level.

1 medium-size ulu (breadfruit), quartered and cored

½ cup macadamia nuts or cashews, soaked for at least 30 minutes and drained

½ cup water

½ cup coconut aminos

¼ cup avocado or sesame oil

1 teaspoon sea salt plus more for finishing

¼ teaspoon cayenne

3 to 6 green onions, thinly sliced

½ small sweet onion or yellow onion, finely diced

1 to 2 cups halved cherry tomatoes

2 to 3 cups limu (ogo) as fresh and crunchy as possible

1 cup inamona (kukui nut), roasted and finely chopped (or toasted macadamia nut pieces)

Steam the ulu until tender, about 40 minutes to an hour.

Cut the steamed ulu into ½- to ¾-inch pieces (discard any browned pieces).

In a high-powered blender, combine the soaked nuts, water, coconut aminos, oil, salt, and cayenne until smooth and creamy. Taste the dressing and adjust the ingredients as necessary.

Pour the dressing over the cubed ulu and mix well to coat every piece.

In a large bowl, combine the green onions, sweet onion, cherry tomatoes, limu, and inamona. Add the ulu mixture and toss gently to combine.

NOTES

• If you don't have ulu, you can substitute cooked kalo (taro), purple or white sweet potatoes, Yukon Gold potatoes, or whatever starchy tuber that may be similar. You will need 8 cups of the cubed tuber for this recipe.

• If you can't find fresh seaweed at your local grocery store, you can use dried seaweed, which can be rehydrated. Use ogo, wakame, or arame.

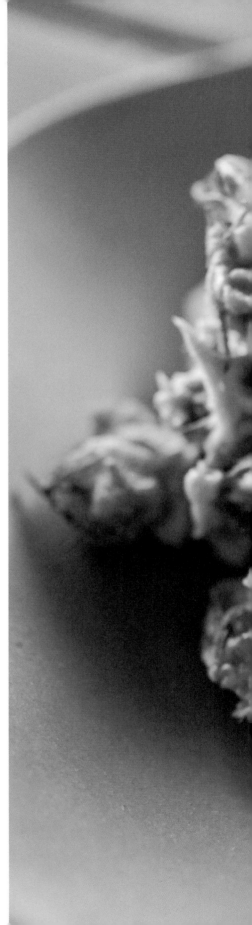

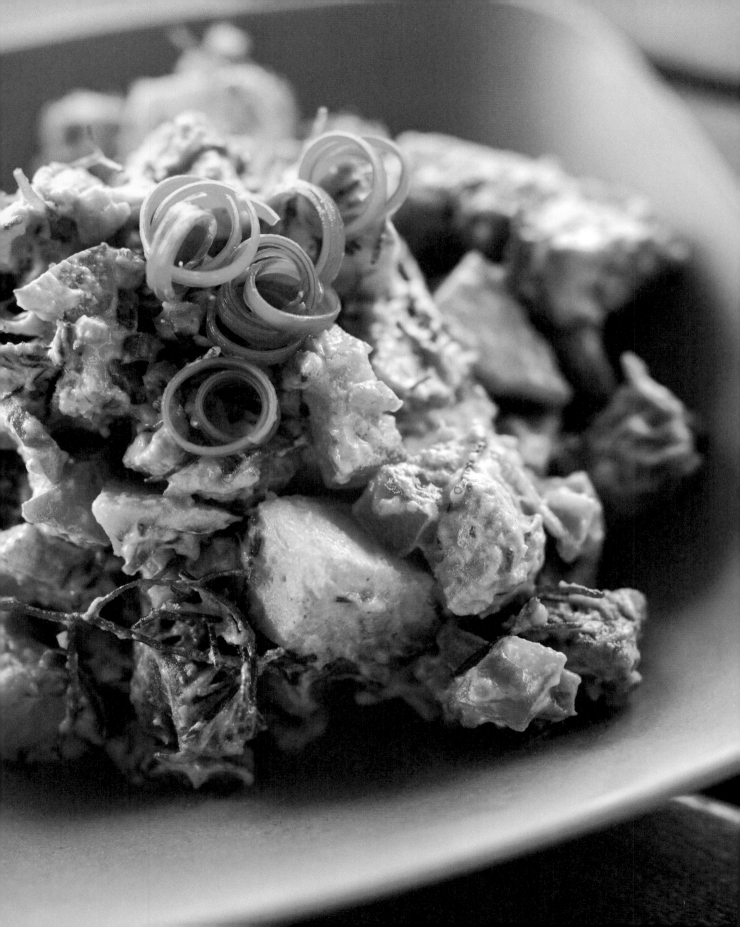

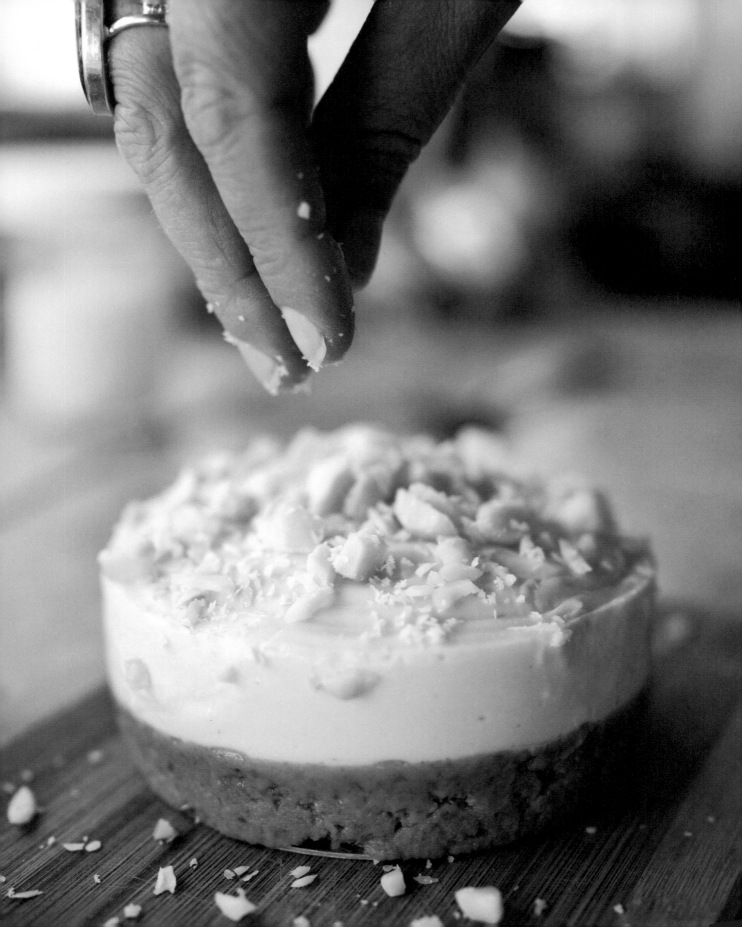

Poi Gravy

TOTAL COOK TIME: 15 MINUTES • MAKES ABOUT 3 CUPS

Poi is a crucial ingredient in this recipe, as it provides the flavor, nutrition, and texture. If you can source fresh taro, you can easily make your own poi by thoroughly cooking the taro, removing the peel, and blending it with enough water to create a pudding-like consistency. If you don't have poi or fresh taro, you can use precooked polenta or grits.

4 ounces shiitake mushrooms, diced

2 celery stalks, diced

1 small yellow onion, diced

Salt

1 cup poi

¼ cup coconut aminos (or soy sauce)

Heat a skillet over medium heat. Add the mushrooms, celery, onion, and salt. Cook, stirring occasionally, until the vegetables are soft and slightly caramelized, about 10 minutes.

Add a splash of water to deglaze the pan.

Use an immersion blender or transfer the vegetables to a countertop blender (cool slightly before transferring to blender) and add the poi and the coconut aminos. Blend until smooth, adding ½ to 1 cup of water as needed to achieve your desired consistency.

Haupia (Hawaiian Coconut Pudding) (left)

TOTAL COOK TIME: 5 TO 7 HOURS OR OVERNIGHT • SERVES 4

Haupia is a Hawaiian coconut pudding that is thickened with cornstarch. It is delicious served alone, or you can make a layered dish with a macadamia nut crust or a layer of mashed purple sweet potato.

FOR THE MACADAMIA NUT CRUST (OPTIONAL):

1 cup raw or dehydrated macadamia nuts

6 to 8 dates, pitted

Dash of vanilla extract

Pinch of salt

FOR THE SWEET POTATO LAYER (OPTIONAL):

1 pound purple sweet potato

Coconut cream or milk, as needed

FOR THE PUDDING:

⅔ cup cornstarch

2 cups sugarcane juice or a mix of ½ cup sugar and 1 cup water

2 (14-ounce) cans unsweetened coconut milk

1 teaspoon vanilla extract (optional)

Line an 8-by-8-inch baking pan with parchment paper.

To make the optional macadamia nut crust, in a food processor, combine the macadamia nuts, dates, vanilla, and salt, and process to the consistency of a coarse meal. Transfer the mixture to the prepared pan and press it into an even layer on the bottom.

To make the optional sweet potato layer, steam or boil the sweet potato until it is very soft, 15 to 20 minutes.

Remove and discard the skin along with any brown spots. Mash the sweet potato by hand or in a food processor while slowly adding the coconut cream, a tablespoon at a time, until you reach a nice, thick consistency—similar to that of mashed potatoes. Spread the mixture over the nut crust or in the bottom of the prepared pan in an even layer.

To make the pudding, in a medium saucepan, combine the cornstarch, sugarcane juice, coconut milk, and vanilla, and mix well to fully incorporate the cornstarch.

Place the saucepan over a medium-low heat and cook, stirring constantly, for 5 to 10 minutes, until the mixture thickens.

Transfer the mixture to the prepared pan.

Refrigerate for 4 to 6 hours or overnight. Serve chilled.

PAULA MARCOUX, ARCHAEOLOGIST, FOOD HISTORIAN, AND LIVE-FIRE COOKING EXPERT

1620s Plymouth Succotash

TOTAL COOK TIME: 20 MINUTES • SERVES 5

A staple of Native diets throughout the region, succotash was a brothy, long-simmered dish consisting primarily of two critical ingredients: dry corn (hulled by steeping in wood ash lye) and dry beans. Upon this savory background was layered an ever varying array of fish, shellfish, meat, roots, nuts, fruits, and leaves. English cooks, also from a broth-cooking culture, viewed this important dish as a conceptual relative of their own oat-based pottage and adopted the hulled-corn-and-beans duo without alteration, applying their own flavorings and garnishes. Over the centuries, the ingredients were altered gradually to suit contemporary conditions, making a full transition from the hunted and gathered foods of the Wampanoag to the barnyard and kitchen-garden stuff of the English. This plant-based succotash is Paula Marcoux's interpretation of a really early English autumnal version.

2 pounds cooked, hulled corn (or reconstituted dry whole hominy, frozen hominy, or pozole)

8 ounces dried cranberry beans (or Jacob's cattle beans or other similar beans), soaked and cooked until just tender

Salt

OPTIONAL ADD-INS:

2 turnips, peeled and chopped

2 carrots, peeled and chopped

1 acorn squash or other winter squash, seeded and sliced

Few handfuls of chopped cabbage, collards, or turnip greens

2 leeks or onions, sliced

Few handfuls of chopped lettuce, spinach, endive, chicory, or arugula (or a combination)

Tender strawberry or violet leaves

1 cup ground walnuts, chestnuts, or hazelnuts

Freshly ground black pepper

Few chives or scallions, chopped

Calendula petals

Fresh mint or parsley

In a large soup pot, stir together the corn, beans, and salt.

Add the optional turnips, carrots, squash, cabbage or other winter greens, and leeks or onions, and simmer until they are almost tender, about 10 minutes. (Add oil, if needed.)

When the above are nearing tenderness, add the leafy greens (lettuce, spinach, endive, chicory, or arugula), strawberry or violet leaves, ground nuts, and pepper, and simmer for a few minutes more.

Stir in the chives or scallions, calendula petals, and mint or parsley.

Serve immediately with toasted Plymouth Meslin Bread (page 64).

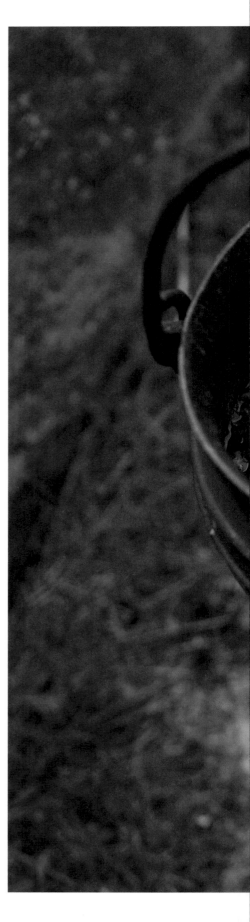

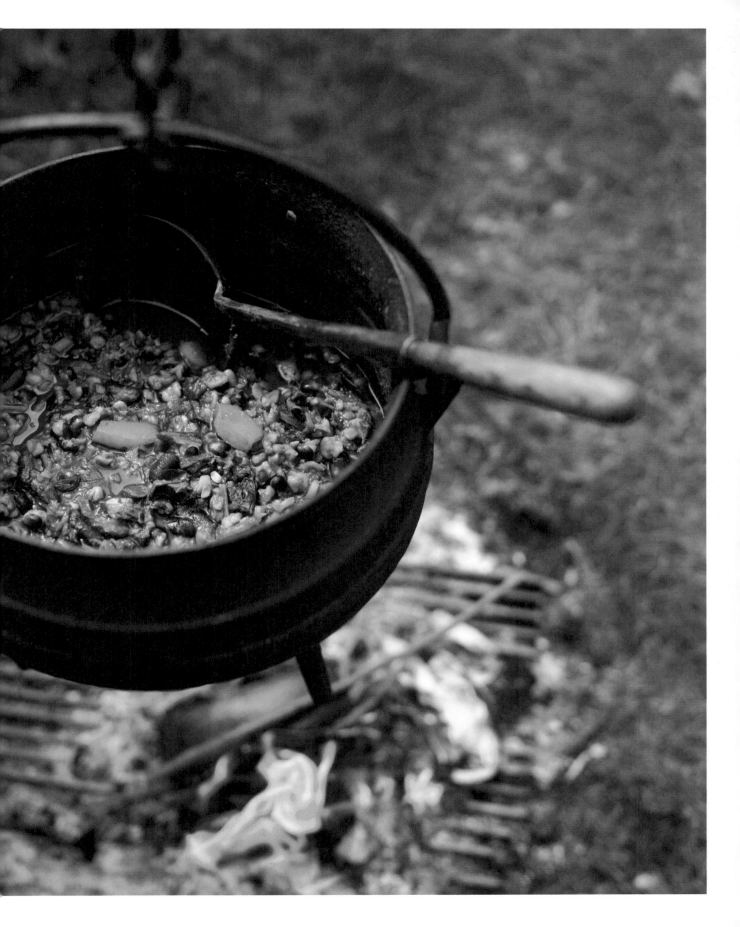

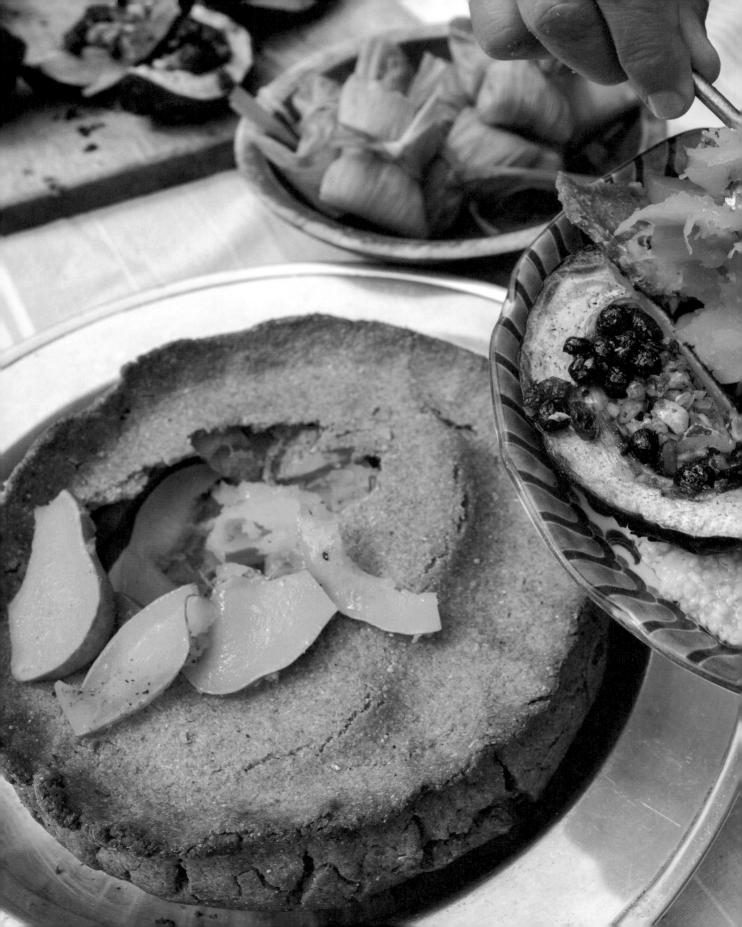

Pompion Pie

TOTAL COOK TIME: 3 HOURS • SERVES 6

For 17th-century Europeans, pompion pie was a meat or vegetable pie enclosed in a self-supporting crust, picturesquely referred to by the English as a "coffin" and cooked in the falling heat of a wood-fired masonry oven. Documents show that American "pompions," which denoted the whole family of pumpkins and squash, had already established themselves in England as suitable candidates for this treatment (sliced and mixed with apples) by the 1590s, a full generation before the departure of the *Mayflower* colonists. A 1620s Plymouth pompion pie would be apple-free, since it was another generation before the commonest and most beloved of English fruits was established in New England.

FOR THE PASTRY CRUST:

1 pound rye flour

5 ounces whole wheat flour

Pinch of salt

8 ounces rendered lard, tallow, or coconut oil

13 ounces water

FOR THE FILLING:

1 pound hard squash (such as acorn or delicata), peeled, seeded, and sliced

3 tablespoons sugar

¼ teaspoon salt

½ teaspoon freshly ground black pepper

½ teaspoon ground cloves

½ teaspoon freshly ground nutmeg

3 tablespoons sherry

½ cup dried currants or raisins (optional)

1 or 2 apples, sliced (optional)

2 tablespoons butter (or vegan butter), cut into small pieces

To make the pastry crust, in a large heatproof bowl, mix the rye flour, wheat flour, and salt.

In a saucepan over medium heat, heat the lard and water together until the fat is melted. Pour the mixture over the dry ingredients and mix thoroughly. Bring it all together into a cohesive lump, working it until it is uniform.

Wrap the ball of dough tightly and allow it to rest for at least 2 hours.

To make the filling, in a large bowl, mix all the filling ingredients.

Cut off about one-quarter of the dough to save for the top, form it into a rough round, and rewrap it.

Preheat the oven to 400°F.

Lightly flour a work surface. Press the larger piece of dough into a flat, round disk. Use your thumbs to make a depression in the center while pushing out and up to raise a smooth circular perimeter wall, about ½ inch thick or less; if any cracks form, push them together. Place your coffin on a baking sheet and fill it with the prepared filling.

On a floured work surface, roll out the reserved dough into a nice round lid, trimming it to fit. Moisten the edge of the top of the coffin wall to "glue" the components together. Place the lid on top and press the lid and the sides together, pinching to seal them. Cut a vent hole in the center of the pie.

Bake for 10 minutes, then reduce the heat to 375°F and bake for another 40 minutes or so, depending on the type of squash used. Poke a sharp knife into a slice of squash through the vent hole to see if it's tender. If the pastry browns too quickly, turn the oven down to 350°F and lay a piece of aluminum foil loosely atop the pie for the last 10 or 15 minutes of baking.

Remove from the oven and let cool a little bit before serving.

NOTES
• Unless you are a professional potter, do not expect perfection the first 9,999 times you make your coffin; rather, appreciate the experience and admire the skill of the bakers who have gone before you.

• If you want to make the pastry crust in advance, make it the day before you plan to use it and store it in the refrigerator. Let it come to room temperature before using.

Plymouth Meslin Bread

TOTAL COOK TIME: 4 HOURS • MAKES 2 LOAVES

English colonists arrived in New England with a range of bread concepts in their heads, and then went about adapting those ideas to local realities. "Meslin" meant wheat and rye that was sown, harvested, and ground together, the mixture having evolved as a bulwark against total crop failure. Fortunately, it's also a delicious combination.

As a primary economic and agricultural imperative, native corn quickly became Plymouth Colony's main crop, and thus the staple foodstuff. Since it was tricky to make into bread that was recognizable as such for the English, they eventually evolved a brown bread that used rye, sometimes wheat, and the native corn together.

3½ ounces flint cornmeal

4½ ounces boiling water

1 pound whole wheat meal

1 tablespoon sea salt

2 cups very warm water

3½ ounces whole rye meal

4½ ounces bread flour

9 ounces ripe rye leavening culture

In a large mixing bowl, stir together the cornmeal and boiling water. Cover and let it stand for at least 30 minutes.

Add the whole wheat meal, salt, and warm water to the mixture, and mix well. Cover again and let it stand for 20 minutes.

Add the whole rye meal, bread flour, and leavening culture, and mix thoroughly—either by hand or using a mixer fitted with a dough hook—until a cohesive, albeit very wet dough forms, about 5 minutes. Cover and let it rest for 40 minutes.

Scrape the dough onto a floured work surface and stretch and work it for a few minutes, incorporating as little new flour as possible. The dough will be pretty sticky and wet, so this requires a light hand.

Let it rest for another 40 minutes.

Divide the dough into two well-shaped loaves and proof it in an airtight container for about 40 minutes more.

Preheat the oven to 400°F. If you have a cast-iron Dutch oven or a baking stone or steel, preheat it in the oven at the same time.

Place each loaf in a Dutch oven (you will have to bake in batches), or place both on a baking stone or baking sheet. Bake the loaves for about 40 minutes, or until the interior temperature reaches 209°F.

NOTE
• Use a balanced kitchen scale to measure dry ingredients in ounces for best accuracy.

Samp

TOTAL COOK TIME: 45 MINUTES • SERVES 3

The staple food of virtually all humans living in the Plymouth region for centuries, samp was a porridge made from the part of flint corn that didn't crush to fine meal and could be sifted free. While the finer cornmeal was put to other uses by both Indigenous and English cooks, these larger "groats" were most easily transformed into food by simple boiling. English commentators described the resulting dish as comparable to another rather exotic food: rice. Samp was eaten on its own or in combination with other foods; for the English, who soon enough also called it hasty pudding, and who were known to lavish it with butter or milk, it may have largely supplanted bread as the anchor of every meal.

3 cups water

½ teaspoon salt

1 cup samp (or grits)

Butter (optional)

In a medium saucepan, bring the water to a boil over high heat, adding the salt. Stir in the samp a little at a time, maintaining a simmer.

Reduce the heat to low and cook, stirring every few minutes, until it thickens considerably.

Stir well, cover, and put the pot on a flame-tamer or super-low burner (or better, in the ashes near a fire) to cook for at least another 30 minutes. Stir it periodically to make sure it doesn't stick.

When the samp is done, it should be perfectly tender and creamy. Taste and add more salt if needed before serving, stirring in a lump of butter, if using.

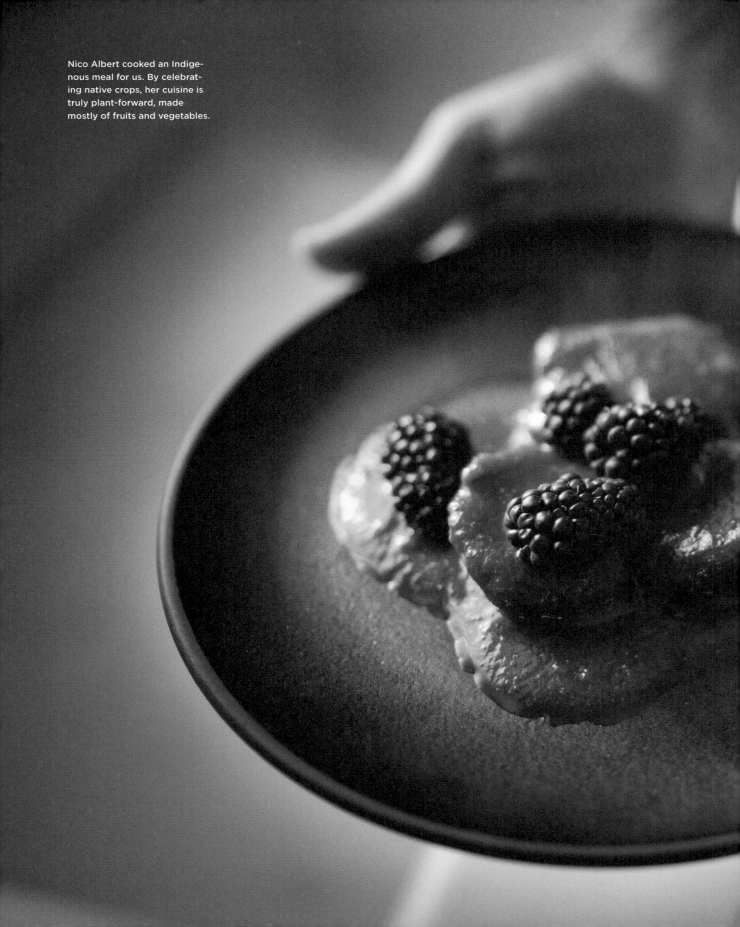

Nico Albert cooked an Indigenous meal for us. By celebrat-
ing native crops, her cuisine is
truly plant-forward, made
mostly of fruits and vegetables.

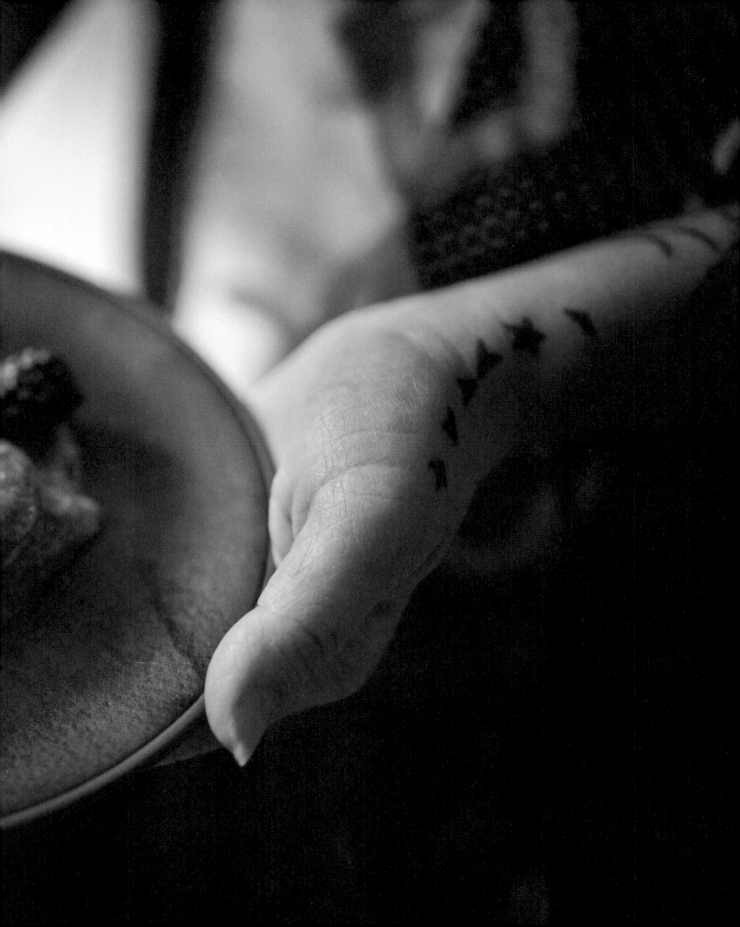

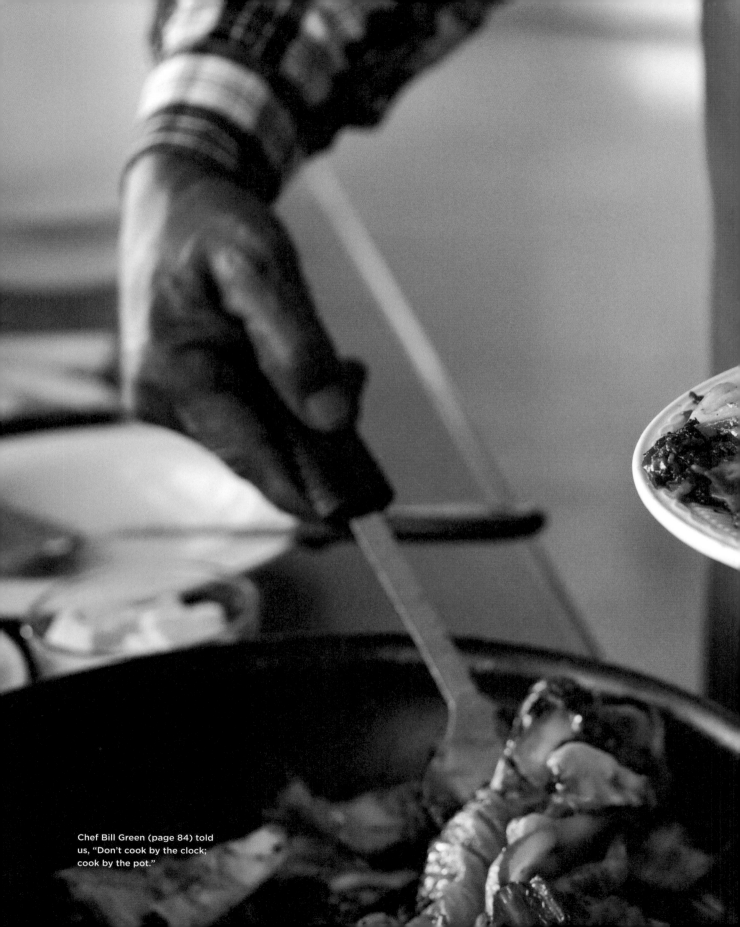

Chef Bill Green (page 84) told us, "Don't cook by the clock; cook by the pot."

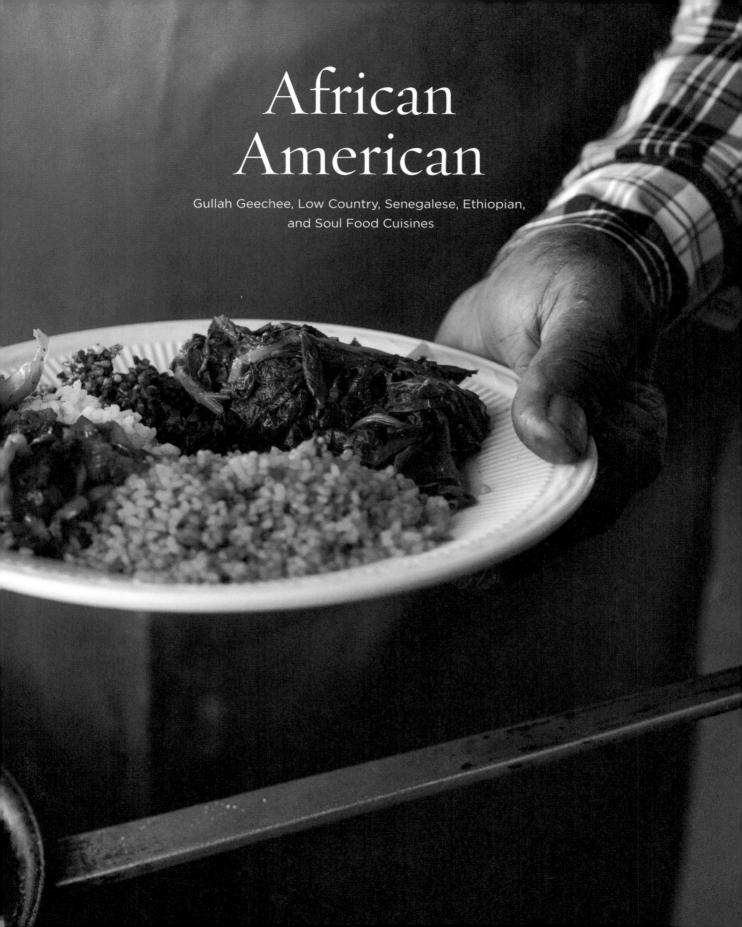

African American

Gullah Geechee, Low Country, Senegalese, Ethiopian, and Soul Food Cuisines

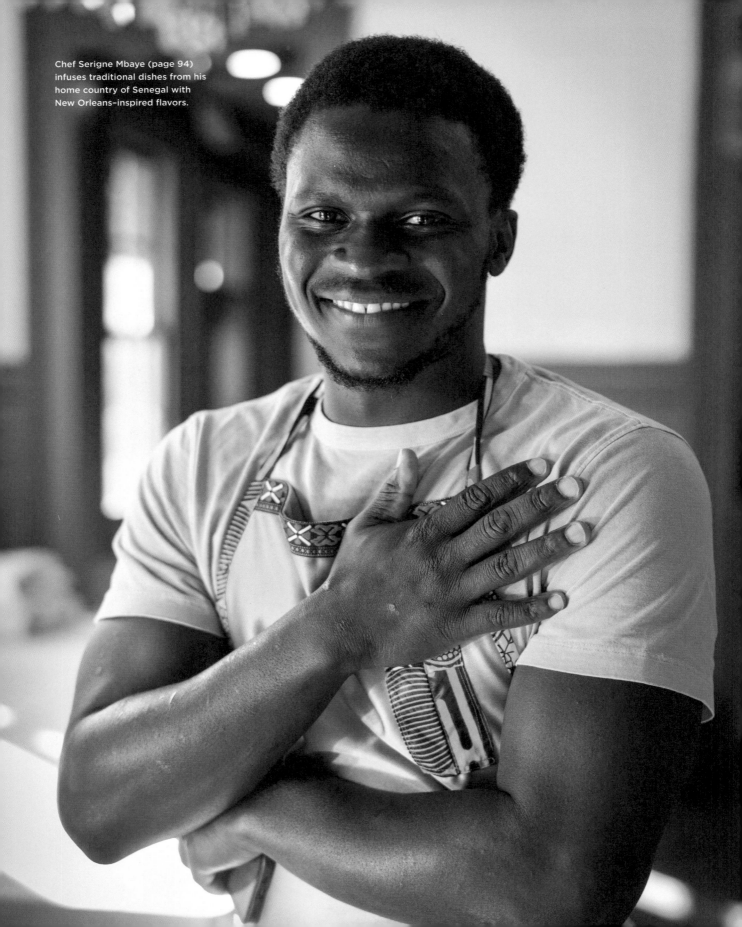

Chef Serigne Mbaye (page 94) infuses traditional dishes from his home country of Senegal with New Orleans–inspired flavors.

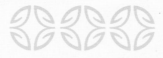

"If you're smiling or laughing, that's going to come out in the food."

~BILL GREEN

It's a steamy September morning in Charleston, South Carolina, and I'm crying tears of joy. We're in chef-historian BJ Dennis's second-story home, huddled around a bubbling pot of Butter Beans With Benne Seeds and Okra (page 83). Garlic, onion, thyme, okra, butter beans (aka lima beans), tomato, searingly hot Scotch bonnet peppers, and the splendid funk of fermented benne seeds fuse New and Old World flavors. My first bite delivers a tsunami of umami followed by an eye-watering spiciness that leaves me with a blush of pure happiness.

BJ, whose round, pleasant face is topped with a floppy golf hat, is on a mission to bring back the cuisine of his rice-growing ancestors. Captured from places like Senegal and Angola, his forebears—the Gullah Geechee—were brought to the Low Country of South Carolina and Georgia to cultivate Carolina Gold rice. Because of their expertise, the Gullah Geechee were allowed to keep private gardens, where they grew African staples along with local ingredients. "We took the rustic soul of the Africans and the Native American techniques and made this special mash-up," says BJ. The resulting cuisine is uniquely American, explosively delicious, and as I've been discovering, it draws from all the ingredients that support longevity.

We know that the world's longest-lived people eat mostly whole, plant-based foods like tubers, greens, grains, nuts, and beans. And so, it seems, did West Africans.

The traditional West African diet consisted mostly of greens, root vegetables, black-eyed peas, okra, benne seeds, and cereals like millet—essentially a vegetarian diet. When enslaved peoples were taken to America, they brought the seeds of their homeland foods with them (occasionally hidden in their hair). In many cases, local Native Americans taught them how to cultivate—and cook with—corn, sweet potatoes, and local bean varieties. The result was a completely new and innovative

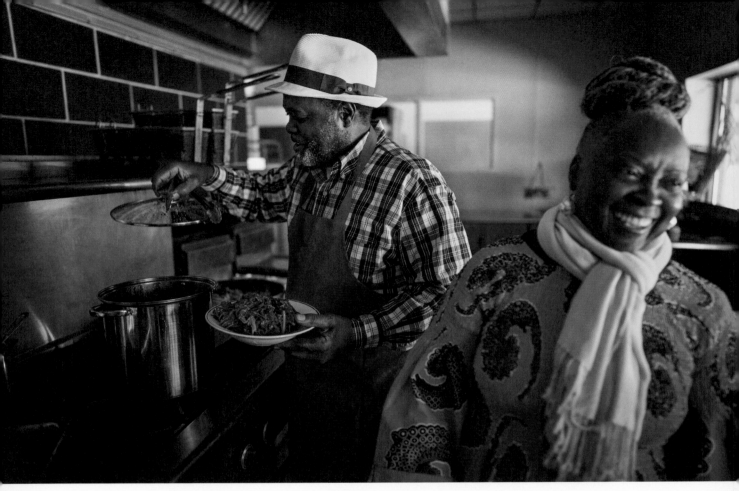

Bill Green and his wife, Sara, have run Gullah Grub on St. Helena Island, South Carolina, for 15 years.

cuisine. For instance, the staple dish Hoppin' John (page 90) blends West African ingredients such as black-eyed peas, rice, and greens with North American accoutrements such as thyme, celery, and corn bread.

Benne seeds (the heirloom ancestor to modern sesame seeds) provided a rich source of nutrients, calories, and flavor to early African American dishes. "Rich in oil and nutty in taste, benne can be eaten raw," and it can also be used as a condiment, flavoring, or thickening agent, University of South Carolina professor David Shields writes in *The Larder: Food Studies Methods From the American South.* "Because it is highly nutritious (25 percent protein, 50 percent fat, yet high in fiber, B vitamins, iron and magnesium), it could provide sustenance with minimal preparation."

According to Herbert C. Covey's *What the Slaves Ate: Recollections of African American Foods and Foodways From the Slave Narratives,* several culinary tendencies that traveled with enslaved people from Africa to the Americas are signature dishes and techniques in the United States, including fritters, boiled greens, rice dishes, and the use of okra, nuts, and seeds as thickening agents. Africans and their American descendants also had a well-deserved reputation for spicy, hot food. Their knowledge of seasonings and spices transformed simple bland foods into zesty meals.

These culinary traditions seemed to survive through the antebellum period to about 1920. W. O. Atwater and his colleagues observed that African Americans in the Deep South ate garden produce such as black-eyed peas, butter beans, okra (fried and stewed), red beans, sweet potatoes, and greens. Other foods included biscuits, chowchow (a spicy pickle relish), corn bread, grits, rice, sorghum, and watermelon. Meat was still largely used only as a seasoning or celebratory food.

That all changed when many African Americans began to migrate from the rural South to big cities in the North between 1920 and 1970. "This was a massive dietary disruption," the James Beard Award–winning culinary historian Adrian Miller tells me. "When African Americans moved to cities, they had nowhere to grow their gardens. So they ate the food that was more readily available, which was cheap cuts of meat and processed foods."

So we seek out chefs like BJ who have kept those pre-1920 culinary traditions alive and are bringing them into the 21st century.

In Savannah, Georgia, we meet Roosevelt Brownlee, a 75-year-old dreadlocked Gullah Geechee chef who has cooked for the likes of Stan Getz and Nina Simone. He converted to Rastafarianism when he met Bob Marley. In a backwoods kitchen, he and his cousin Rollen Chalmers whip up "pink-eyed soup," hoecakes, and red peas—all accompanied by Carolina Gold cracked rice. As his T-shirt proclaims, "Rice Is Life." Who am I to argue?

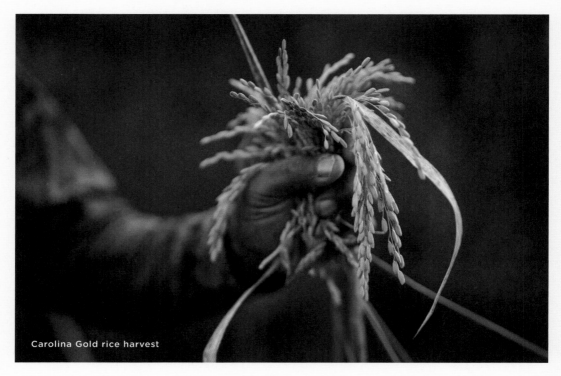

Carolina Gold rice harvest

Matthew Raiford, another celebrated chef who once cooked at the White House, started his training with his great-grandma Florine and honed it at the Culinary Institute of America. He's also an ecological horticulturalist, certified by the University of California's Santa Cruz Center for Agroecology. Today, at the behest of his grandmother, he's taken over the family farm in Brunswick, Georgia. He tours us past his hen-of-the-woods mushrooms, the old truck tires that serve as sweet potato planters, and the vast hibiscus plants he uses to make teas. He prepares exquisitely simple black beans (served with spring greens and pickled cucumbers or wrapped in a tortilla) and collard greens (slow-cooked—never boiled—for 45 minutes with red pepper, white onion, and vinegar). (See Spiced Black Beans on page 79.)

And behind his Gullah Grub Restaurant on St. Helena Island in South Carolina, the ever ebullient Gullah chef Bill Green welcomes us to the community kitchen he uses to prepare 500 meals per week, mostly for kids in need. Wearing a plaid shirt, red apron, and broad-rimmed white hat, and sporting a gray-flecked beard, he shows us how to make Stir-Fried Cabbage and Beets (page 84) and Red Cracked Rice (page 86). "If you're smiling or laughing, that's going to come out in the food. All you have to do is look at a man to know if his food is good or bad," he says. In Bill's case, his smile turns out to be deliciously prescient, because his food couldn't be better.

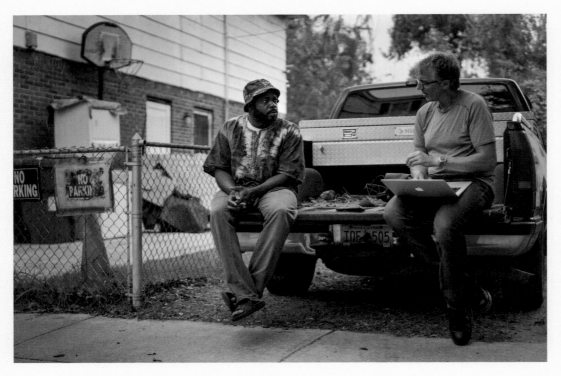

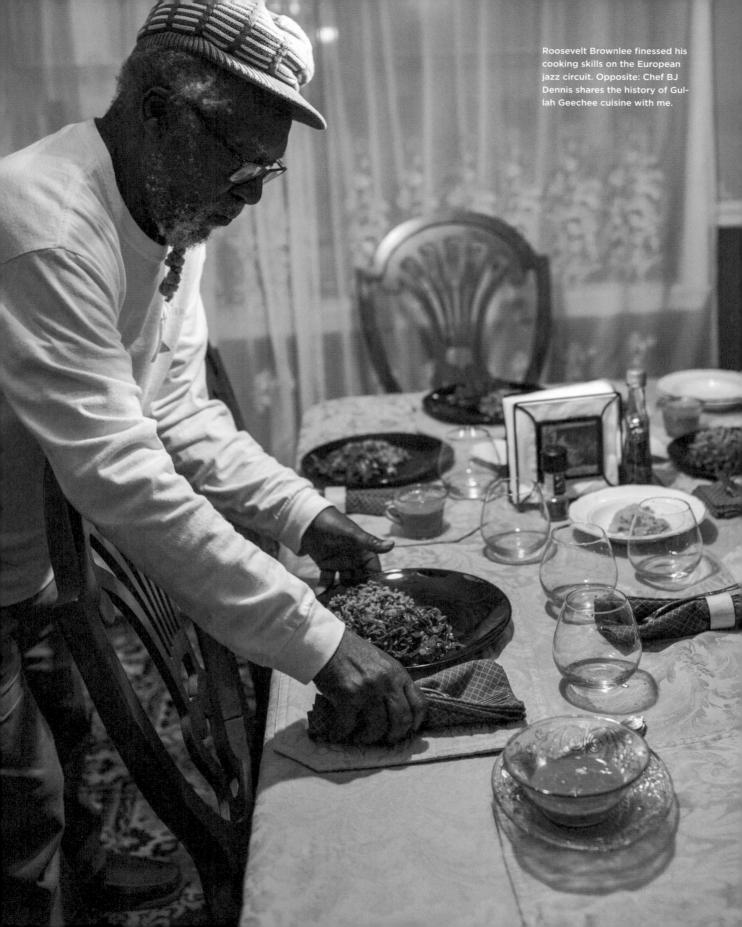

Roosevelt Brownlee finessed his cooking skills on the European jazz circuit. Opposite: Chef BJ Dennis shares the history of Gullah Geechee cuisine with me.

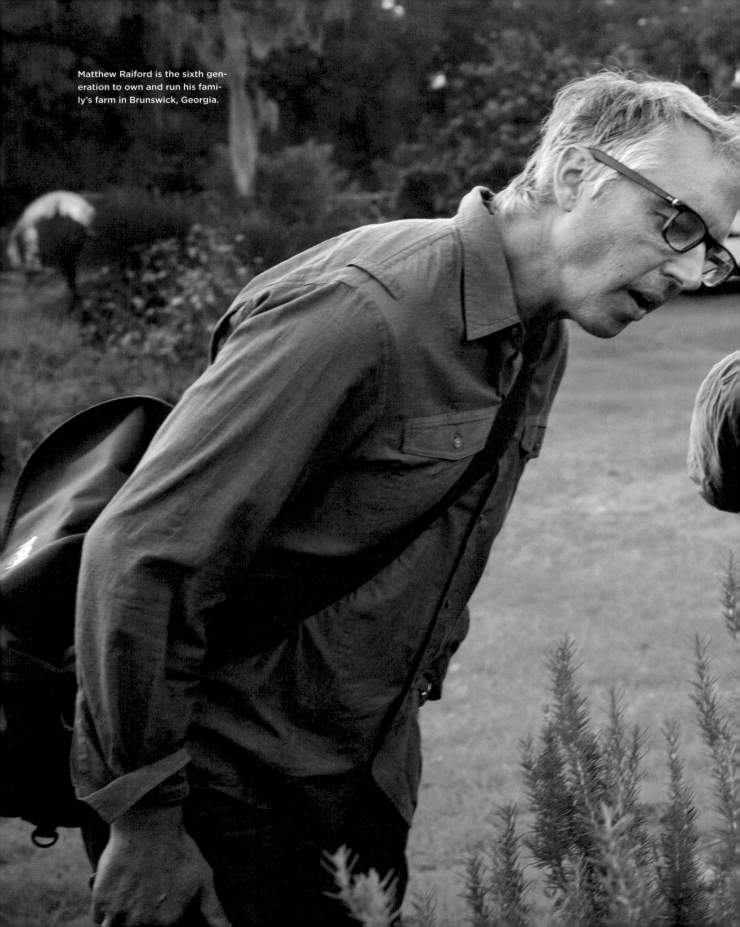

Matthew Raiford is the sixth generation to own and run his family's farm in Brunswick, Georgia.

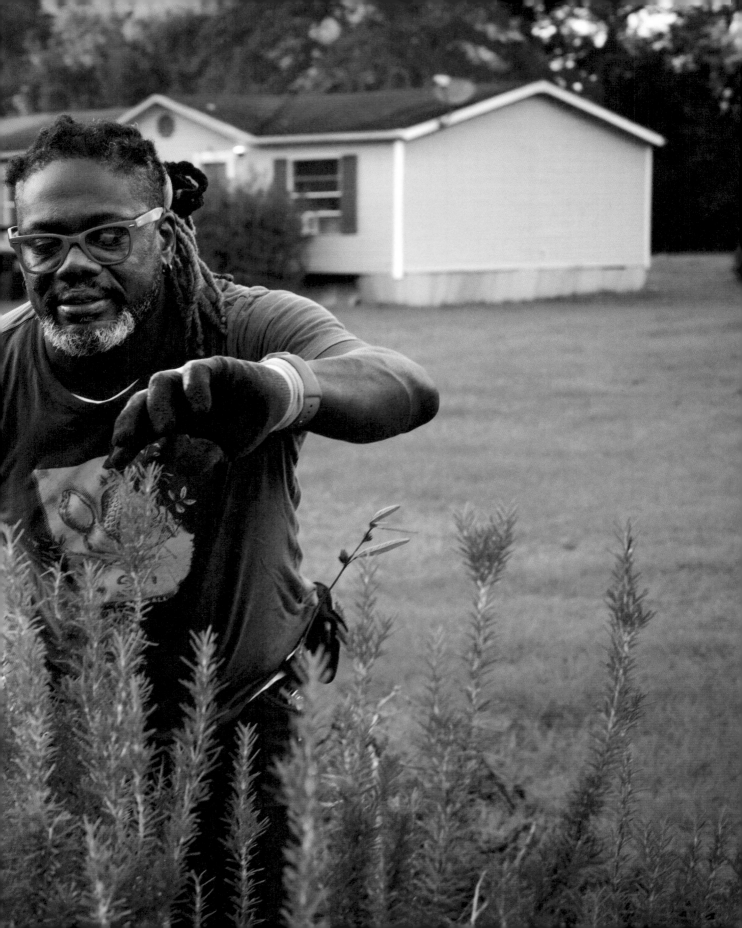

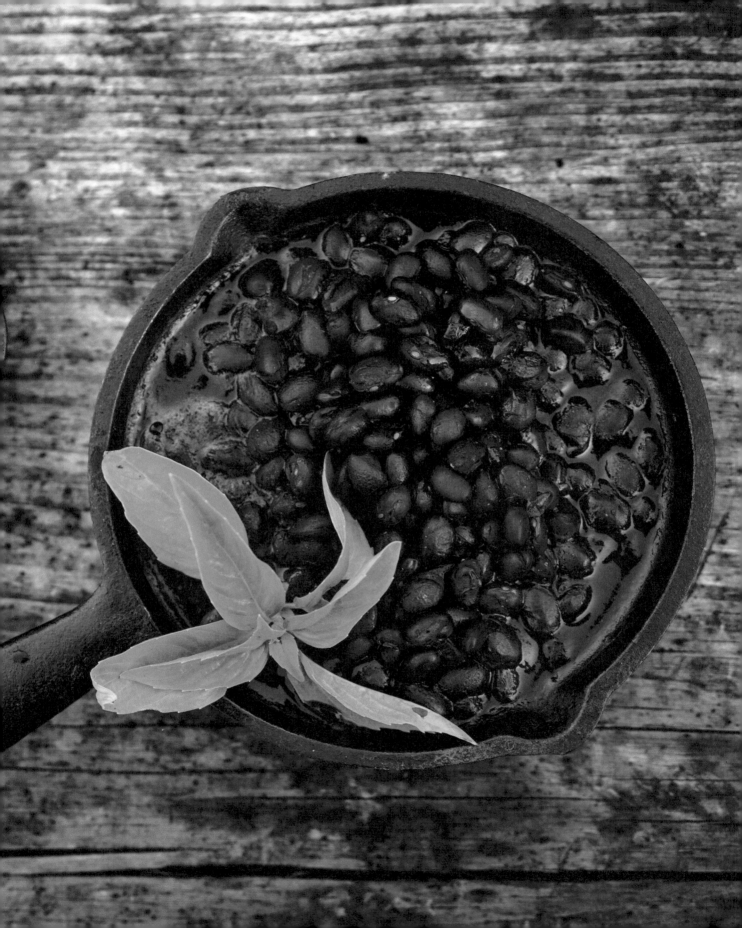

Spiced Black Beans With Rice

TOTAL COOK TIME: 1 HOUR • SERVES 5

Chef Matthew Raiford interprets Coastal Georgia cuisine through the lens of his Gullah Geechee heritage and upbringing on the family farm his great-great grandfather established more than 150 years ago. Matthew trained at the Culinary Institute of America and the University of California, Santa Cruz. Having seen the world, he says that for now he wants to be home on his ancestral land. He enjoys the rhythm of the farm, which he continues to run with his siblings. His farm-to-fork cuisine has won accolades from the James Beard Foundation.

1 pound dried black beans

1 tablespoon pink Himalayan salt

1 teaspoon freshly ground black pepper

1 teaspoon crushed red pepper

1½ teaspoons ground cumin

2 cups white rice

4 cups water

1 teaspoon sea salt

2 teaspoons ground coriander

6 green onions, thinly sliced, for garnish

In a stockpot or large saucepan, combine the beans and plenty of cold water to cover. Bring the pot to a boil over high heat. Once the water boils, remove the pot from the heat and let stand for 30 minutes.

Drain the beans and return them to the pot. Add fresh water to cover the beans by 1 inch. Add the Himalayan salt, black pepper, and crushed red pepper, and bring to a boil.

Reduce the heat so that the water is simmering. Add the cumin and cook for about 30 minutes, until the beans are tender.

While the beans are cooking, make the rice. Combine the rice, water, sea salt, and coriander in a saucepan. Bring to a boil, reduce the heat to low, cover, and let simmer for about 20 minutes, until the rice is tender.

To serve, scoop a small amount of rice onto a plate and then add some of the beans, along with the cooking liquid, over the top. Garnish with the green onions.

Coconut and Spice Chickpeas

TOTAL COOK TIME: 1 HOUR • SERVES 4

This simple spiced-bean dish includes several anti-inflammatory ingredients—turmeric, garlic, olive oil, and red pepper—as well as protein from the chickpeas. Feel free to adjust the seasonings to your liking.

1 pound dried chickpeas, soaked in water overnight

1 tablespoon olive oil

1 medium onion, diced

3 to 4 garlic cloves, mashed

4 cups vegetable stock

1 (14-ounce) can unsweetened coconut milk

1 tablespoon sea salt

1 tablespoon turmeric

1 teaspoon cayenne

Drain the chickpeas.

In a stockpot or large saucepan, heat olive oil over medium heat. Add the onion and garlic and cook, stirring occasionally, until the onion is browned, about 10 minutes.

Add the chickpeas to the onion and stir to coat, then add the vegetable stock, coconut milk, salt, turmeric, and cayenne. Bring up to a hard boil over high heat, then reduce the heat to very low and simmer for 35 to 45 minutes, stirring gently every 10 to 15 minutes, until the chickpeas are tender.

Taste and adjust the seasoning as needed before serving.

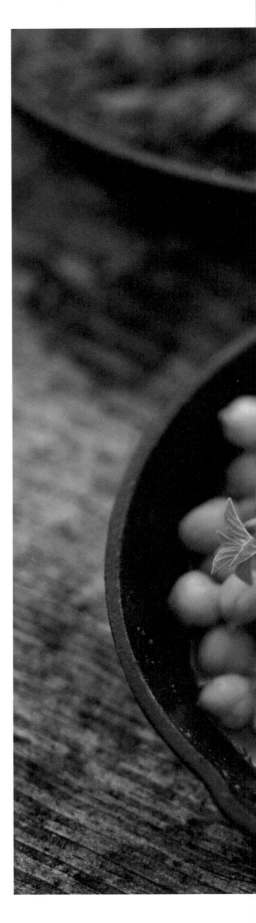

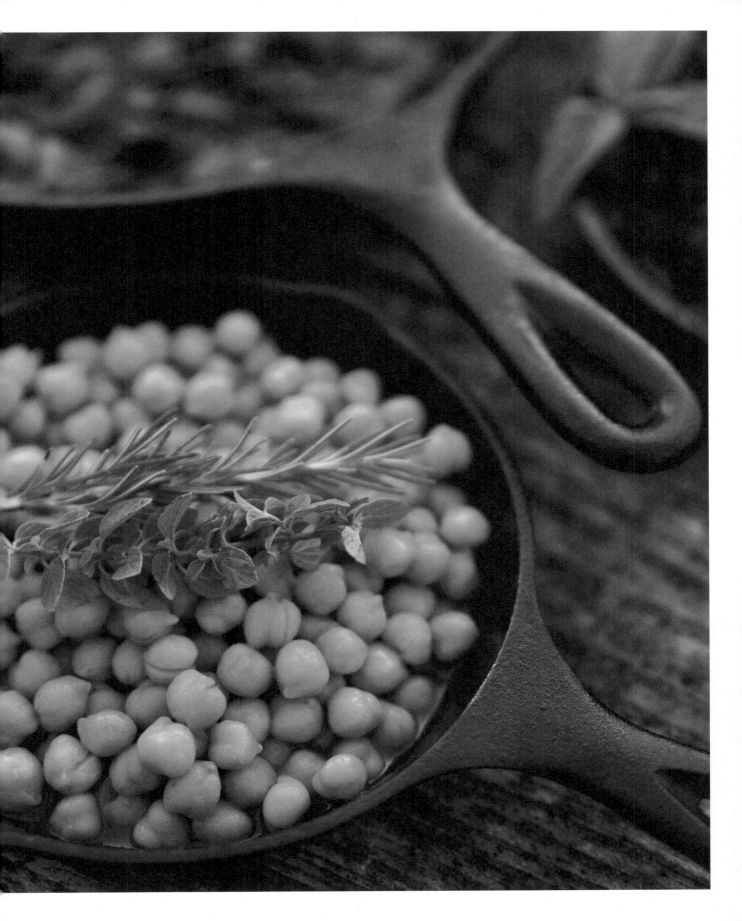

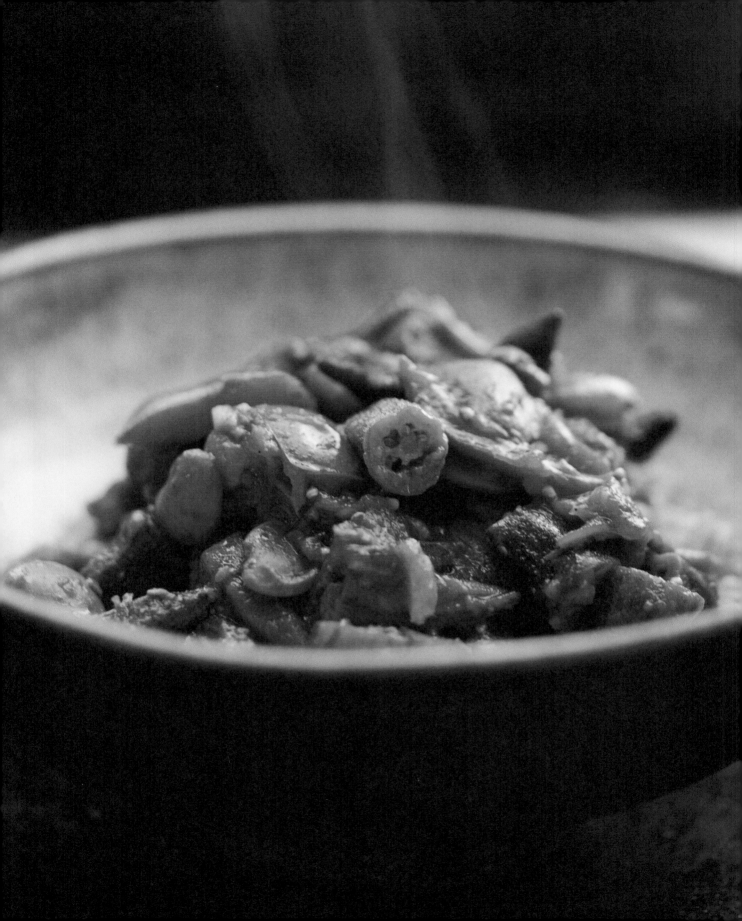

Butter Beans With Benne Seeds and Okra

TOTAL COOK TIME: 45 MINUTES • SERVES 4

Benne seeds are an heirloom variety of sesame seeds that were brought to this country on slave ships from West Africa. In Gullah Geechee cuisine—the cooking style developed by the descendants of enslaved Africans in the Low Country of South Carolina and Georgia—the seeds are used to thicken soups and stews. They also add a deep, slightly bitter, and nutty flavor along with a dose of fat and protein.

1 cup oil

2 pounds fresh tomatoes, diced (or 1 28-ounce can diced tomatoes)

1 small onion

5 garlic cloves, minced

1 hot pepper (such as Scotch bonnet), minced

1 bay leaf

1 cup fermented benne seeds (ogiri) or 1 cup toasted and pounded benne seeds

½ pound butter beans (lima beans)

3 to 4 thyme sprigs

1 quart water or vegetable stock

1 pound okra, cut into ½-inch pieces

Salt

Heat the oil in a stockpot or large saucepan over medium-high heat.

Add the tomatoes, onion, garlic, hot pepper, bay leaf, benne seeds, butter beans, and thyme. Sauté over medium heat for 5 to 7 minutes.

Add the water and cook over medium heat for 20 minutes.

Add the okra to the pot and cook for 10 to 15 minutes more, until the okra is tender.

Add salt to taste and additional water if needed to maintain a stew-like consistency.

Serve hot.

Stir-Fried Cabbage and Beets

TOTAL COOK TIME: 15 MINUTES • SERVES 4

¼ cup vegetable oil

1 large yellow onion, sliced

1 head cabbage, cut into large
  chunks (about 4-inch squares)

3 small beets, peeled and sliced

2 tablespoons brown sugar

½ teaspoon cayenne

1 teaspoon freshly ground black
  pepper

1 teaspoon garlic powder

1 teaspoon ground ginger

1 teaspoon ground sage

Pinch of salt

Heat the oil in a large skillet over
medium-high heat.

Add the onion and cook, stirring,
for about 5 minutes, until
softened.

Add the cabbage, beets, brown
sugar, cayenne, pepper, garlic
powder, ginger, sage, and salt.
Cook until the cabbage and onion
are well browned but not burned,
about 10 minutes.

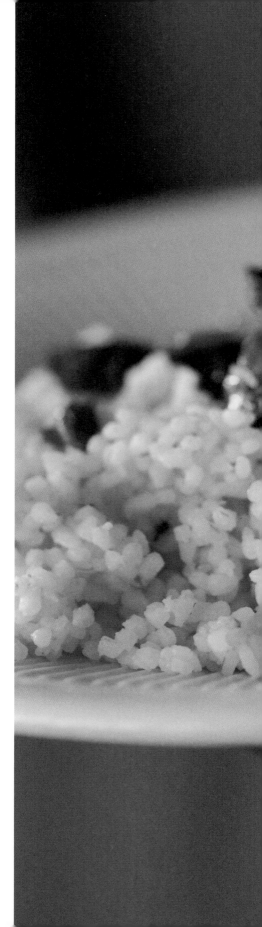

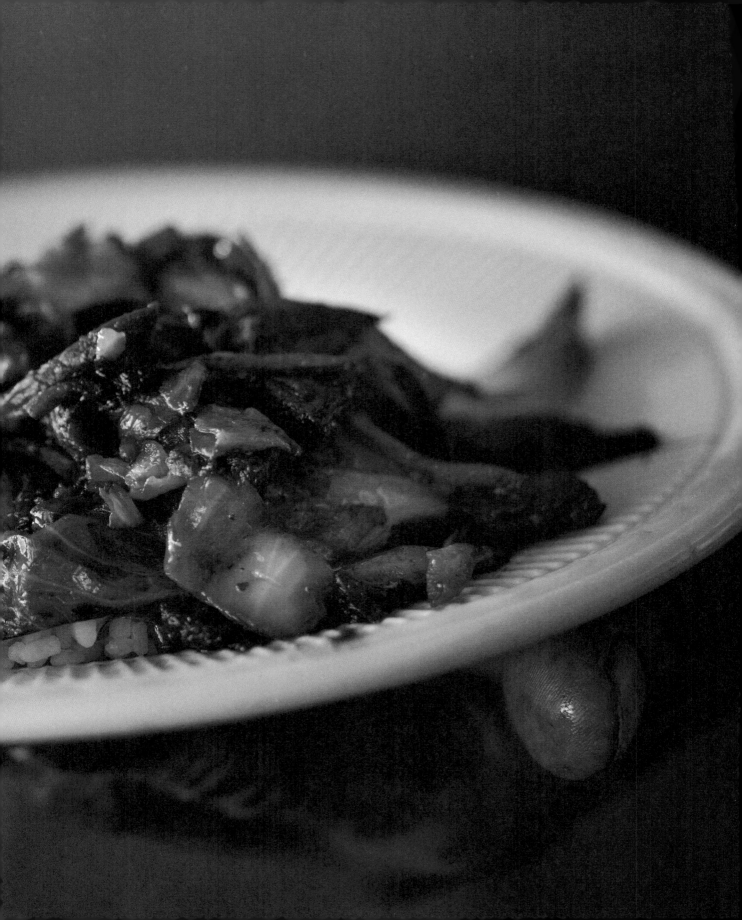

Red Cracked Rice

TOTAL COOK TIME: 1 HOUR 15 MINUTES • SERVES 3

2 cups Carolina Gold rice

⅓ cup oil, plus more for finishing

2 to 3 teaspoons granulated garlic

2 to 3 teaspoons sage

1 quart tomato sauce

3 cups water

Salt

Freshly ground black pepper

Cook the rice according to the package directions.

In a medium saucepan, heat the oil over medium heat. Add the granulated garlic and sage.

Stir in the tomato sauce and water and bring to a boil. Reduce to a simmer and cook for 15 minutes.

Taste and add salt and pepper as needed. Cook for 30 minutes more.

Preheat the oven to 275°F.

Mix the rice and sauce in a pan or Dutch oven, then bake for 30 minutes.

Fluff with a fork and add a splash of oil at the end, if desired.

Lemon and Sage Collard Greens

TOTAL COOK TIME: 1 HOUR 20 MINUTES • SERVES 4

¼ cup oil

1 onion, chopped

2 pounds collard greens

⅓ cup lemon juice

1⅓ teaspoons sage

1½ teaspoons granulated garlic

½ teaspoon cayenne

Salt

3 quarts water

2 teaspoons brown sugar

In a stockpot or large saucepan, heat the oil over medium-high heat. Add the onion and cook, stirring occasionally, until browned, about 10 minutes.

Add the greens, lemon juice, sage, granulated garlic, cayenne, salt, and water. Bring to a boil and then reduce the heat to medium-low and simmer until tender, for about 45 to 90 minutes.

Stir in the brown sugar just before serving.

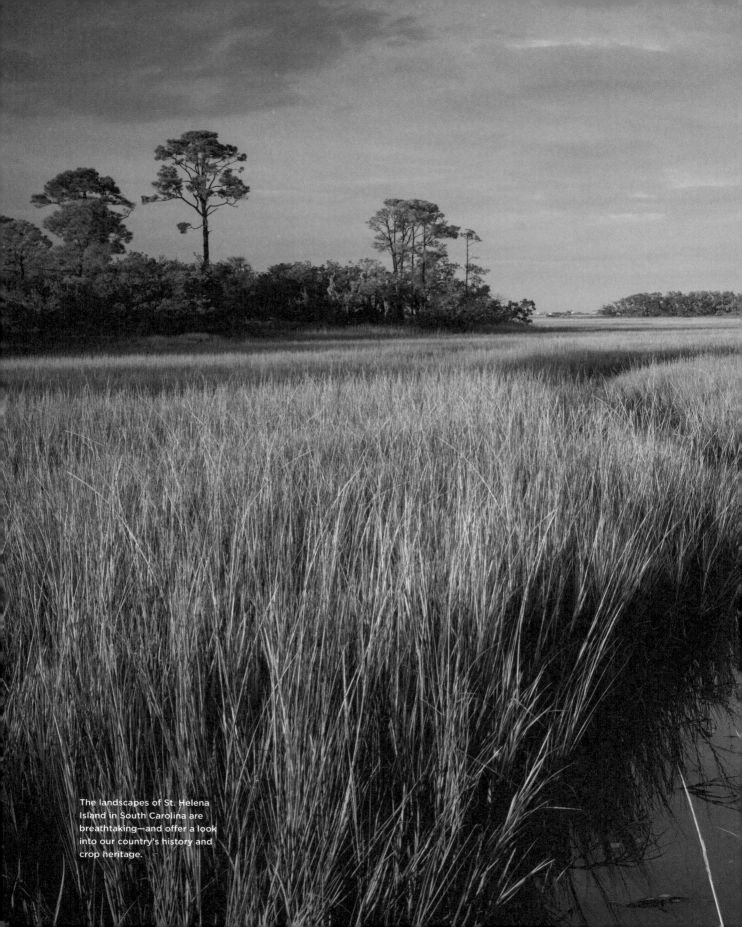

The landscapes of St. Helena Island in South Carolina are breathtaking—and offer a look into our country's history and crop heritage.

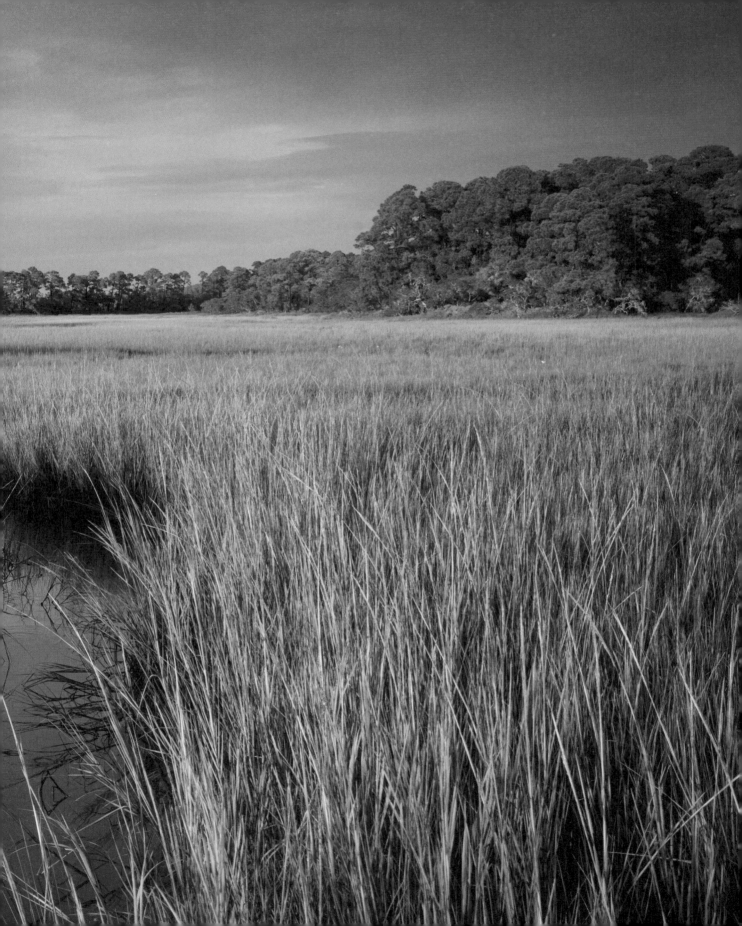

Hoppin' John With Carolina Gold Rice and Sapelo Red Peas

TOTAL COOK TIME: 1 HOUR • SERVES 6

Carolina Gold rice is a unique heirloom grain that's unlike the supermarket rice most of us are used to. A West African strain, it was first grown, cultivated, and cooked on American soil by enslaved peoples on plantations. In the 19th century, it became the dominant rice in the U.S. market, only to all but completely disappear after the Great Depression. Though you couldn't find it on grocery store shelves for decades, it was legendary in the Low Country for its unique starchiness and earthy, nutty flavor. Thanks to a handful of industrious growers like Rollen Chalmers who are reviving such heirloom grains, you can now find Carolina Gold rice again on grocery store shelves and online.

1 cup Sapelo red peas

1 teaspoon salt

½ teaspoon freshly ground black pepper

1 teaspoon smoked paprika

3 cups water

2 cups Carolina Gold rice

Preheat the oven to 350°F.

In a large pot, combine the peas, salt, pepper, and paprika. Add the water and bring to a boil.

Reduce the heat to low and simmer for 30 minutes.

Put the rice in a 9-by-13-inch baking dish, and pour the pea mixture over the top. Cover the baking dish with aluminum foil and bake for 30 minutes.

Serve hot.

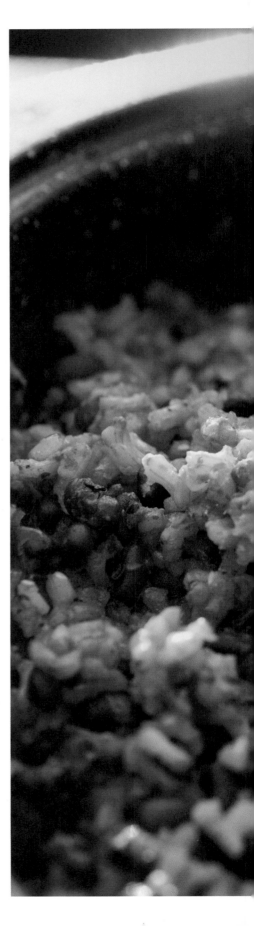

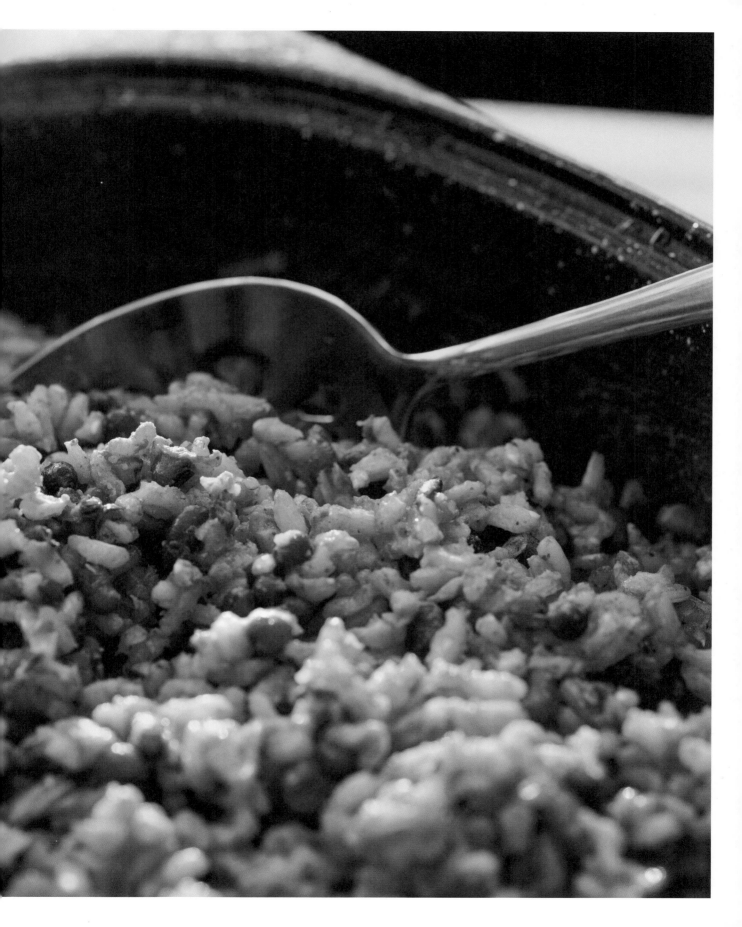

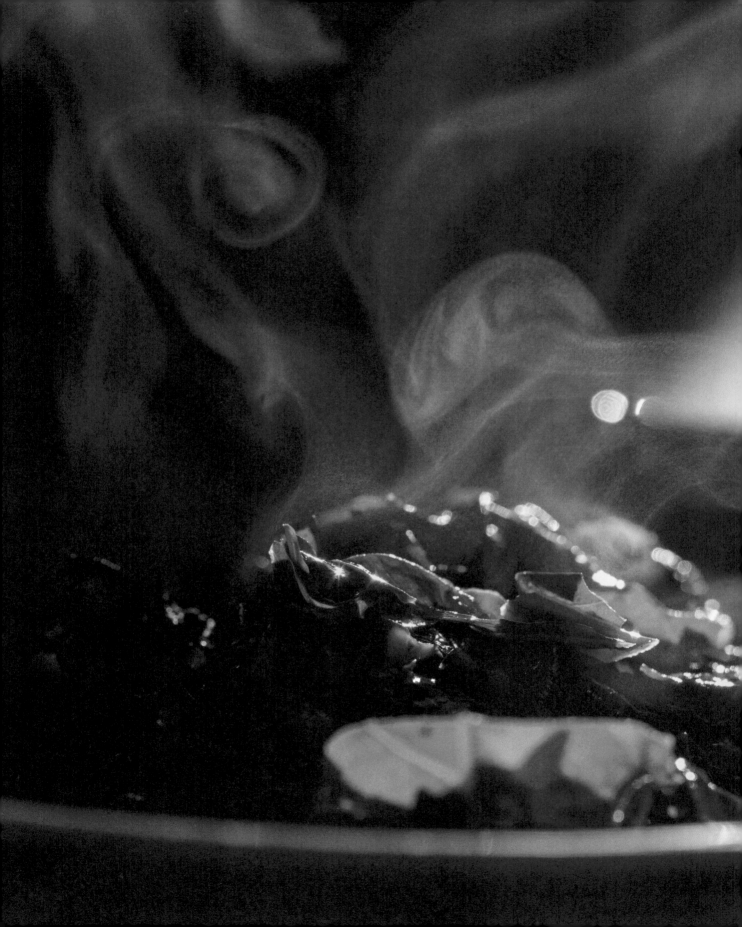

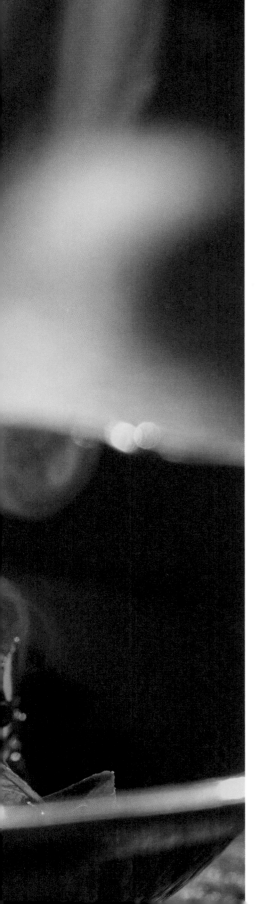

Smoky Collard Greens

TOTAL COOK TIME: 1 HOUR • SERVES 6

3 tablespoons benne oil (or sesame oil)

1 garlic clove, minced

1 onion, sliced

2 pounds collard greens, chopped

1 tablespoon salt

1 teaspoon freshly ground black pepper

1 teaspoon crushed red pepper

1 teaspoon smoked paprika

Heat the oil in a large pot over medium heat. Add the garlic, onion, collard greens, salt, black pepper, red pepper, and paprika. Stir to mix the ingredients, and cook until the greens reach the desired tenderness, about 45 to 60 minutes.

Serve hot.

Senegalese Fonio Grain Salad With Mango and Avocado

TOTAL COOK TIME: 25 MINUTES • SERVES 4

Serigne Mbaye, an award-winning Senegalese American chef, got his start in Michelin-starred restaurants. After settling in New Orleans, he created a pop-up that connects the cuisines of New Orleans and Senegal. Serigne cites West African food as the grandparent of New Orleans cooking, since the city was a major slave port from the Senegal and Gambia regions.

Fonio is a type of millet that has been cultivated in West Africa for thousands of years. It's been described as having a texture between quinoa and couscous with a delicious earthy, nutty flavor. It's also full of protein and other nutrients. In Senegalese cuisine, it's often served as a base for stew.

FOR THE FONIO:

½ cup fonio

½ cup water

Salt

FOR MANGO VINAIGRETTE:

1 mango, peeled and diced small

Salt

1 teaspoon Dijon mustard

2 tablespoons sugar

2 teaspoons lemon juice

1 tablespoon cayenne

½ vegetable oil

FOR THE SALAD:

½ head cabbage, julienned

½ red onion, sliced and pickled
  (page 119)

1 avocado, diced

2 tomatoes, diced

1 tablespoon chopped pecans

1 sprig parsley, for garnish

To make the fonio, wash the fonio in running water five times, straining it through a fine-mesh sieve in between.

In a medium saucepan, boil the water with a pinch of salt. Add the fonio and cook, stirring, for 3 minutes. Remove from the heat, cover, and let stand for 10 minutes. Fluff with a fork.

To make the mango vinaigrette, in a blender, add the mango, a sprinkle of salt, Dijon mustard, sugar, lemon juice, and cayenne. Blend with the oil until it has a smooth and thick consistency. Add more seasoning to taste.

To assemble the salad, in a medium bowl, add the prepared fonio, cabbage, pickled red onion, avocado, tomatoes, and pecans. Mix everything, and toss with a little bit of mango vinaigrette until you find the right balance.

Garnish with the parsley and serve immediately.

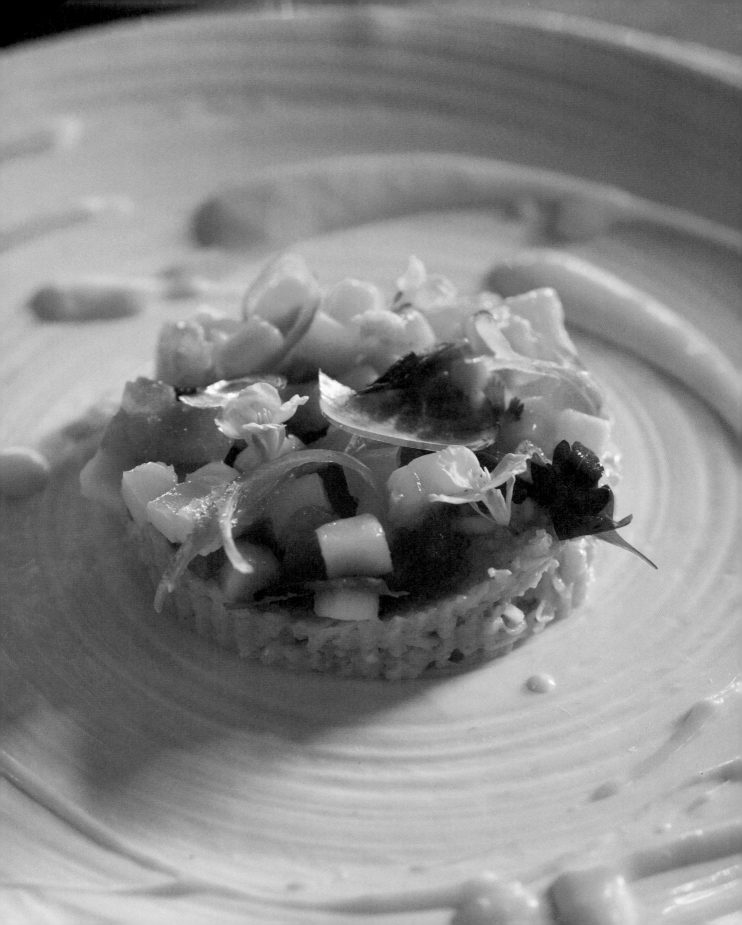

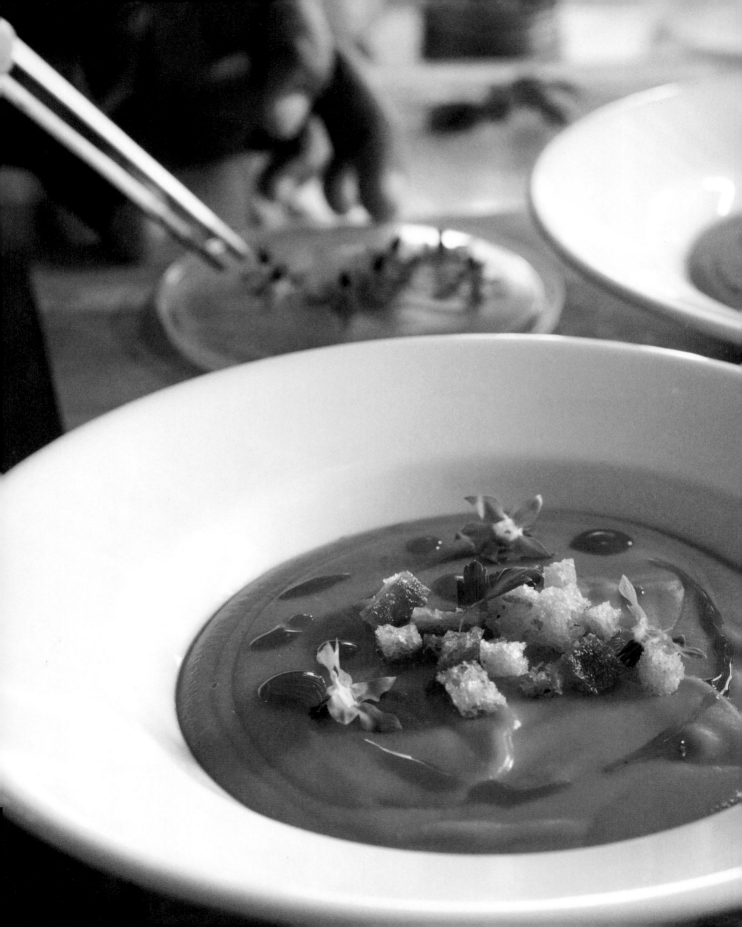

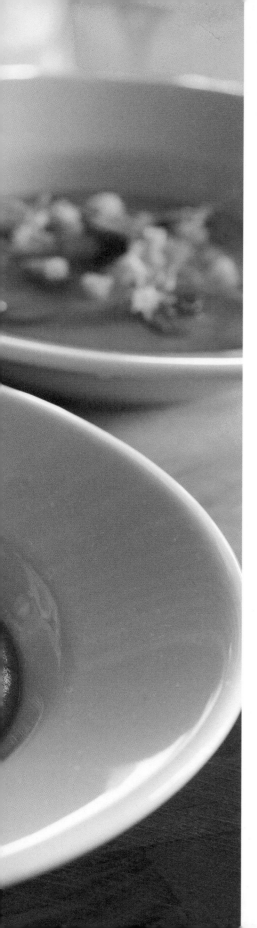

The Last Meal: Sweet Potato and Black-Eyed Pea Soup

TOTAL COOK TIME: 20 MINUTES • SERVES 4

Serigne Mbaye tells the story of his enslaved ancestors who were fattened up with black-eyed peas and palm oil by traders who needed them to reach a minimum weight of 125 pounds to put them on a ship. The food wasn't meant for them to enjoy—if they didn't eat it and gain weight, they would be shot. Serigne has chosen to reclaim this combination, making his own version of "the last meal." He makes it taste good by using fresh vegetables, aromatics, and spices. Now, this last meal is made for pure enjoyment.

1 cup black-eyed peas, soaked in water for 3 hours

¼ cup vegetable oil

1 large onion, diced

2 garlic cloves, minced

1 green pepper, diced

3 tomatoes, diced

½ teaspoon cayenne

Salt

1 tablespoon white wine vinegar

3 large sweet potatoes, peeled and diced

2 cups water

3 tablespoons palm oil (or coconut oil)

Drain and rinse the black-eyed peas.

Heat a stockpot or large saucepan over medium heat. Add the vegetable oil, onion, garlic, green pepper, tomatoes, cayenne, and a pinch of salt. Cook, stirring occasionally, until the onion is caramelized, about 10 minutes.

Add the vinegar to the pot to deglaze it.

Add the black-eyed peas, sweet potatoes, and water, and bring to a simmer. Cook until the black-eyed peas are very soft. Add the palm oil and more seasoning if needed. Remove from the heat and let cool for a few minutes.

Using an immersion blender, or in batches in a countertop blender, puree the soup until smooth.

Reheat the soup just before serving and serve hot.

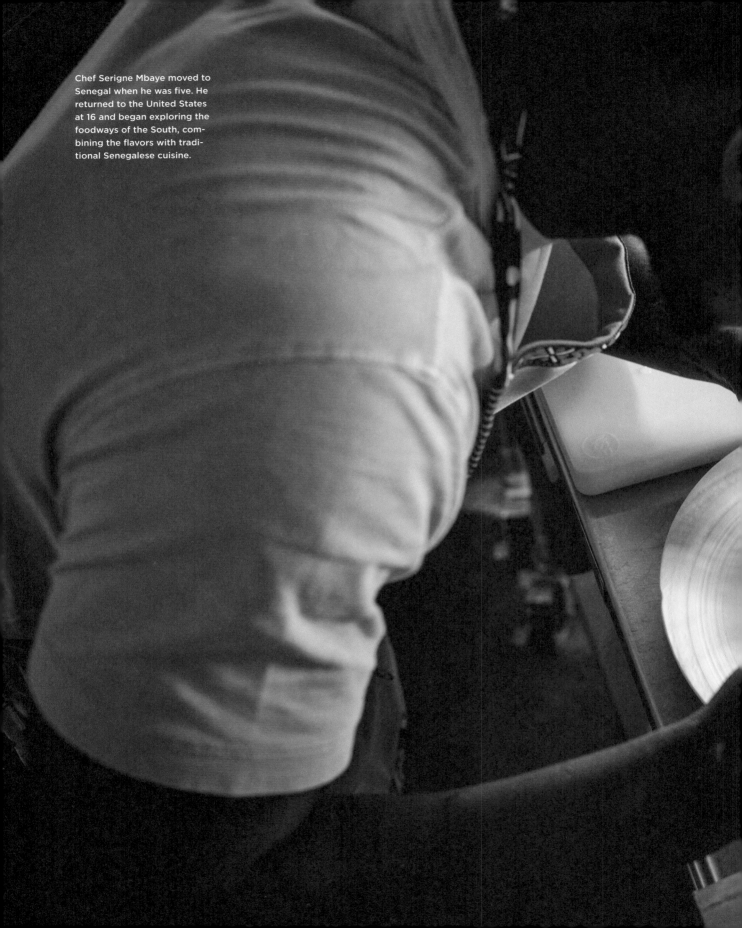

Chef Serigne Mbaye moved to Senegal when he was five. He returned to the United States at 16 and began exploring the foodways of the South, combining the flavors with traditional Senegalese cuisine.

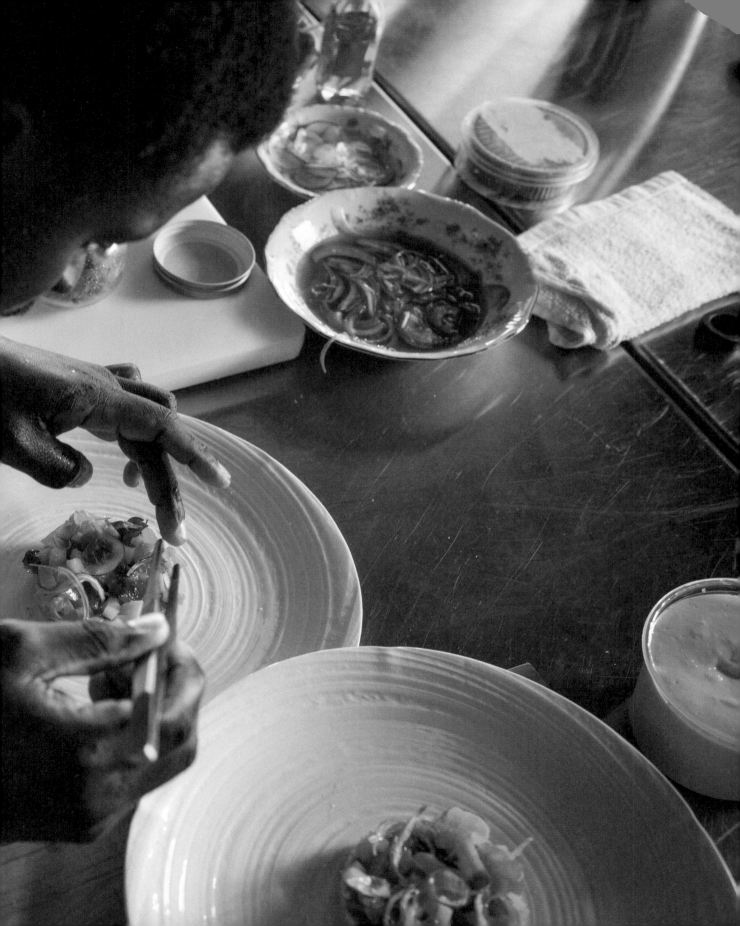

Spicy Cabbage Salad

TOTAL COOK TIME: 10 MINUTES • SERVES 4

Chef and owner Tenagne Belachew opened Lalibela in the Little Ethiopia neighborhood of Los Angeles with her six daughters in 2016. She started the family affair with recipes handed down to her from her grandmother and mother, and the restaurant has been in demand for its flavor-filled, communal, family-style meals.

3 tablespoons vegetable oil

1 onion, sliced

2 carrots, peeled and sliced

1 jalapeño pepper, seeded and finely diced

1 head cabbage, chopped

1½ tablespoons minced garlic

Salt

Freshly ground black pepper

In a large skillet, heat the oil over medium-high heat. Add the onion and cook until softened, about 5 minutes.

Add the carrots and jalapeño and cook a few more minutes.

Add the cabbage, garlic, and salt and pepper to taste, and cook a few minutes more, until the cabbage wilts.

Plant-Based Kitfo

TOTAL COOK TIME: 5 TO 10 MINUTES • SERVES 4

Mitmita is a ground spice mixture used in Ethiopian cooking. It contains African bird's eye chili peppers, which give it its orange-red color, along with other spices such as cardamom, cloves, and salt, and sometimes seasonings including cumin, cinnamon, and ginger. Here it's used to season a ground plant-based mixture that's served with traditional injera bread.

3 tablespoons spiced oil

¾ pound plant-based ground meat substitute

1½ to 2 tablespoons mitmita

1 teaspoon black cardamom

1 tablespoon minced onion

1 tablespoon minced garlic

1½ teaspoons salt

1 tablespoon freshly ground black pepper

Heat the oil in a skillet over medium-high heat. Add all the remaining ingredients and cook, stirring and mixing the ingredients together with a spatula.

To serve the kitfo raw, cook just until the plant-based meat is warmed and the ingredients are thoroughly mixed.

To serve the kitfo cooked, continue cooking and mixing until the plant-based meat is either partially or thoroughly cooked through.

Serve the kitfo immediately, preferably with injera bread.

NOTE
• Kitfo is typically made with niter kibbeh, a clarified butter infused with herbs and spices. To avoid butter, you can infuse oil with spices such as cardamom, fenugreek seeds, cumin, ginger, nutmeg, oregano, basil, and turmeric. The longer infused oil sits, the more intense the flavor of the spices.

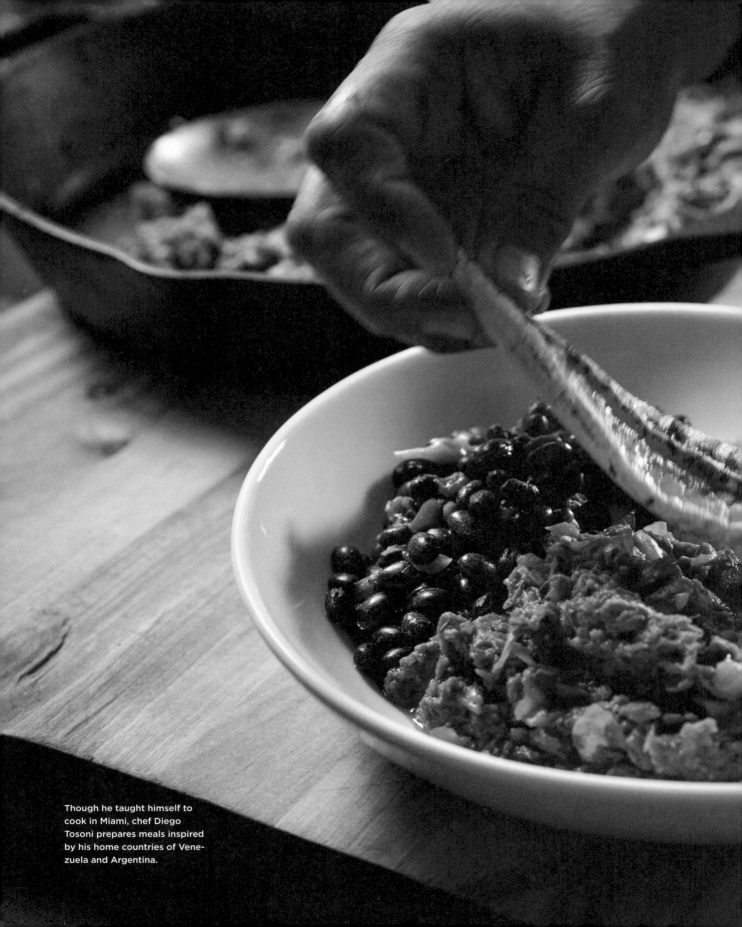

Though he taught himself to cook in Miami, chef Diego Tosoni prepares meals inspired by his home countries of Venezuela and Argentina.

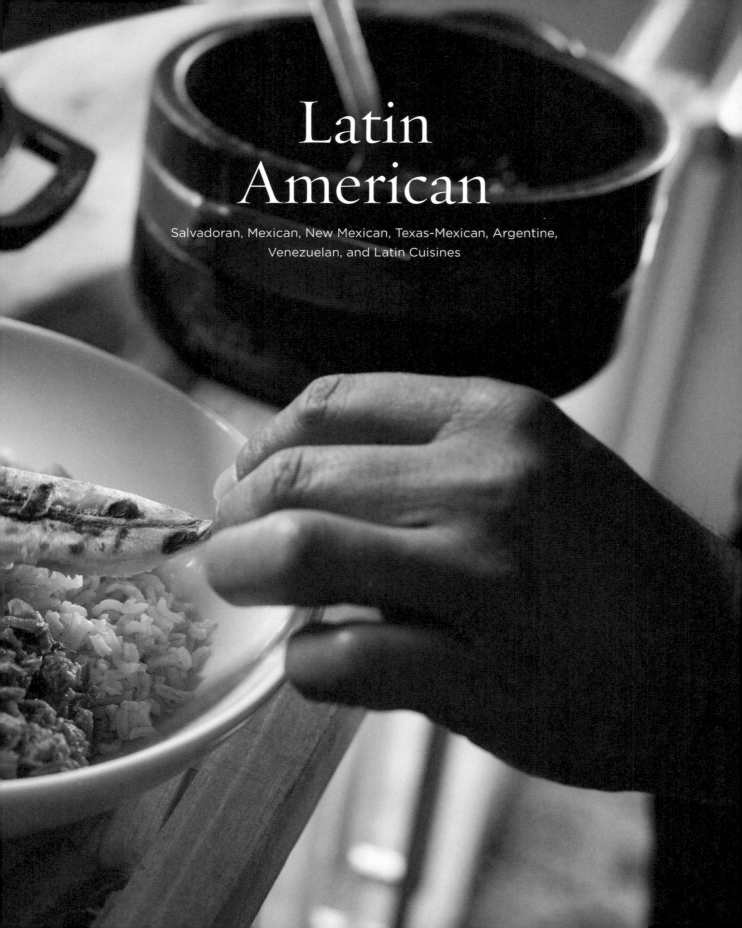

Latin
American

Salvadoran, Mexican, New Mexican, Texas-Mexican, Argentine,
Venezuelan, and Latin Cuisines

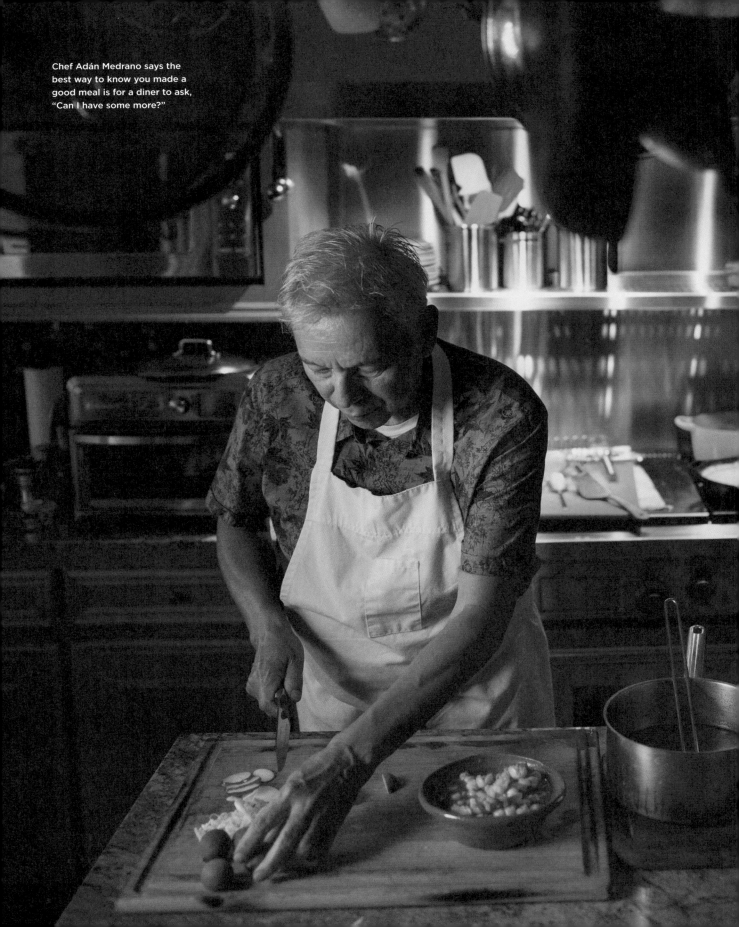

Chef Adán Medrano says the best way to know you made a good meal is for a diner to ask, "Can I have some more?"

"Greasy, cheesy Tex-Mex food was largely an Anglo invention."

~ADÁN MEDRANO

It's midday on Tuesday, and we're standing in chef-historian Adán Medrano's Houston kitchen as he destroys the myth of Tex-Mex cooking. In one pot he stirs a savory pozole (a traditional Mexican stew) and in another a tomato-stewed rice, both dishes flavored with the Texas-Mexican "holy trinity" of garlic, cumin, and pepper. "Greasy, cheesy Tex-Mex food was largely an Anglo invention," he tells me. "Our traditional enchiladas were not slathered with cheese. We fill ours with carrots and potatoes."

Medrano, 73, wears a crisp white apron over a floral shirt, his silver hair swept boyishly to one side. He was born in San Antonio, which was the capital of New Spain and later the Mexican province of Tejas, until 1845, when Texas was made a U.S. state. He grew up eating cactus, beans, corn, chilis, potatoes, onions, mushrooms, portulaca, amaranth, sunflowers, Jerusalem artichokes, berries, and occasionally wild game. These were the authentic foods of Texas-Mexican cuisine, a far cry from "Tex-Mex" culinary corruptions like steak fajitas and overstuffed quesadillas with sour cream.

After 23 years of traveling and working throughout Latin America, Europe, and Asia, Adán made a career 180 and enrolled in the Culinary Institute of America at age 61. There he found his teachers had misguided ideas of Mexican cuisine, which spurred him to launch a crusade to set the record straight. In the documentary *Truly Texas Mexican,* he argues that his people mainly ate plant-based foods. Proof comes from "archaeological evidence from areas like the [Richard] Beene site near San Antonio . . . that confirms that earth-oven technology was used mainly to cook plant foods, including tubers and roots," he tells me. "The earliest written records, including Cabeza de Vaca and Gonzalo Fernández de Oviedo y Valdés [both 1500s], indicate the prevalence of plant foods."

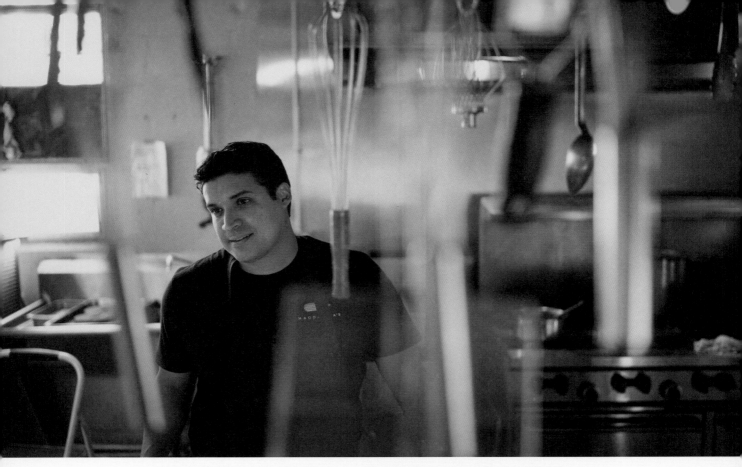

Above and opposite: In Fort Worth, Texas, chef Juan Rodriguez prepares moles and tostadas, among other traditional recipes, inspired by the dishes his grandmother made when he was a child—but with a modern twist.

It turns out, authentic Mexican American cuisine in the southwestern United States was also largely whole food and plant-based. In 1895, Arthur Gross, a chemistry professor, collected food dietaries from three families living near Las Cruces, New Mexico. He found one household ate absolutely no animal protein over the course of two weeks. The others consumed just three eggs over the course of 165 meals.

So what did they eat? Mostly corn tortillas and beans, always cooked in an earthen pot, often with lard or vegetable oils, and always with chilis. Though on average they only consumed about eight different foods per week, seasonal foods like green onions, dried tomatoes, and apples crept into their diet too.

Colonel John R. Brooke, an ethnographer with the U.S. Army, published *The Folk Foods of the Rio Grande Valley and of Northern Mexico* in 1895. In it he offered a purely descriptive account of the traditional foods of the Mexican-American border region. While he found that flour and cornmeal made up the bulk of diets, he also described 45 indigenous fruits and vegetables. Lentils, peas, onions, corn tortillas, *fideos* (noodle soups), spicy grape jam, parsnips, pumpkin, cabbage, scarlet prickly pears, and custard apples also made their way into the diet.

Luis Martinez, the chef behind Tequio Foods in Asheville, North Carolina, remembers growing up eating similar foods in a small village with neither roads nor refrigeration in Oaxaca, Mexico. "We were poor and ate beans and tortillas every day," he tells me. "I remember my grandma occasionally killed a rabbit, but otherwise I was pretty much vegetarian. We loved pickles, ramps, and wild garlic."

In 2006, at age 20, he left the austerity of Mexico and found new hardship in the United States, where he took lowly jobs in restaurants. Armed with passion and a genius for blending flavors, he taught himself how to cook.

When we meet him at his restaurant, El Gallo, he's wearing running shoes, blue jeans, and an apron embroidered with "Chef Luis." He prepared his marquee dish, *chimol,* a creative upgrade to guacamole that blends butternut squash, onions, and chilis with avocados and is topped with toasted corn, which delivers a crunchy, percussive finish.

When I ask his inspiration for his wildly inventive food, he responds, "Austerity gives you a certain inventiveness that you never get when you're used to frying a piece of meat or sautéing your food in butter."

In every city on our sweep across America, we found chefs ingeniously riffing on home-country staples. Chef Diego Tosoni grew up in Argentina and Venezuela but taught himself how to cook in Miami. Together with his wife, Veronica, he opened Love Life Café, which is one of the Wynwood neighborhood's most popular lunch

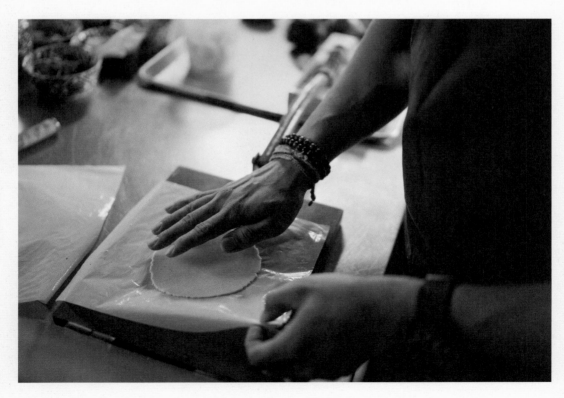

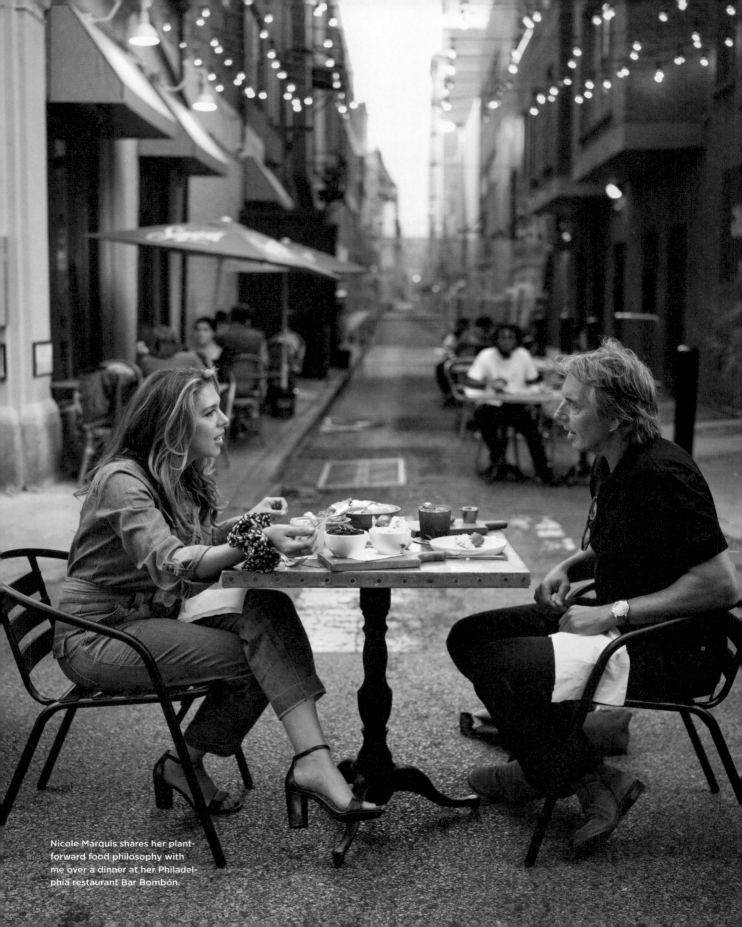

Nicole Marquis shares her plant-
forward food philosophy with
me over a dinner at her Philadelphia restaurant Bar Bombón.

spots. On any given day, you might see the mayor and besuited businesspeople sitting shoulder to shoulder with vegan yoginis as they tuck into Diego's veggie burger (voted number one in America by the Seed Food and Wine Festival in 2016).

Like Luis's, Diego's passion for traditional ingredients fuels his inventiveness. One evening in his simple home in North Miami, we gather around a huge industrial stove. Diego is sporting a T-shirt, flip-flops, and a cap that reads, "Give a f*ck about what you eat." Fiercely focused, he jockeys three pots, each with a different dish based on rice, beans, corn, plantains, and avocados—common foods in his native South America. His chlorophyll-and-chia-seed-infused arepa (page 135), a thick taco-like shell sliced like a bun and filled with black beans, transforms a typical meat-and-cheese-filled dish into a healthy pocket.

We also meet Puerto Rican entrepreneur Nicole Marquis, who runs three of Philadelphia's hottest restaurants including HipCityVeg and Bar Bombón; Mexican American Juan Rodriguez, who has helped make plant-based Mexican food mainstream in Fort Worth, Texas; and Claudia Lopez, who operates Mama's International Tamales in Los Angeles, where she serves up the best plant-based Salvadoran food. All these chefs have deep roots in the traditional cuisine of their home countries, which they have imaginatively and healthfully Americanized— similar to the Blue Zones way.

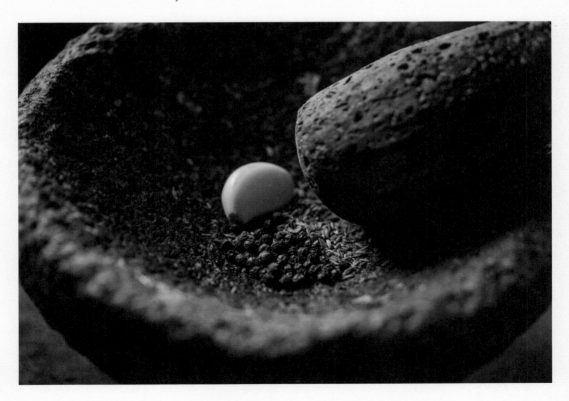

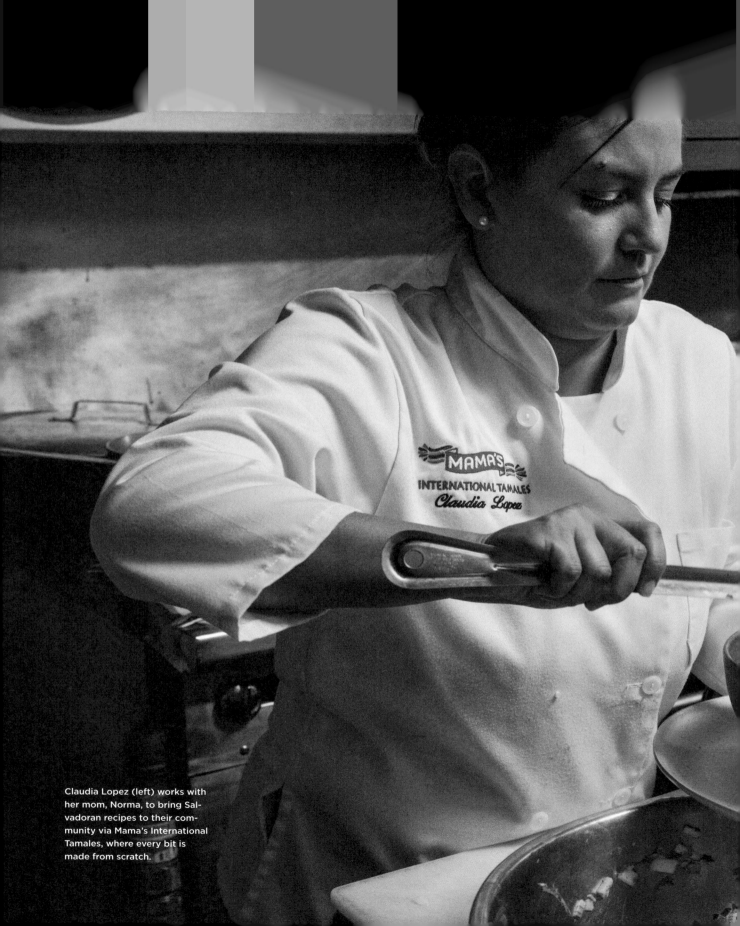

Claudia Lopez (left) works with her mom, Norma, to bring Salvadoran recipes to their community via Mama's International Tamales, where every bit is made from scratch.

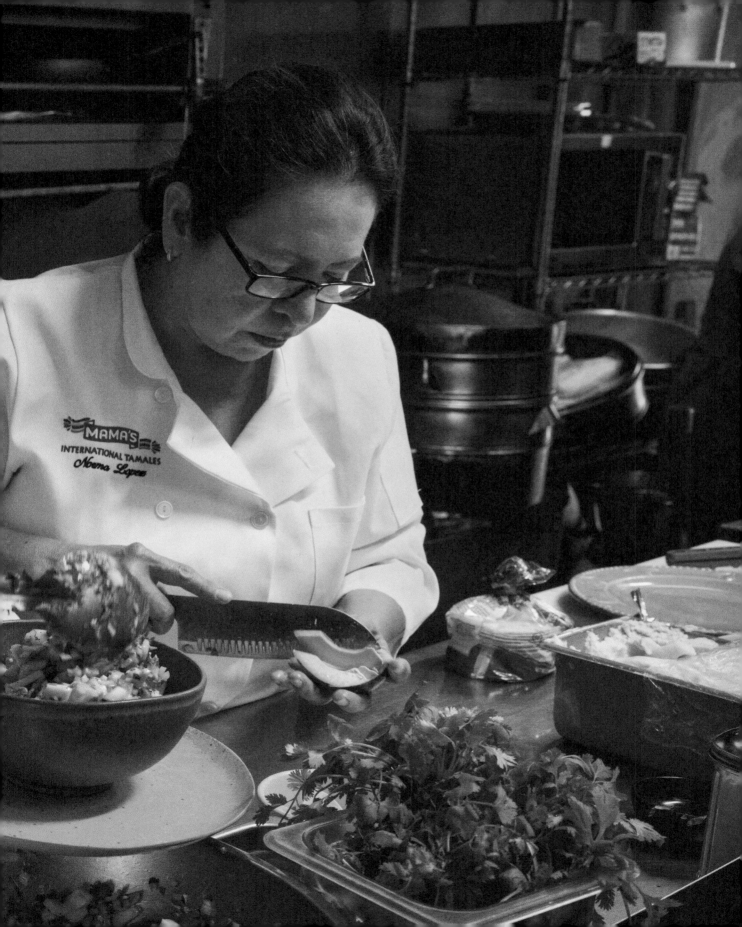

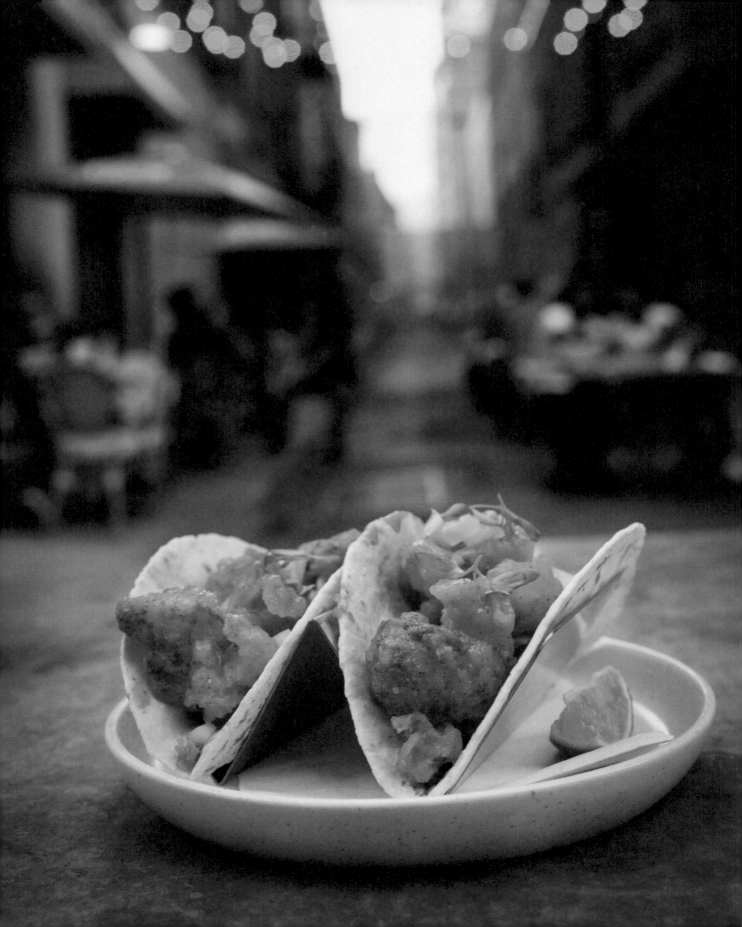

Buffalo Cauliflower Tacos

TOTAL COOK TIME: 15 TO 20 MINUTES • MAKES 8 TACOS

Chef Nicole Marquis has created award-winning plant-based restaurants. She is driven to make delicious food that is both good for people's health and good for the environment. This vegan take on street tacos is an example of the food that she serves at her Philly hot spot Bar Bombón.

TO MAKE THE CAULIFLOWER:

Vegetable oil for frying

1 head cauliflower, washed and patted very dry, cored and quartered, then broken down into small florets

½ cup tempura flour

½ cup club soda

TO MAKE THE BUFFALO SAUCE:

¾ cup vegan butter

1½ cups hot sauce (such as Frank's RedHot)

1 tablespoon Dijon mustard

½ teaspoon fine sea salt

1 teaspoon freshly ground black pepper

TO MAKE THE TACOS:

8 flour tortillas

1 avocado, sliced

Cuban Black Beans (page 116)

Green Goddess Sauce (page 114)

¼ cup finely diced white onion

Micro cilantro (optional)

2 limes, cut into wedges (optional)

To make the cauliflower, heat the oil to 350°F in a large stockpot over medium-high heat. Adjust the heat to maintain the oil at 350°F.

In a medium mixing bowl, gently whisk the tempura flour and club soda together until just combined. Do not over-whisk.

In batches, add the cauliflower to the tempura batter and toss to fully coat. Drop the cauliflower pieces into the hot oil for 5 to 6 minutes, rotating them by carefully stirring about halfway through, until they are golden brown. Work in batches, being careful not to overcrowd the pot.

Using a slotted spoon, transfer the fried cauliflower to a plate lined with paper towels.

To make the buffalo sauce, in a small saucepan, melt the butter over low heat. Don't allow it to come to a boil.

Add the remaining sauce ingredients and, using an immersion blender or in a countertop blender (let cool slightly before adding to blender), blend on high speed for 30 to 45 seconds, until smooth. Transfer the sauce to a medium bowl.

After the fried cauliflower rests for a couple of minutes, add it to the bowl with the buffalo sauce and toss to fully coat.

To make the tacos, warm the tortillas on a griddle or in a skillet. Then place a tortilla on a plate. Top it with some of the avocado, black beans, green goddess sauce, buffalo cauliflower, and, if using, the onion, micro cilantro, and a squeeze of lime juice. Repeat to make 8 tacos.

Guacamole Fresca (right)

TOTAL COOK TIME: 5 MINUTES • SERVES 4

3 avocados, halved and pitted

¼ cup plum tomatoes, seeded and finely diced

¼ red onion, finely diced

1 jalapeño, seeded and finely diced

2 tablespoons minced cilantro

Juice of ½ lime

½ teaspoon fine sea salt

In a medium bowl, mash the avocados. Fold in the remaining ingredients. Taste and adjust the seasonings as needed.

Green Goddess Sauce

TOTAL COOK TIME: 5 MINUTES • SERVES 4

1 tablespoon chopped fresh cilantro or dill

1 tablespoon chopped fresh parsley

1 teaspoon chopped garlic

1½ cups plant-based mayonnaise

2 tablespoons horseradish

1½ tablespoons whole-grain mustard

1 tablespoon capers

1½ tablespoons water

To make the green goddess sauce, in a blender, combine all the ingredients. Process until smooth and well combined.

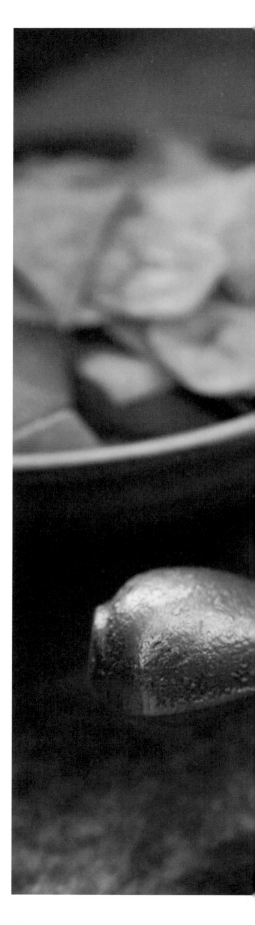

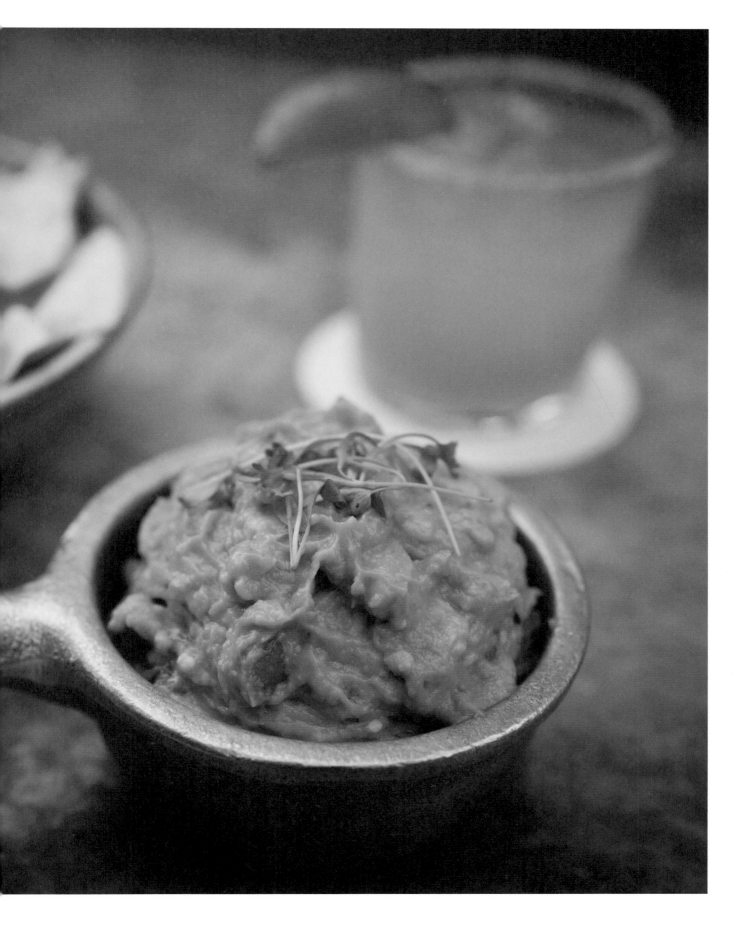

Cuban Black Beans

TOTAL COOK TIME: 20 MINUTES • SERVES 6

2 teaspoons olive oil

½ onion, finely diced

2 garlic cloves, minced

2 tablespoons minced green bell pepper

3 tablespoons chopped fresh cilantro

1 (15-ounce) can black beans, with their liquid

½ cup water, or more if needed

1 bay leaf

⅛ teaspoon ground cumin

⅛ teaspoon dried oregano

1 teaspoon red wine vinegar

¼ teaspoon salt

⅛ teaspoon freshly ground black pepper

In a medium saucepan, heat the oil over medium heat.

Add the onion, garlic, bell pepper, and cilantro, and sauté for about 3 minutes, until soft.

Add the beans, water, bay leaf, cumin, oregano, vinegar, salt, and pepper, and bring to a boil.

Turn the heat to low and cover the pot. Simmer for about 15 minutes, stirring occasionally. Add additional water, about ¼ cup at a time, if the beans are drying out.

Season with the salt and pepper to taste.

Serve on top of Coconut Rice (page 117).

Coconut Rice

TOTAL COOK TIME: 35 MINUTES • SERVES 6

2 tablespoons dried coconut shreds

3 cups long-grain rice

2 cans unsweetened coconut milk

2½ cups water

2 teaspoons cane sugar

In a small sauté pan over medium-low heat, sauté the dried coconut until golden brown throughout. Set aside.

In a rice cooker, combine the rice, coconut milk, water, and sugar. Cover and turn on the rice cooker. (Alternatively, cook the rice in a covered pot.)

Once the rice is cooked, fold in the toasted coconut.

Serve with Cuban Black Beans (page 116).

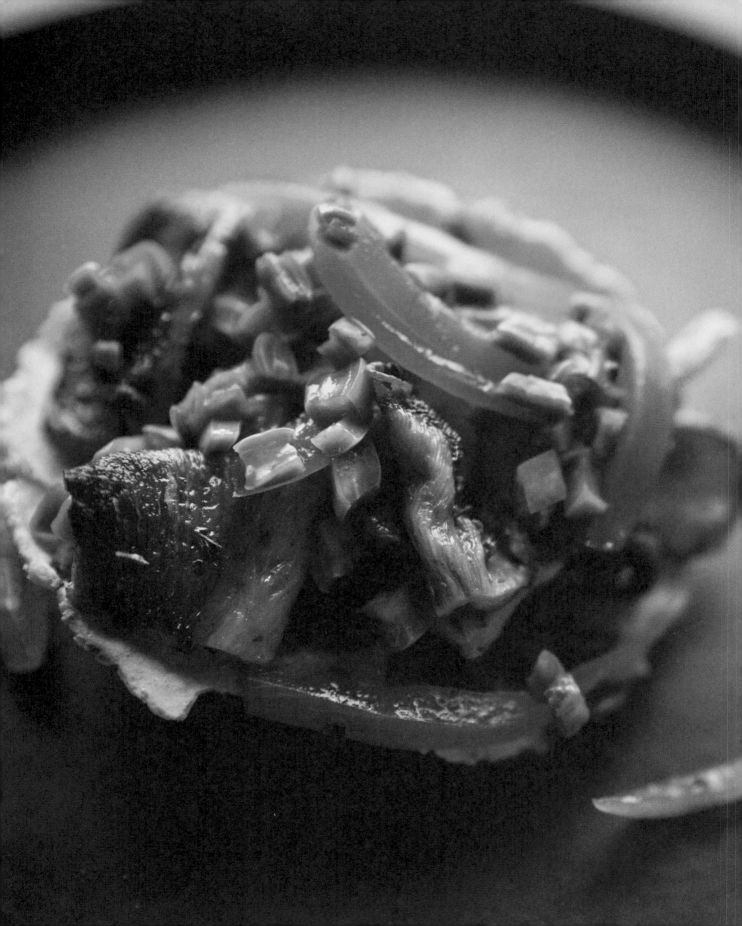

Black Bean and Nopalitos (Cactus) Tostadas With Pickled Red Onions

TOTAL COOK TIME: 2 HOURS • MAKES 4 TOSTADAS

Chef Juan Rodriguez's Fort Worth supper club has a waiting list, and getting a seat at the gourmet dinner is a source of pride. Juan wanted to re-create his grandmother's tradition of bringing people together through food. The communal tables mean people rub elbows with other diners and make new connections and friends.

Fort Worth is currently the largest certified Blue Zones Community in the United States. Since the launch of the initiative, the city has gone from one of the least healthy to one of the healthiest cities in the country. As part of his commitment to the community, Chef Juan gives free Blue Zones Project cooking demonstrations, teaching people how to make delicious, plant-slant dishes. Juan's black bean and nopalitos tostadas are a good example. Everyone knows beans and crispy tortillas, but Juan throws in a sauté of nopalitos, a type of cactus that's a bit like okra in texture, with a tart, citrusy flavor.

FOR THE BLACK BEANS:

1 cup dried black beans

6 cups water

1 tablespoon oregano

2 tablespoons epazote

1 teaspoon ground cumin

1 tablespoon salt

FOR THE NOPALITOS:

1 tablespoon olive oil

1 nopal (cactus) paddle, trimmed to remove any thorns and finely diced

½ cup finely diced onion

1 tomato, diced

FOR THE PICKLED RED ONION:

½ cup red wine vinegar

½ cup water (or prickly pear juice)

1 tablespoon sugar

1 tablespoon kosher salt

1 teaspoon dried oregano

1 red onion, thinly sliced

FOR THE TOSTADAS:

4 corn tortillas

Oil for brushing

¼ head green cabbage, shredded

To make the beans, in a stockpot, combine the beans, water, oregano, epazote, cumin, and salt, and bring to a boil. Reduce the heat and cook until the beans are tender, about 1 hour 20 minutes. Taste and adjust the seasoning as needed.

To make the nopalitos, heat the oil in a skillet over medium-high heat. Add the cactus, onion, and tomato, then cover, reduce the heat to low, and cook for about 20 minutes, until the cactus is tender.

To make the pickled red onion, in a saucepan, bring the vinegar, water, sugar, salt, and oregano to a boil over medium-high heat.

Place the onion in a heatproof bowl. When the liquid is boiling, remove it from the heat and pour it over the onion in the bowl.

Let it cool.

To make the tostadas, preheat the oven to 400°F.

Brush the tortillas lightly with oil and arrange them in a single layer on a baking sheet.

Bake for about 10 minutes, until the tortillas are lightly browned and crisp.

Top each tortilla with a generous spoonful of beans, a generous spoonful of the nopalitos, some of the pickled onion, and a handful of shredded cabbage.

NOTES

• You can find epazote, an aromatic herb, in Mexican grocery stores or online.

• To reduce the cooking time of your beans, you can soak the beans in water overnight. Drain the soaking water and add fresh water to cook.

• Pickled onion can be stored in the refrigerator for up to a month.

Enmoladas de Calabacitas (Squash Enmoladas)

TOTAL COOK TIME: 2 HOURS • MAKES 6 ENMOLADAS

FOR THE CALABACITAS:

½ cup vegetable oil

2 to 3 cups half-moon slices Mexican squash

1 cup finely diced onion

2 garlic cloves, minced

1 cup diced Roma tomatoes

1 cup fresh or frozen corn kernels

1 tablespoon chopped fresh Mexican oregano

2 tablespoons chopped cilantro

Salt

Freshly ground black pepper

2 cups vegetable stock

FOR THE DARK MOLE SAUCE:

8 dried pasilla chilis, stemmed and seeded

4 dried chile de arbol, stemmed and seeded

4 dried ancho chilis, stemmed and seeded

1 (16-ounce) can crushed tomatoes

⅓ cup chopped yellow onion

2 garlic cloves

1 corn tortilla, toasted in the oven

3 tablespoons roasted almonds

3 tablespoons raw peanuts

1 tablespoon toasted sesame seeds

¼ cup raisins

5 whole cloves

1 cinnamon stick

1 tablet (90 grams) Mexican chocolate

4 cups vegetable stock

½ cup oil

FOR THE ENMOLADAS:

6 corn tortillas

Mexican pickled vegetables (cabbage, carrots, jalapeños)

To make the calabacitas, in a large skillet, heat the oil over medium-high heat. Add the squash, onion, garlic, and tomatoes, and cook, stirring occasionally, for 2 to 3 minutes.

Stir in the remaining calabacitas ingredients and bring to a simmer. Reduce the heat to medium-low and simmer, uncovered, for about 20 minutes. The mixture should retain some moisture, so if the stew becomes too dry, add a bit more vegetable stock or water.

Taste and adjust the seasoning if needed.

To make the mole sauce, toast the dried chilis in a 350°F oven for 5 minutes.

In a large saucepan, combine the toasted chilis, crushed tomatoes, onion, garlic, toasted tortilla, almonds, peanuts, sesame seeds, raisins, cloves, cinnamon stick, and chocolate. Add the vegetable stock and bring to a simmer over medium heat, stirring with a wooden spoon.

Let the sauce simmer and reduce for about 30 minutes over medium-low heat.

Using an immersion blender, puree the mixture until smooth and then transfer it to a bowl; you can use a countertop blender, but let the mole cool down for an hour before transferring it to the blender. If the puree is too thick, add water as needed to achieve the desired consistency.

In the same saucepan, heat the oil over medium heat. Slowly add the pureed mole back to the pan. Bring it to a simmer and let it cook, covered, for 30 to 45 minutes. Add additional vegetable stock, if needed, to maintain a saucy consistency.

Taste and adjust the seasonings if needed.

To make the enmoladas, heat the corn tortillas on a griddle, on a skillet, or in the oven.

Spread a bit of the calabacitas on half of a tortilla and fold the other half over the filling. Repeat with the remaining tortillas. Spread the mole evenly across the enmoladas; you can go heavy on the mole and cover the tortillas, or you can put just a little bit of mole over them, depending on your preference.

Top with pickled vegetables and serve immediately.

NOTES
• You can buy premade mole at a Mexican grocery store or at many supermarkets.

Jicama "Scallop" Aguachile

TOTAL COOK TIME: 10 MINUTES • SERVES 4

Aguachile is a spicy Mexican recipe that's similar to ceviche, in that the ingredients are "cooked" in lime juice and it usually features shrimp. This version uses jicama for a bright, light, and flavorful plant-forward dish.

½ cup freshly squeezed lime juice

½ cup English cucumber, peeled and seeded

1 serrano chili

1 teaspoon sugar

¼ cup cilantro, plus additional for garnish

1 teaspoon salt

½ clove garlic

1 jicama, peeled, sliced ½ inch thick, and cut into rounds with a cookie cutter

1 grapefruit, cut into supremes

½ avocado, diced

½ red onion, thinly sliced, for garnish

In a blender or food processor, combine the lime juice, cucumber, chili, sugar, cilantro, salt, and garlic, and puree until smooth. Taste and adjust the seasoning if needed. Transfer to a medium bowl.

Add the jicama and grapefruit and toss to combine. Top with the avocado.

Serve garnished with cilantro and sliced red onion.

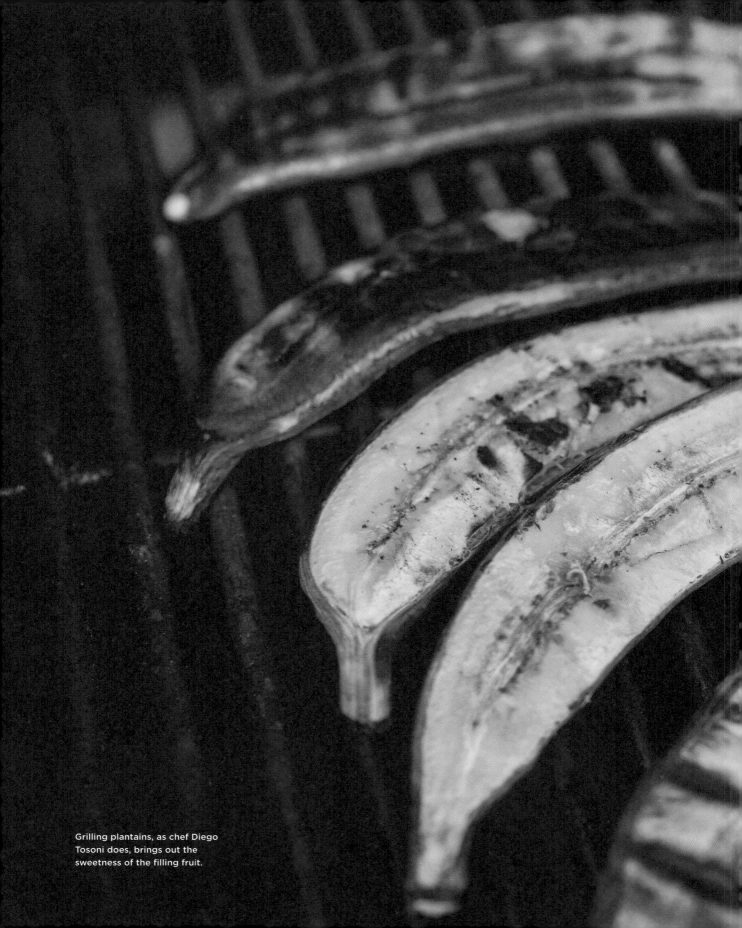

Grilling plantains, as chef Diego Tosoni does, brings out the sweetness of the filling fruit.

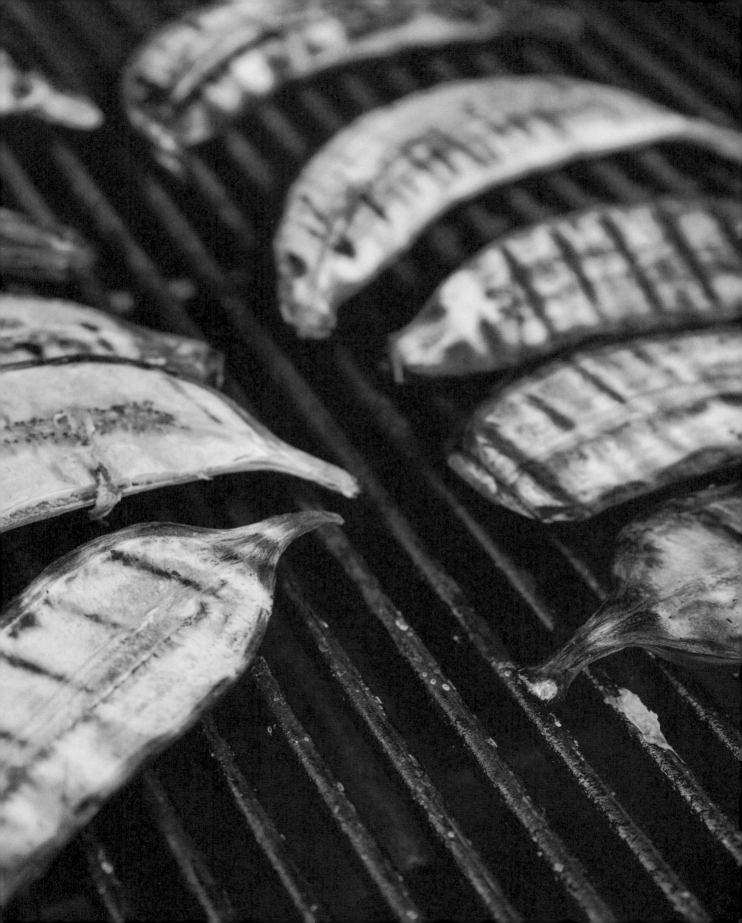

ADÁN MEDRANO, CHEF AND AUTHOR OF *TRULY TEXAS MEXICAN*

Frijoles Borrachos (Drunken Beans)

TOTAL COOK TIME: 2 HOURS 20 MINUTES TO 8 HOURS 20 MINUTES • SERVES 8 TO 10

Chef Adán Medrano first learned this recipe from his sisters María and Esther when they were both in their 20s. It was a delight to have entered the grown-up world and to cook a recipe that included beer.

Served piping hot in a small bowl, this dish is just plain delicious. It also serves as a key memory of the Chicano experience. Adán says that his non-Chicano friends tell him they've made these for parties and the "borrachos" are a hit.

Like all Texas-Mexican family foods, this one, adapted from his book *Truly Texas Mexican: A Native Culinary Heritage in Recipes,* depends on fresh ingredients and timing. Adán urges you to follow his sisters' advice: Avoid overcooking the tomato and onion, and add the cilantro at the very end to enjoy the aromatic oils of the herb.

1 pound pinto beans, picked over for debris and rinsed

1 cup dark beer

2 tablespoons salt

1 cup finely diced white onion

4 cups chopped tomatoes (about 4 medium tomatoes)

1½ tablespoons finely diced serrano chili (remove seeds for *menos picante*—less heat)

1 bunch cilantro, coarsely chopped

Place the beans in a stockpot or Dutch oven and cover them with water until it is 2 inches above the beans. Add the beer and salt. Bring to a boil, then reduce the heat to a slow simmer and cook for 2 to 4 hours, until the beans are completely soft. Add more water during cooking as needed to keep the pot from drying out. Alternatively, you can cook them in a slow cooker on medium or high for 6 to 8 hours.

When the beans are cooked, add the onion, tomatoes, and chili, and cook for 20 minutes.

Just before serving, add the cilantro.

Serve in small bowls and just watch the smiles on everyone's faces.

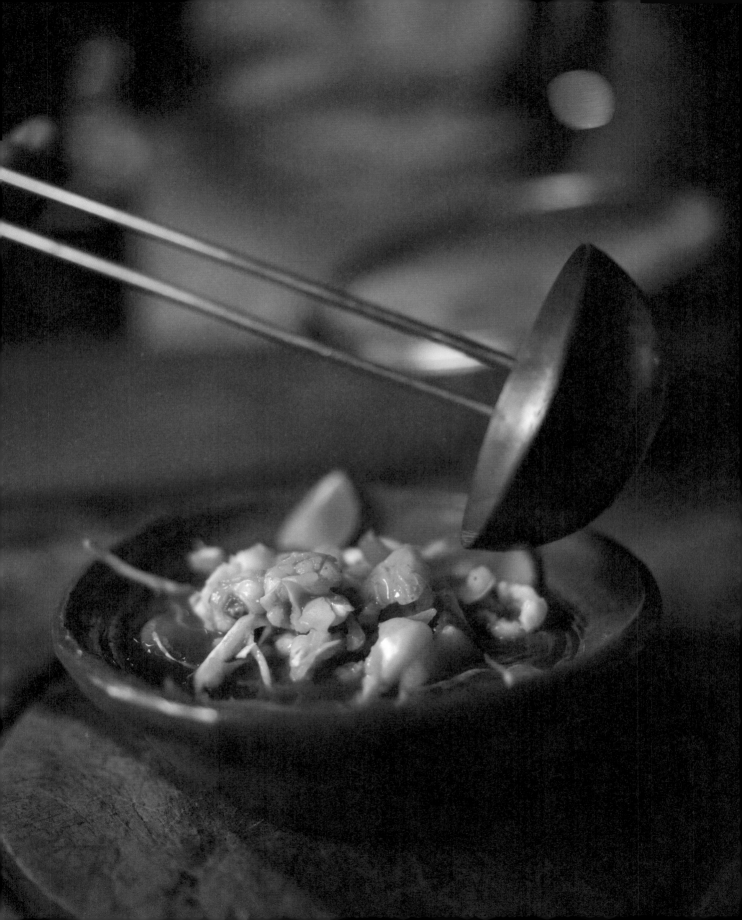

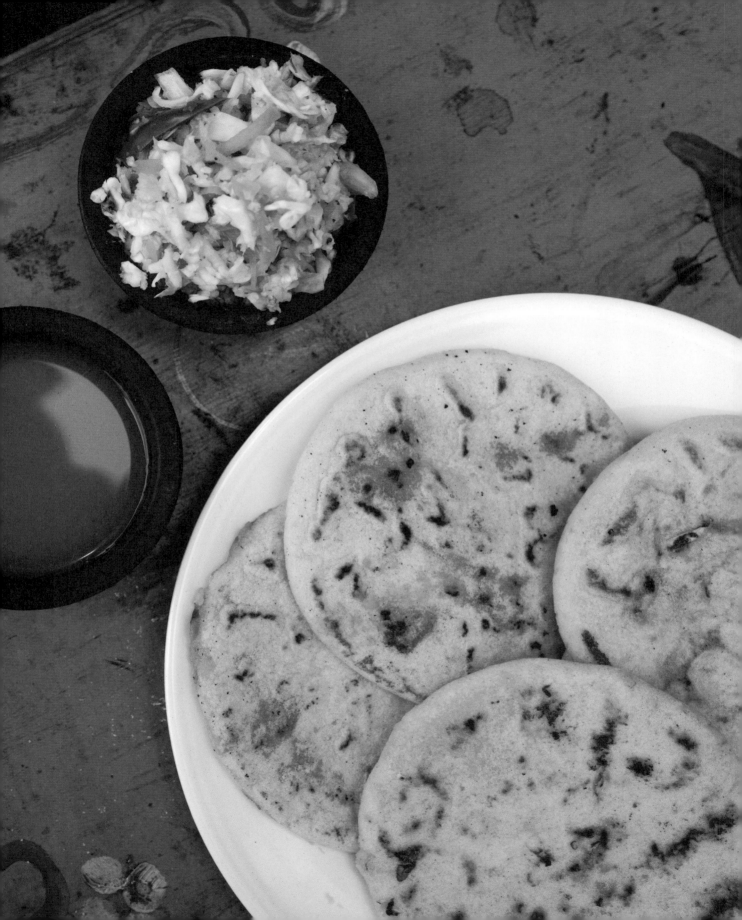

Mama's Zucchini Pupusas

TOTAL COOK TIME: 25 MINUTES • MAKES 12 PUPUSAS

Salvadoran chef Claudia Lopez and her mom, Norma, watched the *Forks Over Knives* documentary about plant-based eating and had an epiphany. Their restaurant, Maria's International Tamales in downtown Los Angeles, is now an oasis of healthy food in a jungle of fast food. Claudia's excellence and skill mean that her pupusas and tamales are in high demand and well loved by veggie and meat lovers alike.

Her pupusas are filled with zucchini and easy to make at home. Once you get the hang of whipping up the dough, you can experiment with alternative fillings like beans, jackfruit, and other vegetables. Masa harina, used in the dough, is a finely ground cornmeal that is made from nixtamalized, dried corn.

FOR THE DOUGH:

3 cups masa harina

1 cup warm water, plus additional as needed

Pinch of salt

FOR THE FILLING:

2 zucchini, grated on the large holes of a box grater, sprinkled with a pinch of salt, and squeezed to remove excess water

FOR SERVING:

Hot sauce

Salsa

Curtido (pickled cabbage)

To make the dough, in a large bowl, add all the ingredients and mix to combine. You may need to add a bit more water, 1 tablespoon at a time, to get the dough to come together. Let stand for about 10 minutes before forming the pupusas.

Wet your hands with a bit of water and/or oil to keep the dough from sticking.

Make a ball of dough about the size of an ice-cream scoop and flatten it between the palms of your hands into a round that's about ¼ inch thick. Add 2 to 3 tablespoons of the zucchini filling to the center of the dough. Wrap the dough around the filling and then flatten it again between the palms of your hands, until it is about ¼ inch thick and 4 inches across. Repeat with the remaining dough and filling.

To cook, heat a nonstick skillet over medium-high heat. Cook each pupusa until lightly browned, about 5 minutes per side.

Serve with the hot sauce, salsa, and curtido.

Hearts of Palm Ceviche

TOTAL COOK TIME: 5 MINUTES • SERVES 4

1 (8-ounce) jar or can hearts of palm, drained and diced

1 large cucumber, diced

2 tomatoes, diced

½ red onion, diced

¼ cup chopped cilantro

2 limes

1 teaspoon salt

¼ freshly ground black pepper

1 avocado, diced (optional)

Tortilla chips

In a medium bowl, combine the hearts of palm, cucumber, tomatoes, red onion, and cilantro. Squeeze the two limes over the top, add salt and pepper, and toss to mix well.

Top with the avocado, if using, and serve with tortilla chips.

Salvadoran-Style Tofu Scramble

TOTAL COOK TIME: 20 MINUTES • SERVES 4

Serve this quick scramble with a side of black beans and fried plantains.

1½ teaspoons oil

1 tomato, diced

¼ onion, diced

½ green bell pepper, diced

1 (16-ounce) package firm tofu, drained and diced

¼ teaspoon turmeric

¼ teaspoon salt

⅛ teaspoon freshly ground black pepper

In a skillet, heat the oil over medium-high heat. Add the tomato, onion, and bell pepper, and cook, stirring occasionally, until they're soft and beginning to brown, about 8 minutes.

Add the tofu and cook, stirring occasionally, for 5 minutes more. Stir in the turmeric, salt, and pepper, and simmer for a few minutes more until the vegetables are very tender.

Serve hot.

Texas-Mexican Holy Trinity

TOTAL COOK TIME: 5 MINUTES • MAKES 4 TEASPOONS

Sylvia Casares is Houston's "Enchilada Queen," and she has won numerous accolades and awards for her restaurants. A former food scientist, she makes and celebrates Texas border cuisine, which has been passed down from her mother and grandmother and the women before them.

3 garlic cloves, peeled

1½ teaspoons cumin seeds

1¼ teaspoons whole black peppercorns

1 tablespoon water

Combine all the ingredients in a molcajete, a mortar and pestle, or a spice or coffee grinder.

Grind and process until it's a smooth paste.

Calabacitas y Maiz Enchiladas
(Squash and Corn Enchiladas)

TOTAL COOK TIME: 1 HOUR • SERVES 6

FOR THE CHILI SAUCE AND TORTILLAS:

7 guajillo chilis, rinsed, stemmed, and seeded

2 chiles de arbol, rinsed and stemmed

1¾ cups water

FOR THE FILLING:

2 tablespoons vegetable oil

½ onion, chopped

1 tomato, coarsely chopped

3 cloves garlic, minced

5 calabacitas (small green Mexican squash) or zucchini, cut into small pieces

1 cup corn kernels (cut from 2 ears of corn or use frozen)

½ cup tomato sauce

1½ cups chicken stock or vegetable stock

2 teaspoons Texas-Mexican Holy Trinity (page 129)

½ teaspoon salt

FOR THE ENCHILADAS:

1 cup vegetable oil

12 corn tortillas

¾ cup very finely diced tomato, rinsed and drained well to remove the seeds

Cilantro, chopped

¼ cup finely diced onion

To make the chili sauce, in a medium saucepan over high heat, combine the guajillo chili and chile de arbol with the water. Bring it to a boil and then reduce the heat and let simmer for 15 minutes. Remove from the heat and let stand for another 10 minutes.

Put the chilis and the liquid in a blender or food processor and process until smooth. Strain the mixture through a fine-meshed sieve into a bowl, pressing on the solids with the back of a spoon to remove as much liquid as possible. Discard the solids.

To season the tortillas, dip each tortilla into the chili sauce and then let the excess run off into the bowl. Stack the dipped tortillas on a plate. Cover the stack with a plate or plastic wrap and refrigerate.

To make the filling, in a large skillet over medium heat, heat the oil until it shimmers. Add the onion, tomato, and garlic. Cook, stirring occasionally, until the onion is soft and translucent but not browned, about 3 minutes.

Add the squash, corn, tomato sauce, stock, Texas-Mexican Holy Trinity, and salt. Cook over medium heat until the squash is tender, about 10 minutes. Drain in a colander, discarding the liquid.

When you are ready to make the enchiladas, soften the tortillas. Heat the cup of vegetable oil in a medium skillet until it shimmers (375°F). Using a nonstick spatula, slide one tortilla at a time into the oil. Let it cook for 2 to 3 seconds, then turn it over and let it cook for 1 to 2 seconds more; the tortillas should soften but not brown or crisp. As the tortillas are softened, transfer them to a plate, stacking them on top of each other.

Once all the tortillas have been softened, cover the plate with plastic wrap or aluminum foil and let cool for about 10 minutes.

To make the enchiladas, preheat the oven to 425°F and spray a 9-by-11-inch baking dish with cooking spray.

Place about 3 tablespoons of the filling in the center of a softened tortilla. Roll the tortilla around the filling and place it seam-side down in the prepared baking dish. Repeat until all the tortillas are filled, arranging them in the baking dish with about ⅛ inch in between.

Pour ¼ cup of the chili sauce over each enchilada. Bake for 7 to 10 minutes, until the sauce is bubbling.

Garnish each enchilada with about 1 tablespoon of the diced tomato and serve immediately.

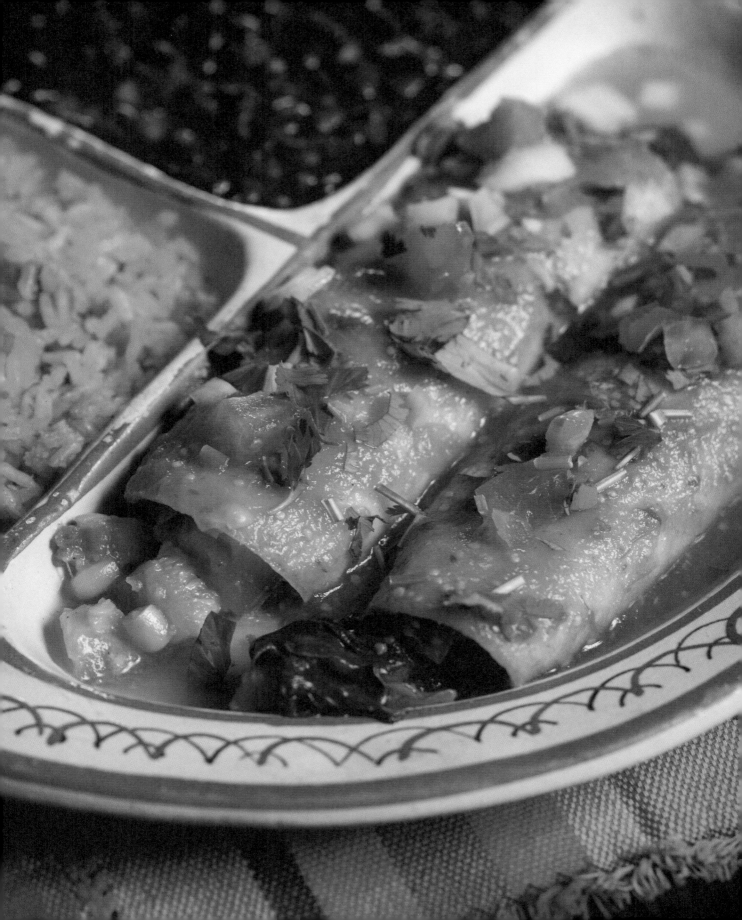

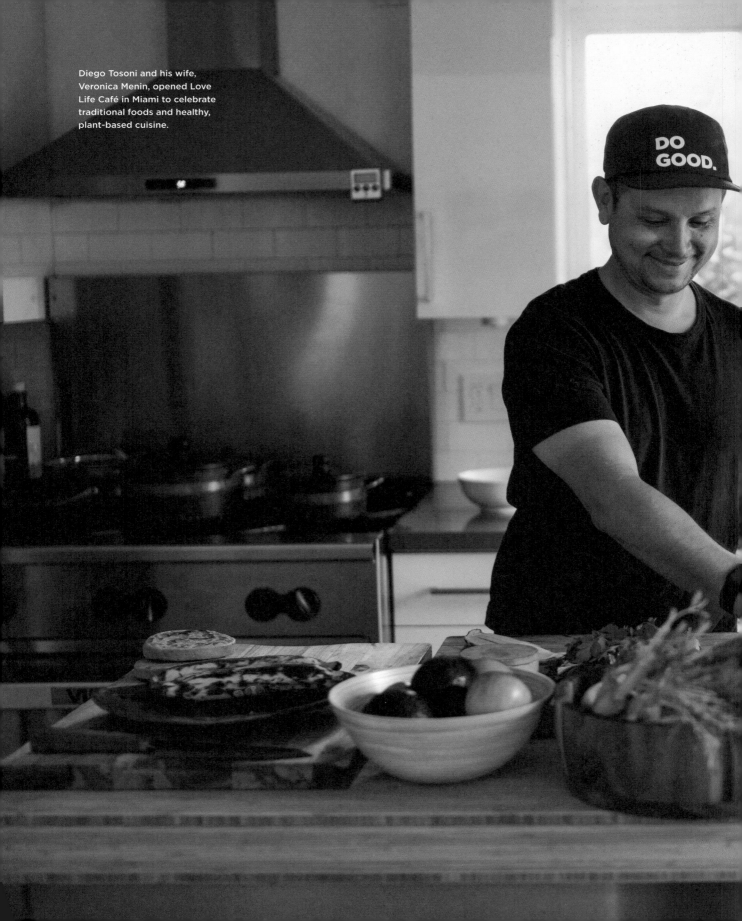

Diego Tosoni and his wife, Veronica Menin, opened Love Life Café in Miami to celebrate traditional foods and healthy, plant-based cuisine.

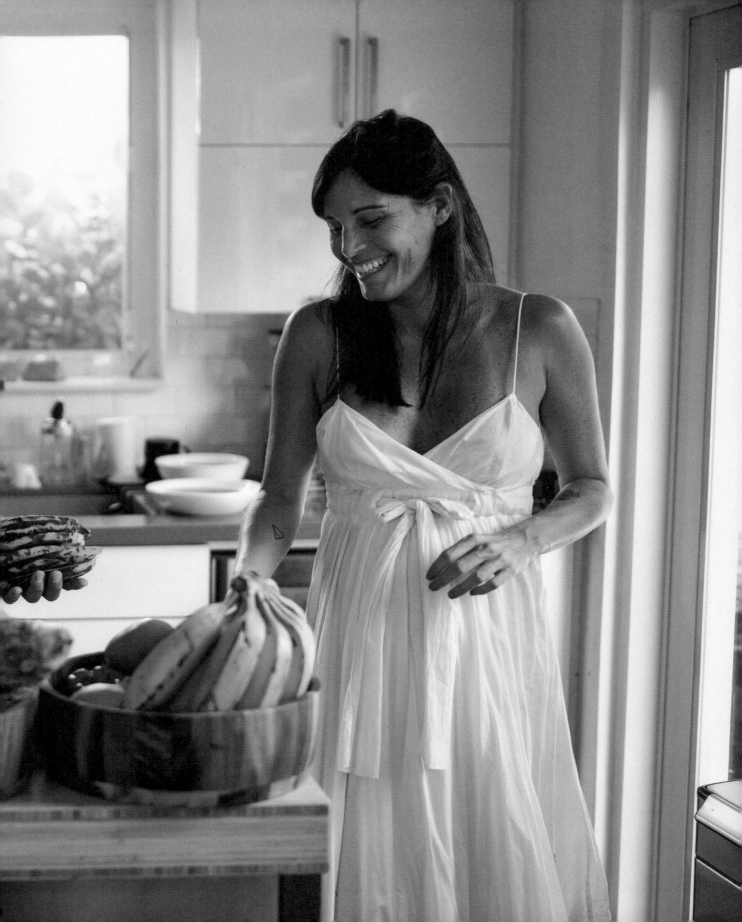

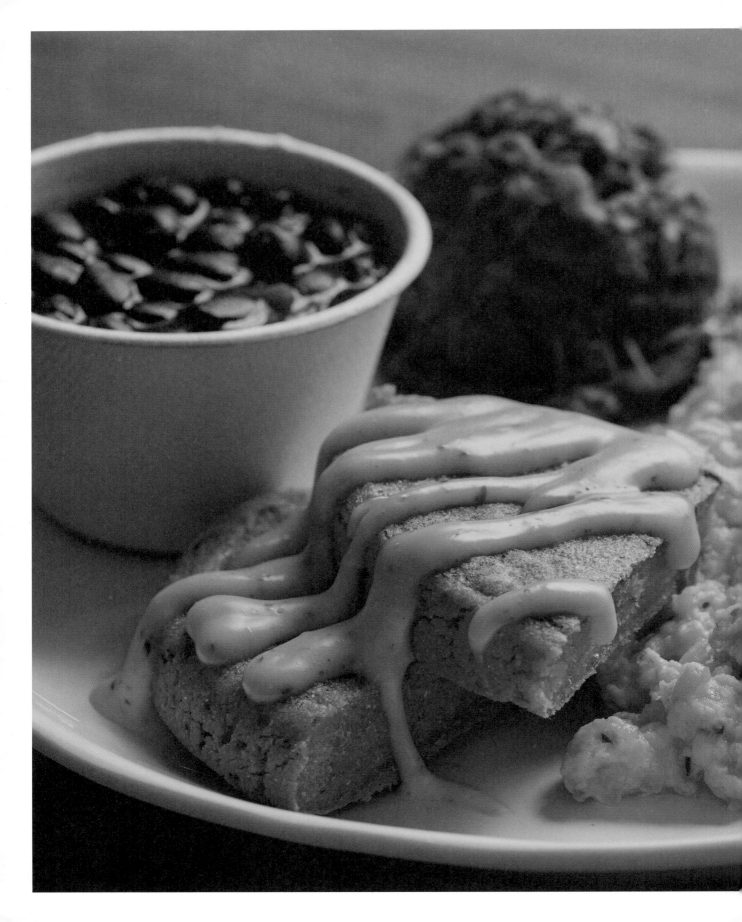

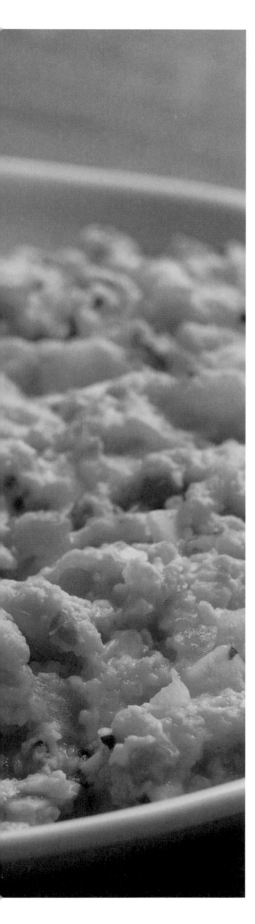

Plant-Powered Arepa

TOTAL COOK TIME: 15 MINUTES • MAKES 6 AREPAS

An arepa is like a thick corn tortilla. You can slice it open and stuff it with whatever fillings you like.

2½ cups warm water

½ cup spinach

1 teaspoon salt

3 tablespoons olive oil, divided

1 teaspoon chlorophyll

3 tablespoons chia seeds

1½ cups masarepa corn flour

In a blender, combine the water, spinach, salt, 2 tablespoons of the olive oil, and the chlorophyll, and blend until smooth.

In a large mixing bowl, combine the blended mixture and the chia seeds, and mix well. Slowly add the corn flour to the mixture in the bowl, mixing well using your hands until a loose dough forms. Once the dough is mixed completely, let it rest for 5 minutes.

Scoop out fist-size portions of the dough and shape each into a ball. You should have six equal-size balls. Pat each ball out into a round disk about 1 inch thick. If the dough cracks or feels too dry, add a little more water to moisten it.

In a skillet or on a griddle over medium heat, heat the remaining 1 tablespoon of olive oil. Add the arepas in a single layer (you'll need to cook in batches if you're using a skillet) and cook for 5 to 7 minutes on each side, until golden brown.

Serve hot.

NOTE
• You can omit the chlorophyll from this recipe if you can't find it in your local health food store.

Grilled Plantains

TOTAL COOK TIME: 25 MINUTES • SERVES 4

2 ripe plantains, halved lengthwise
   but not peeled

1½ tablespoons avocado oil or
   melted vegan butter

Preheat a grill to high heat or the oven to 400°F.

Brush the cut sides of the plantains with the oil.

Place the plantains cut side down on the grill, or if using the oven, cut side up on a baking sheet.

Grill or bake until they are golden brown, about 10 minutes. Turn the plantains on the grill over and baste them with more of the oil. If using the oven, brush more oil onto the cut-side-up plantains.

Cook for about 15 minutes more, until the plantains are very soft and caramelized.

Serve hot.

Sancocho Soup (right)

TOTAL COOK TIME: 45 MINUTES • SERVES 4

2 tablespoons olive oil

1 sweet onion, diced

1 tomato, diced

½ cup chopped cilantro, plus additional for garnish

1 red bell pepper, grated

2 cloves garlic, minced

½ teaspoon freshly ground black pepper

2 teaspoons ground cumin

1 tablespoon no-salt seasoning

1 green plantain, cubed

8 cups vegetable stock

1 large potato, cubed

1 ear corn, cut into 1-inch-thick rounds

1 pound yucca pieces, cubed

In a Dutch oven or stockpot, heat the oil over medium heat. Add the onion, tomato, cilantro, bell pepper, and garlic, and cook until the vegetables are softened, 5 to 7 minutes.

Add the black pepper, cumin, no-salt seasoning, and plantain, and cook, stirring occasionally, for another 5 minutes.

Add the stock along with the potato, corn, and yucca. Bring to a simmer and then reduce the heat to low. Let simmer for 25 to 30 minutes.

Serve hot, garnished with cilantro.

NOTE
• You can substitute 1 cup of frozen corn kernels if you don't have fresh corn on the cob.

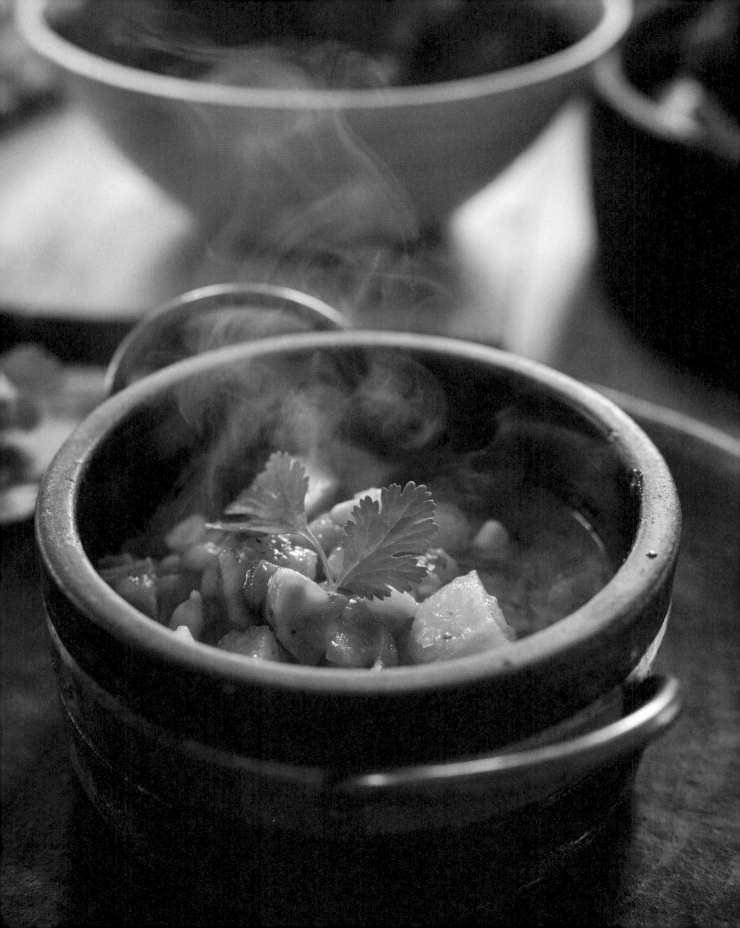

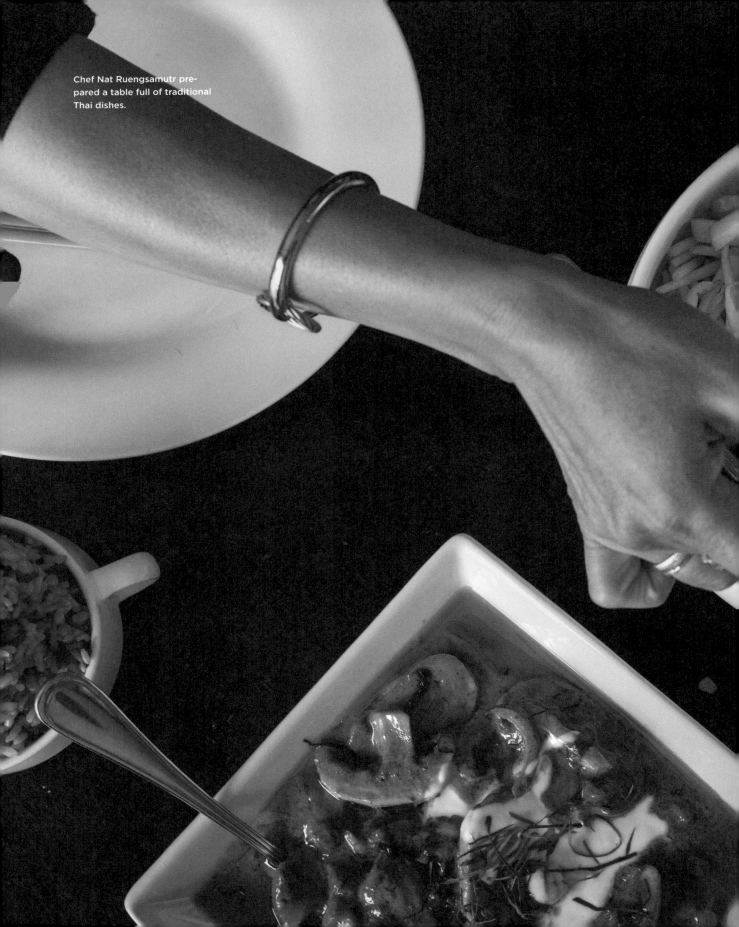

Chef Nat Ruengsamutr pre-
pared a table full of traditional
Thai dishes.

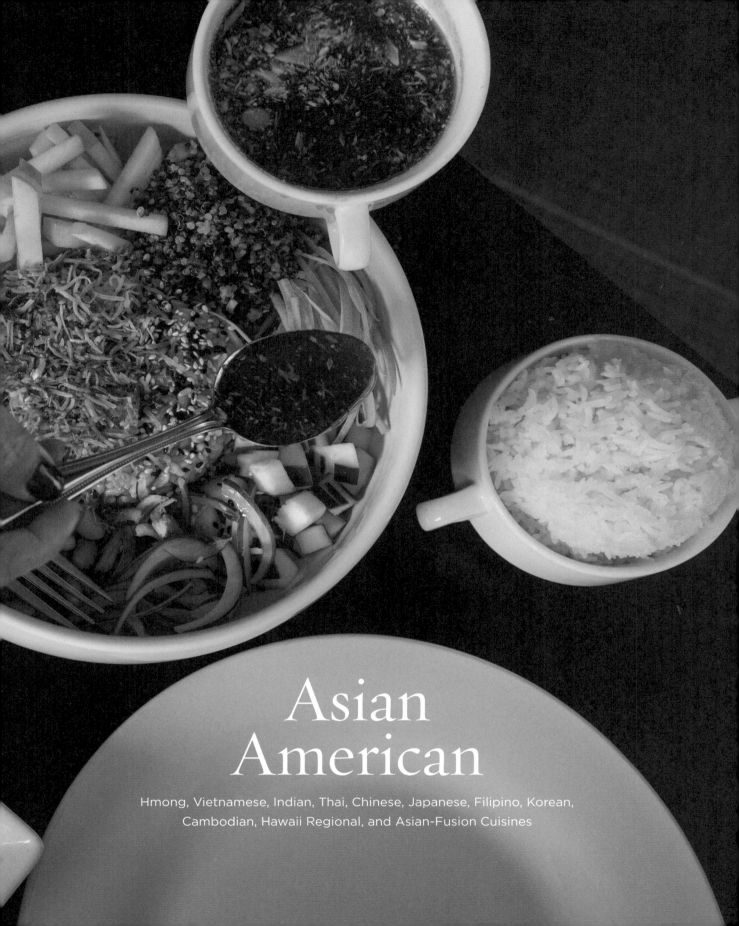

Asian American

Hmong, Vietnamese, Indian, Thai, Chinese, Japanese, Filipino, Korean,
Cambodian, Hawaii Regional, and Asian-Fusion Cuisines

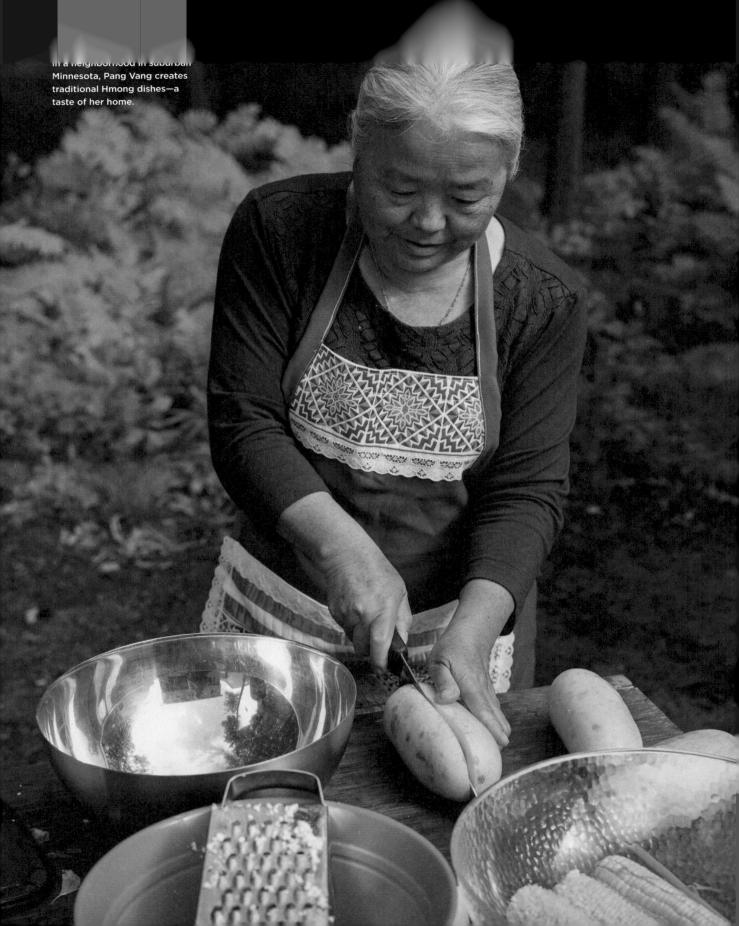

In a neighborhood in suburban Minnesota, Pang Vang creates traditional Hmong dishes—a taste of her home.

"It was Asian immigrants who taught Americans how to eat greens."

~DR. KRISHNENDU RAY

I t's a sultry Friday afternoon in suburban Honolulu, where 95-year-old Ruth Chang prepares lunch. With an enormous cleaver in each hand, she vigorously minces root vegetables. The menacing blades clash with her mother-of-pearl earrings and leopard-print loafers. "I cook every day," she informs me matter-of-factly, her silver bob bouncing to the staccato beat of her chopping. "Once you stop, you lose it."

I'm here thanks to my old friend Dr. Bradley Willcox, who, along with his brother, Craig, and economist Makoto Suzuki, authored *The Okinawa Program*. Dr. Willcox is currently a professor and director of research at the Department of Geriatric Medicine at the University of Hawaii at Manoa. When I asked him to introduce me to an older Chinese American woman who might be willing to cook with me, he instantly replied, "Ruth is the one. I'll join you."

Ruth shuttles food from the kitchen to a lazy Susan on her dining room table with a Chihuahua's energy and a ballerina's grace. Steaming, delicious-smelling platters of Savory Garlic Tofu With Minced Mushrooms (page 160) and Veggie Noodle Stir-Fry (page 163) arrive. Craig, David, my dad, and I look on hungrily. "This food has maybe a fifth the caloric density of a hamburger and 10 times the nutrients," Craig says, rotating the garlic tofu in his direction. "So you can eat to your stomach's content and never gain weight."

Ruth represents a demographic that may be the longest-lived in the world. According to a study by professor of public health and social work Kathryn Braun and her colleagues at the University of Hawaii at Manoa, Chinese American women living in Hawaii enjoy 90 years of life expectancy. That's two years longer than women in Hong Kong (currently the longest-lived country in the world) and 3.1

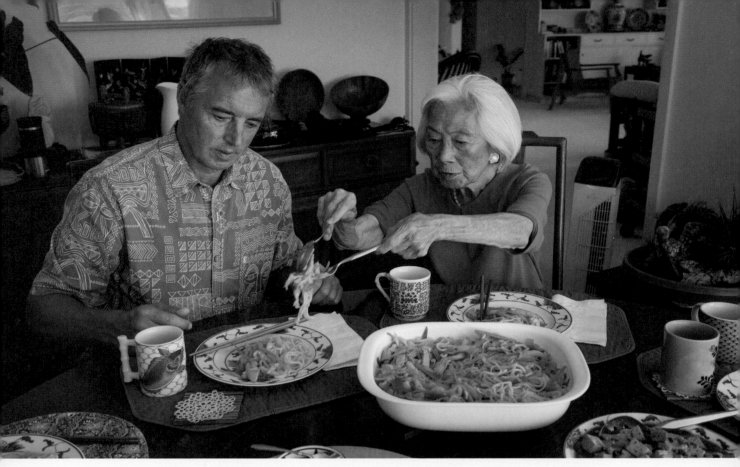

Above: Ruth Chang made me a lunch of dishes from her childhood in China, including her Veggie Noodle Stir-Fry (page 163). Opposite: Alan Wong marries Chinese and Hawaii Regional cuisines, with ingredients like purple taro.

years longer than women in Okinawa (previously the world's longest-lived). Part of the explanation lies in the unique diet of Chinese Americans living in Hawaii.

By 1830, Chinese immigrants began arriving in Hawaii as contract agricultural laborers (and later to the continental United States largely to work in gold mines). Japanese and Korean immigrants came later, and in the early 20th century so did Filipinos. Each group brought their own dishes and ingredients with them. The Chinese brought leafy cabbage, soybean products, and teas. The Japanese contributed miso and their own version of tofu. Filipinos introduced seaweed (for umami) and tender tips of plants such as squash, pumpkin, cow peas, and sweet potato vines, which they add to stews. Meanwhile, Dr. Krishnendu Ray, a food studies scholar at New York University and the author of *The Migrant's Table,* tells me that immigrants from central Europe brought their cows, pigs, and pickles. "It was Asian immigrants who taught Americans how to eat greens," he says. "In their countries, they couldn't afford meat, so they learned how to make vegetables taste good, largely through cooking technique and use of herbs."

East Asians have immigrated to the United States for more than 250 years, and the U.S. experienced enormous Southeast Asian migrations in the late 20th century.

Only a handful of dietary studies were recorded before World War II. Between 1896 and 1903, the University of California, Berkeley, professor Myer Edward Jaffa and his students studied the food consumption of 10 Chinese laundry workers, a dozen fieldworkers, and a dentist's family living in and around San Francisco. He found their diets consisted largely of rice, noodles, and tofu. The laundry workers consumed yams, wheat bread, sprouts, mustard greens, dried fungus, and water chestnuts. Though their hard labor had them consuming more that 4,200 calories daily, less than 25 percent of those calories came from animal products, and only 5.5 percent came from sugar.

Today, Hawaii is arguably the best place in America to experience Asian-fusion cuisine. Many traditional Asian herbs and vegetables thrive in the fertile soil and mild climate of Hawaii. And throughout the island state, plantation systems—where several ethnicities shared a communal kitchen—became de facto fusion laboratories that have influenced the cuisine of today.

Alan Wong, a New York–trained chef and the son of a Japanese mother and a Chinese Hawaiian father, is considered one of the founding fathers of Hawaii Regional Cuisine (an organization that put traditional Hawaiian food on the map) and is one of the first chefs to popularize Asian fusion. At his hugely popular restaurant, Alan Wong's Honolulu, he plays up his influences, creating dishes like ginger-crusted onaga (long-tailed red snapper) and soy-braised short ribs. Lately, his vegetarian better half, Alice, has him expanding his repertoire into healthier plant-based domains. When we visit him, he prepares wildly inventive dishes like Sweet Potato Gazpacho With Lomi Tomato Relish (page 274)—a creamier, sweeter version of the

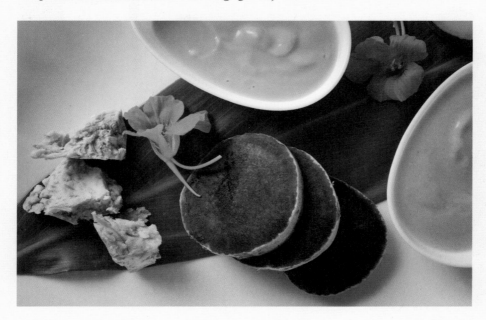

cold Spanish soup—and his symphonic Grains, Beans, Nuts, and Moromiso Moringa Salad (page 270) made with rye berries, barley, spelt, bulgur, moringa, cherry tomatoes, moromiso, sesame, walnuts, pumpkin seeds, and nutritional yeast.

Throughout Hawaii's Big Island and Oahu, we meet chefs who brilliantly express their culinary genius through their Asian roots, including Lynette Lo Tom (author of *A Chinese Kitchen: Traditional Recipes With an Island Twist*), Guatemalan-Filipino chef Henry Pineda, and Tess Villegas-Rumley, who runs Barefoot Zone in Kona, Hawaii.

In New Orleans, the Vilkhu family, of Saffron Nola restaurant fame, treats us to an Indian feast and shares recipes for three of their best-selling plant-based dishes.

We then explore a more contemporary flowering of Asian cooking in Los Angeles. The Korean and Vietnam Wars and the end of exclusionary immigration laws brought waves of immigrants from Korea, Cambodia, and Vietnam to California, and with them new creations. We seek out Korean chefs Krissy Song and Suzan Lee Paek and Thai restaurateur Narintr "Nat" Ruengsamutr. We also meet with the amazing Cambodian cooks Chad Phuong and Laura Rhatmeny Som, who gather regularly at Laura's MAYE Center in Long Beach, where former Khmer Rouge refugees converge around traditional cooking and cultivate healing and wellness.

All these chefs blend their homegrown knack for plant-based cooking with a flair for incorporating American influences and ingredients. What they produce is nothing short of a culinary revolution.

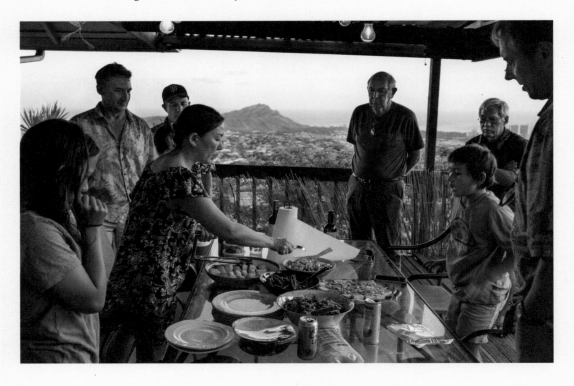

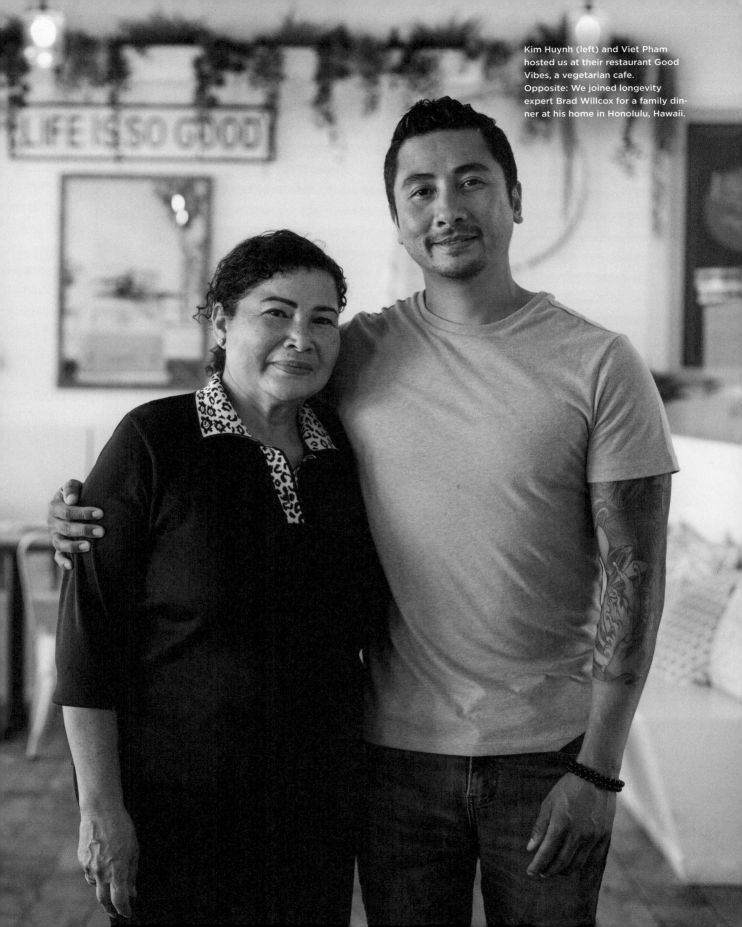

Kim Huynh (left) and Viet Pham hosted us at their restaurant Good Vibes, a vegetarian cafe. Opposite: We joined longevity expert Brad Willcox for a family dinner at his home in Honolulu, Hawaii.

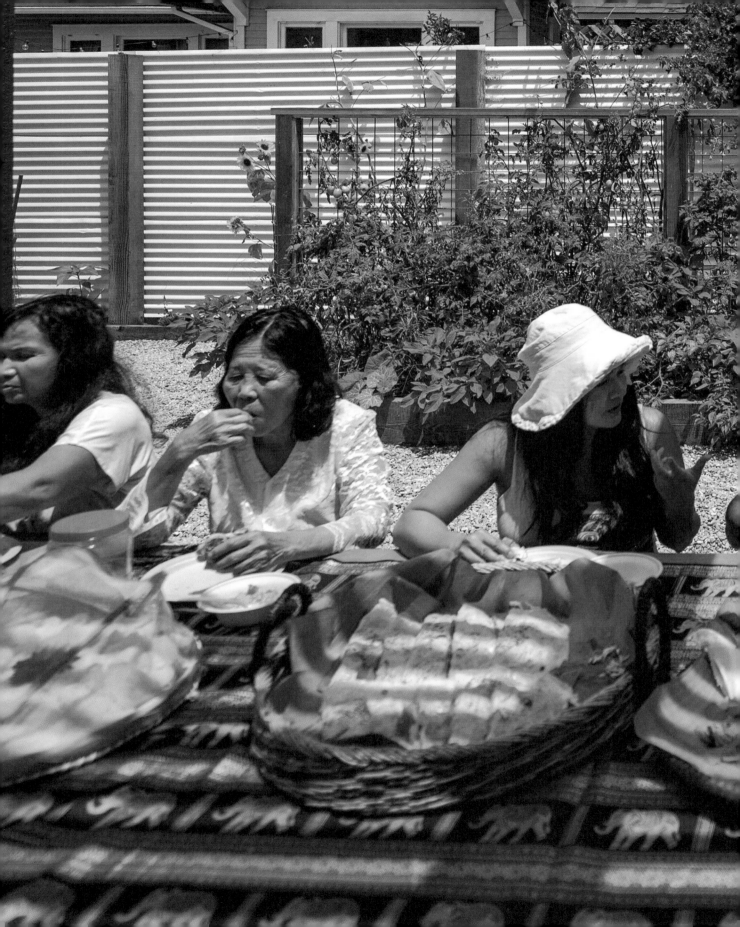

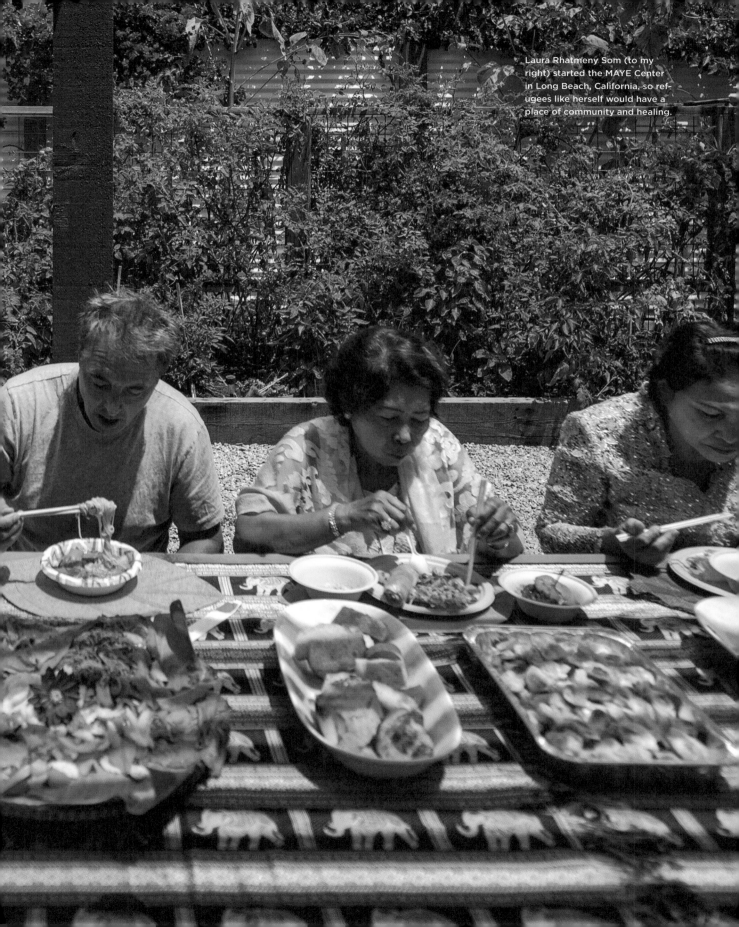

Laura Rhatmeny Som (to my right) started the MAYE Center in Long Beach, California, so refugees like herself would have a place of community and healing.

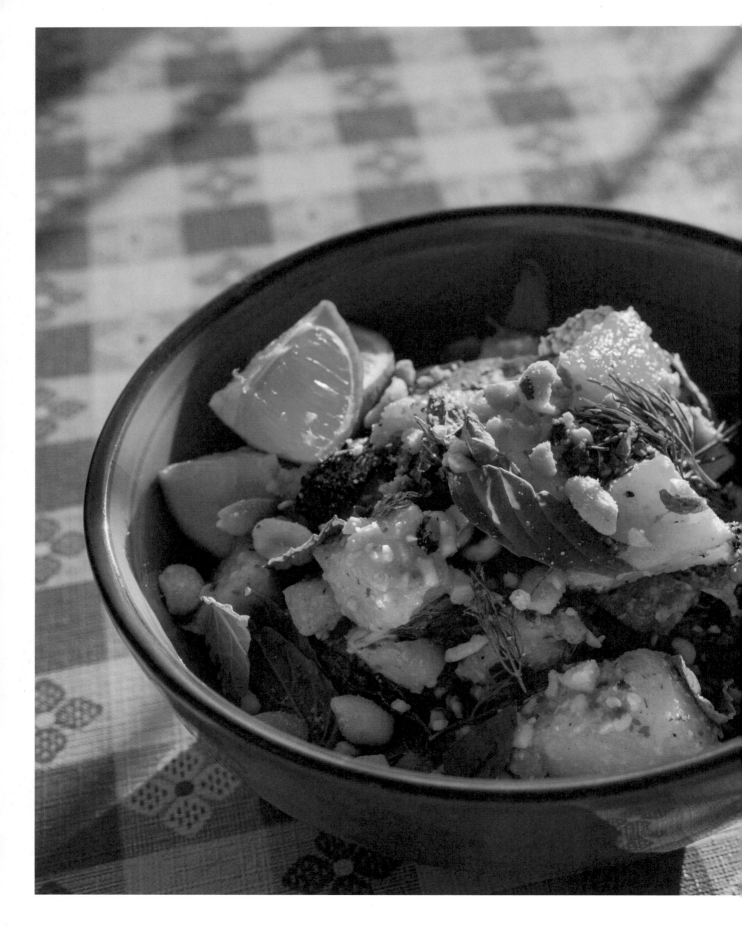

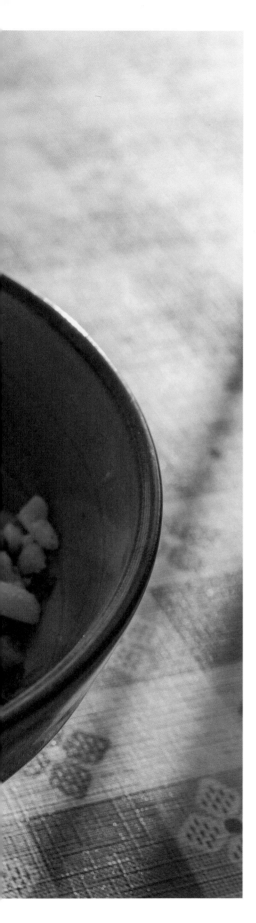

Mint Mango Salad With Peanuts and Lime

TOTAL COOK TIME: 5 MINUTES • SERVES 6 • SEASONING MIX MAKES 1½ CUPS

FOR THE SEASONING MIX:

1½ tablespoons tamarind powder

½ teaspoon tomato powder

½ teaspoon onion powder

1 teaspoon paprika

⅓ cup crushed dried Thai chili

⅓ cup salt

½ cup sugar

FOR THE MANGO SALAD:

1 pineapple, peeled, quartered, cored, and cut into 1-inch-thick slices

1 unripe mango, peeled and diced

6 crabapples, peeled, cored, and diced

¼ cup chopped fresh mint

¼ cup chopped fresh Thai basil

¼ cup roasted unsalted peanuts, chopped

½ teaspoon lime zest

Juice of 1 lime

Salt

Freshly ground black pepper

To make the seasoning mix, combine all the ingredients in a bowl or jar and mix well.

To make the mango salad, heat a grill to high heat and then grill the pineapple slices for about 45 seconds per side, until they caramelize.

In a large bowl, combine the grilled pineapple, mango, and crabapple.

Top with the seasoning mix, to taste.

Add the mint, basil, peanuts, lime zest, and lime juice. Toss to combine and add salt and pepper to taste.

NOTE
• Look for tamarind powder in an Asian grocery store or online.

Brown Rice Pudding With Nuts and Cardamom

TOTAL COOK TIME: 1 HOUR 20 MINUTES • SERVES 4

3 cups unsweetened, unflavored, plant-based milk, such as almond, soy, cashew, or rice

1 cup uncooked brown rice

¼ cup chopped dates

¼ cup pure cane sugar or pure maple syrup

1½ cup room-temperature water plus ¼ cup hot water

2 pinches of saffron, plus additional for garnish

1 tablespoon raisins

1 tablespoon toasted slivered or sliced almonds, plus additional for garnish

1 tablespoon chopped roasted pistachios, plus additional for garnish

1 teaspoon ground cardamom

In a large saucepan, combine the milk, rice, dates, sugar, and 1 cup of the room-temperature water over medium-high heat. Bring to a boil and then reduce the heat to low. Simmer uncovered, stirring frequently, for about 45 minutes, or until the rice is completely cooked; there should still be plenty of liquid in the pot.

Meanwhile, in a small bowl, combine the saffron and the ¼ cup of hot water. Let stand for 10 to 15 minutes.

Add the saffron with its soaking liquid, the raisins, almonds, pistachios, cardamom, and the remaining ½ cup of room-temperature water to the pot with the cooked rice. Cook for 10 to 20 minutes more, stirring occasionally, until the rice is creamy.

Serve hot, garnished with a few threads of saffron, sliced almonds, and chopped pistachios.

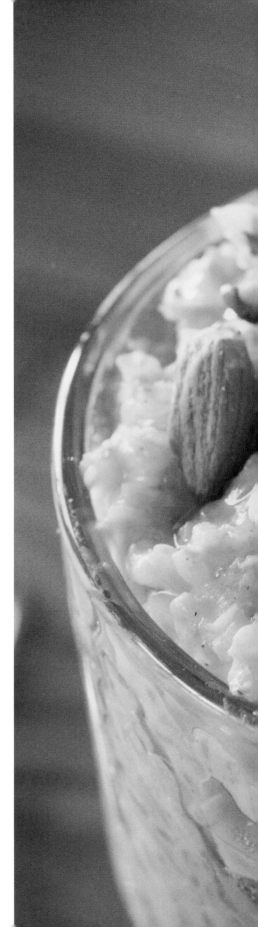

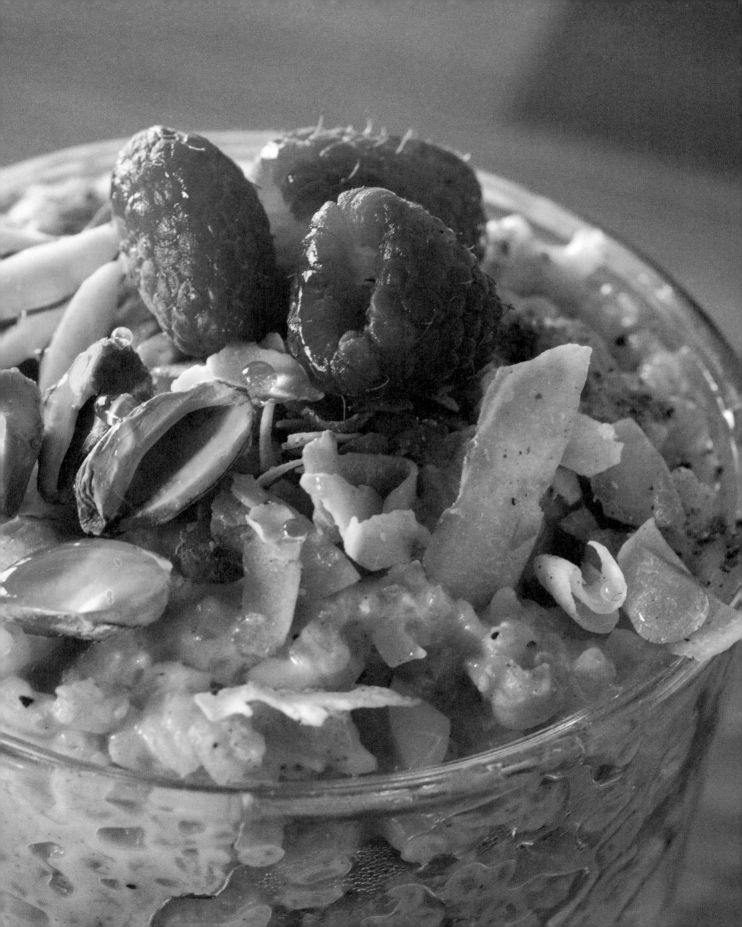

Sprouted Spicy Bean Salad

TOTAL COOK TIME: 35 MINUTES + 1 DAY FOR SPROUTING • SERVES 4

1 cup dried mung beans

3 cups water

1 heaping tablespoon grated ginger

2 hot chili peppers, finely chopped (use more or less depending on your taste)

¼ cup finely chopped cilantro

Salt

Freshly ground black pepper

Juice of 2 large lemons

To sprout the mung beans, place the beans in a large bowl with the water. Let stand for 12 to 14 hours. Drain and rinse the beans and return them to the bowl.

Cover the bowl of soaked beans with a kitchen towel and let them stand for an additional 12 to 24 hours to sprout. The time it takes for the beans to sprout will depend on the freshness of the beans and the temperature in your kitchen. Once you see small sprouts growing, refrigerate the beans until ready to use.

To make the salad, add the ginger, chili peppers, cilantro, salt, and pepper to the bowl of sprouted beans and toss to mix. Sprinkle the lemon juice over the top. Taste and adjust the seasoning if necessary.

Refrigerate for at least 30 minutes before serving.

Sautéed Japanese Eggplant With Thai Basil

TOTAL COOK TIME: 10 MINUTES • SERVES 4

Sophy Khut escaped the Khmer Rouge in Cambodia with her family when she was eight years old. They walked 100 miles to Thailand with the threat of execution hanging over them at every turn. At her Cambodian restaurant in Long Beach, Sophy calls on the only things she brought with her from her homeland—her memories of how her mother and grandmother cooked.

1 tablespoon oil

1 teaspoon crushed garlic

1 teaspoon crushed Thai chili

3 Japanese eggplants, sliced into rounds

½ green bell pepper, seeded and cut into ½-inch chunks

½ red bell pepper, seeded and cut into ½-inch chunks

2 tablespoons soy sauce

1 tablespoon sugar

Small handful Thai basil leaves

In a medium skillet, heat the oil over medium-high heat. Add the garlic and chili and cook, stirring, for 30 seconds.

Add the eggplant and bell pepper. Cook, stirring occasionally, until the vegetables begin to soften and brown, about 3 minutes.

Add the soy sauce and sugar, reduce the heat to low, and let simmer for 5 minutes, until the vegetables are soft.

Just before serving, stir in the basil leaves.

Neoum Salad (Khmer Coleslaw)

TOTAL COOK TIME: 10 MINUTES • SERVES 4

FOR THE SAUCE:

¼ cup palm sugar

¼ cup vegan fish sauce

1 tablespoon lime juice

1 tablespoon white vinegar

FOR THE SLAW:

4 cups shredded white cabbage

1 cup shredded purple cabbage

½ cup bean sprouts

1 cup shredded carrots

1 cup room-temperature clear rice noodles or bean thread, cooked according to package directions

Minced roasted peanuts, for garnish

Thai basil, for garnish

Mint, for garnish

To make the sauce, in a small saucepan over low heat, heat the sugar and fish sauce together until the sugar melts. Add the lime juice and vinegar and stir to mix. Remove from the heat and set aside to cool.

To make the slaw, in a large bowl, combine the white cabbage, purple cabbage, bean sprouts, and carrots with the sauce and toss to mix. Let it stand for about 5 minutes.

Add the noodles and toss to combine. Garnish with the roasted peanuts, basil, and mint.

Serve immediately.

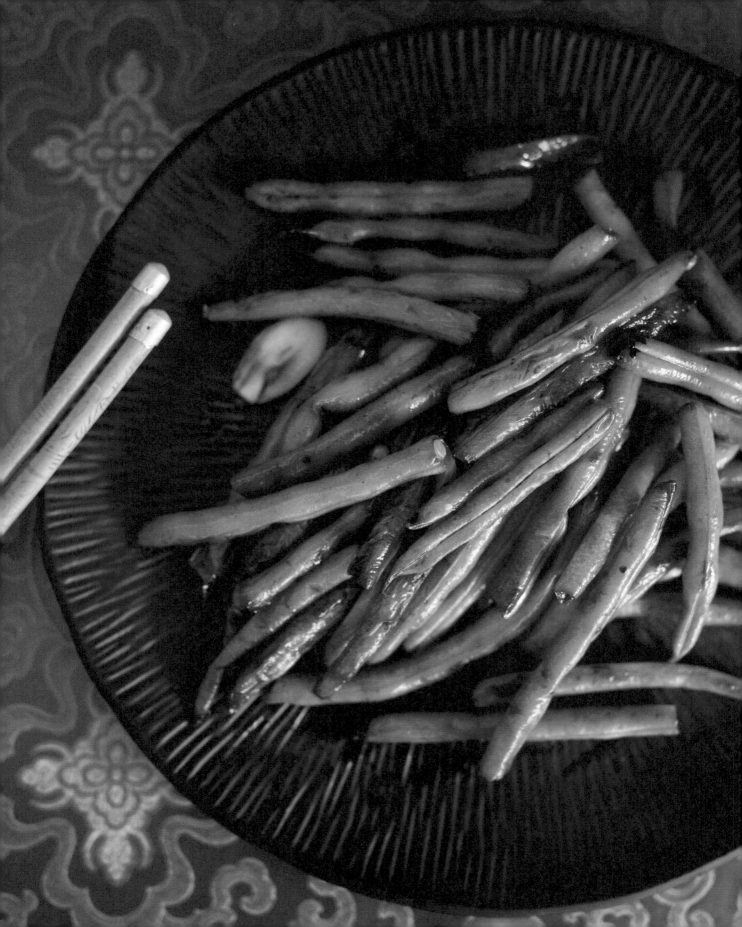

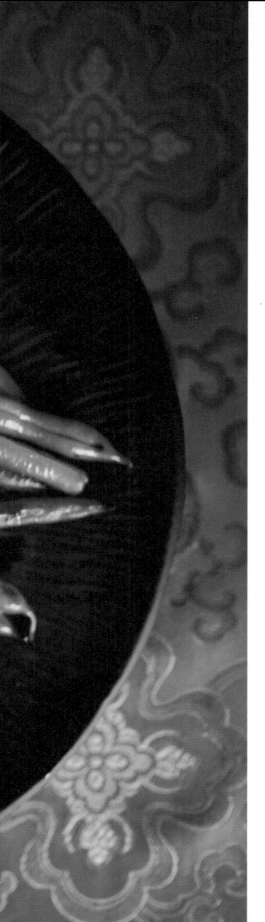

Crispy Stir-Fried Green Beans

TOTAL COOK TIME: 6 MINUTES • SERVES 4

Food columnist and author Lynette Lo Tom is known for sharing some of Hawaii's most loved comfort foods. Lynette, a Hawaii-born, fifth-generation Chinese American, captures the cooking of her mother, family, and the wider Chinese community in Hawaii (most of whom came from the area in China formerly called Canton, now Guangzhou).

This recipe proves you don't need a wok to cook classic Chinese-style crisp yet tender green beans. You can use a very hot cast-iron skillet to cook the green beans to the texture you enjoy. You can substitute other vegetables—try Broccolini, asparagus, or snap peas—and cook them the same way.

2 tablespoons vegetable oil

1 pound green beans (such as haricots vert), ends trimmed and strings removed

2 tablespoons soy sauce

1 tablespoon Shaoxing wine, dry sherry, or dry white wine

1 teaspoon vegan fish sauce

½ teaspoon salt

½ teaspoon sugar

½ teaspoon toasted sesame seeds, for garnish

In a wok or cast-iron skillet (or other heavy-bottomed skillet), heat the oil over high heat. When the oil begins to smoke, add the beans and cook, stirring continuously for 1 minute.

Add the soy sauce, wine, fish sauce, salt, and sugar. Cook for 3 to 5 minutes more, until the beans are charred in places and the sauce has thickened to a glaze.

Serve hot or at room temperature, garnished with the sesame seeds.

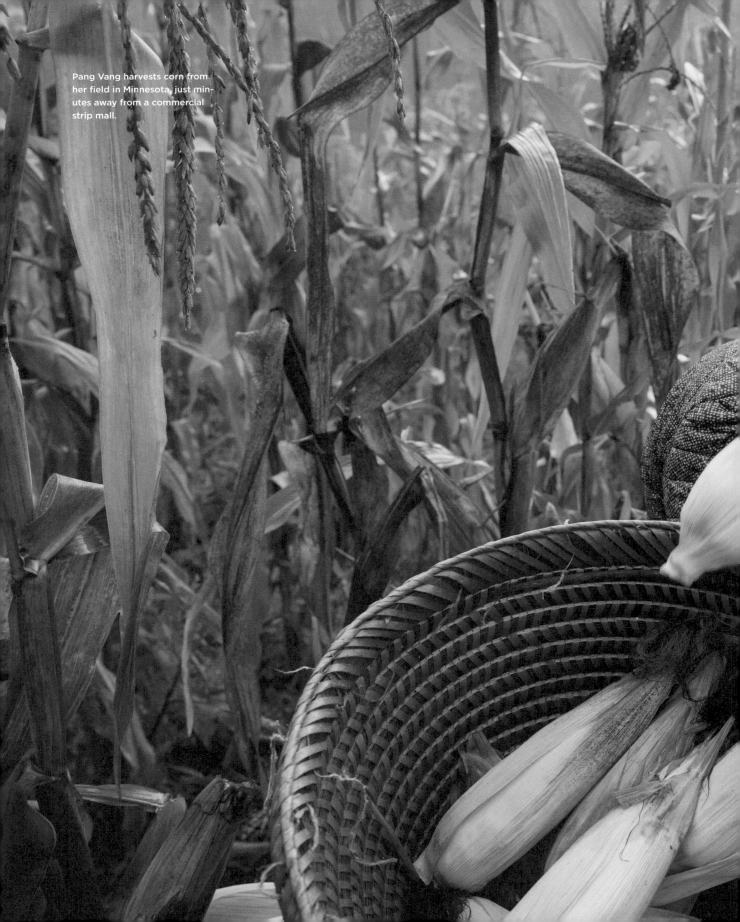

Pang Vang harvests corn from her field in Minnesota, just minutes away from a commercial strip mall.

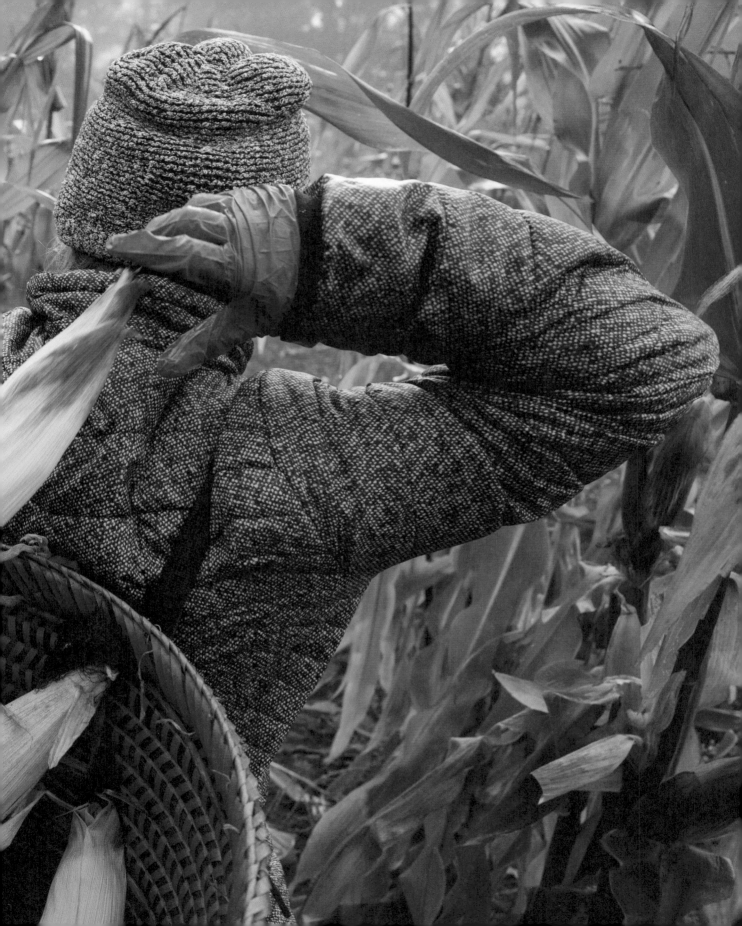

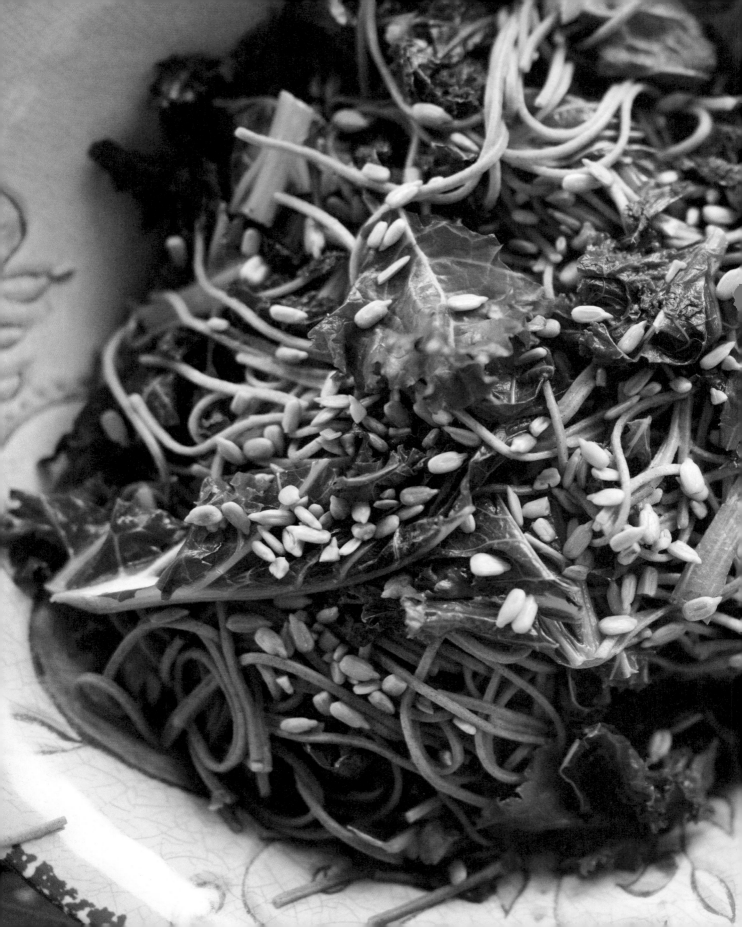

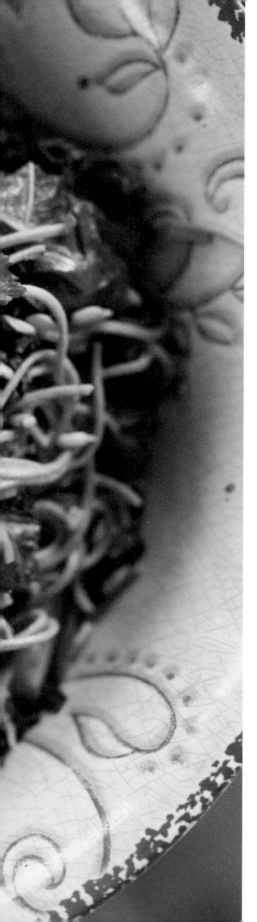

Kale Soba Salad

TOTAL COOK TIME: 10 MINUTES • SERVES 4

Soba noodles are made of buckwheat flour (and also usually a smaller amount of wheat flour), a nutritious grain that is unrelated to wheat. They have a stronger, nuttier flavor and are less chewy than other Japanese noodles like ramen or yakisoba. They're often served in soups, chilled with a dipping sauce, or in salads like this one.

4 ounces soba noodles (Japanese buckwheat noodles)

1 tablespoon sesame oil

3 garlic cloves, thinly sliced

4 cups chopped kale

1 tablespoon low-sodium soy sauce or your favorite soy sauce (tamari, mentsuyu, etc.)

3 tablespoons sunflower seeds

Cook the soba noodles according to the package directions. Drain in a colander and immediately rinse with cold running water. Transfer them to a salad bowl.

In a large skillet over medium heat, heat the sesame oil. Add the garlic and cook, stirring, until it is fragrant and golden, about 1 minute.

Raise the heat to high and add the kale. Cook for 30 seconds to 1 minute, until the kale is tender. Add the soy sauce and toss to mix.

Add the kale to the soba noodles and stir gently. Sprinkle with the sunflower seeds and serve.

Savory Garlic Tofu With Minced Mushrooms

TOTAL COOK TIME: 10 MINUTES • SERVES 4

Serve this vegetarian dish over rice with a dish of chilis in vinegar on the side.

1 tablespoon oil

5 large garlic cloves, chopped

6 to 8 fresh mushrooms, finely chopped

¼ onion, chopped

2 tablespoons cooking wine

1 tablespoon hoisin sauce

1 tablespoon black bean garlic sauce

1 teaspoon chili garlic sauce, or more to taste

1½ cups vegetable broth

¼ teaspoon ground white pepper

½ teaspoon white vinegar

1 teaspoon sugar

1 teaspoon sesame oil

1 tablespoon cornstarch mixed with 1 tablespoon cold water

1 pound firm tofu, drained and cut into ¾-inch cubes

1 green onion, chopped

Heat the oil in a wok or large heavy skillet over medium heat. Add the garlic and cook, stirring, until the garlic begins to turn golden brown on the edges, 1 to 2 minutes.

Add the mushrooms and onion and cook, stirring, for another 5 minutes, until the onion is soft and translucent.

Add the wine, hoisin sauce, black bean garlic sauce, and chili garlic sauce, and cook for 1 minute.

Add the broth, white pepper, vinegar, sugar, and sesame oil, and bring to a simmer. With the mixture bubbling, stir in the cornstarch mixture and cook, stirring, for 1 minute, until the sauce thickens.

Stir in the tofu and simmer for another 2 minutes, stirring gently.

Serve hot, garnished with the green onion, over rice.

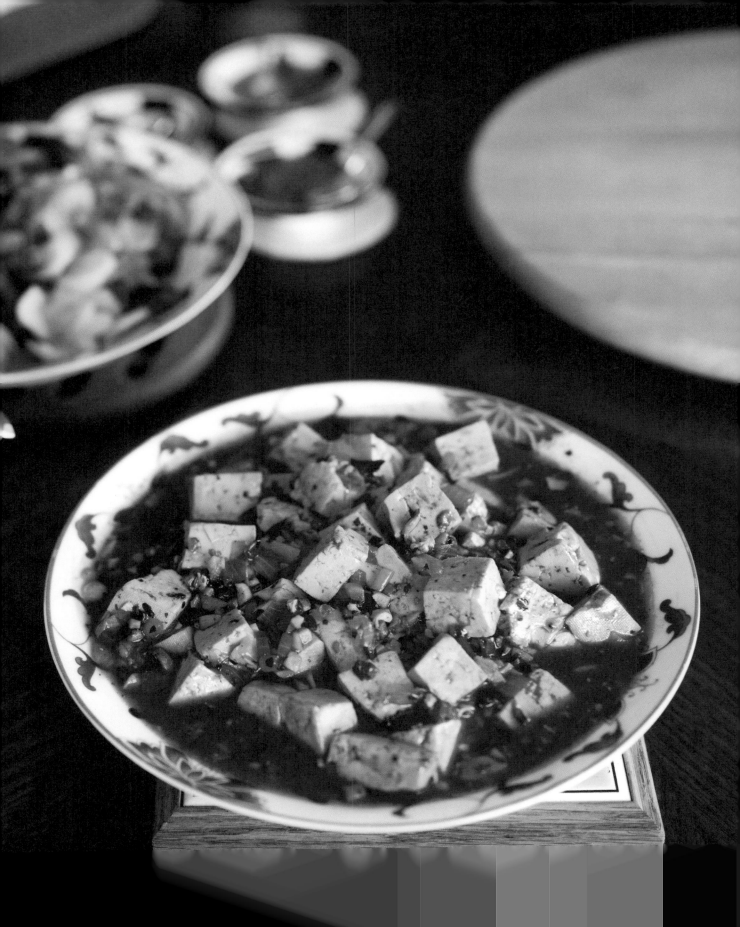

Bean Thread Noodles With Bok Choy and Shiitake Mushrooms

TOTAL COOK TIME: 40 MINUTES • SERVES 3

5 dried shiitake mushrooms

1 cup warm water

1 ounce clear bean thread noodles

1 tablespoon plus ½ tablespoon oil

2 to 3 garlic cloves, minced

8 to 10 water chestnuts, sliced

12 ounces baby bok choy or regular bok choy, cut into 1½-inch strips, stems and leaves separated

1 tablespoon vegetarian oyster sauce, or 1 teaspoon vegetable bouillon (such as Better Than Bouillon)

½ teaspoon sugar

¼ teaspoon salt, or to taste

Soak the dried mushrooms in the 1 cup of warm water until soft, about 30 minutes.

Remove the mushrooms from the soaking liquid, reserving the liquid. Cut the stems off the mushrooms (discard the stems), and slice the mushrooms into strips.

Place the bean thread noodles in a heatproof bowl and pour hot water over them. Soak them for at least 5 minutes, until the noodles are soft. Drain the noodles and cut them in half with scissors.

Heat 1 tablespoon of the oil in a wok or large skillet over high heat. Add the mushrooms, garlic, and water chestnuts, and cook, stirring, until fragrant, about 1 minute. Remove the mushroom mixture from the wok.

Add the remaining ½ tablespoon of oil to the wok and heat over high heat. Add the bok choy stems and stir-fry for 1 minute, until stems start to soften. Then add the bok choy leaves and cook, stirring, for another minute, until the leaves are bright green.

Add the mushroom mixture back to the skillet along with the noodles.

Add the reserved mushroom-soaking liquid, oyster sauce, sugar, and salt. Cover and reduce the heat to low. Simmer until the vegetables are crisp-tender.

Serve immediately.

NOTE
• You can use fresh shiitake mushrooms. Use 1 cup of mushroom broth in place of the mushroom-soaking liquid.

Veggie Noodle Stir-Fry

TOTAL COOK TIME: 10 MINUTES • SERVES 8

1 cup plus 1½ teaspoons water

¼ cup soy sauce, divided

1 tablespoon hoisin sauce

1 teaspoon vinegar, plus more for serving

1 teaspoon Shaoxing wine, dry sherry, or dry white wine

2 (8-ounce) packages tofu gan (firm pressed tofu) or fried tofu, cut into small strips

20 ounces fresh Chinese noodles (or yakisoba, vermicelli, or linguine noodles)

2 tablespoons oil, divided

3 garlic cloves, minced

6 mushrooms (button, cremini, shiitake, or portobello), sliced

12 to 15 (about 3 ounces) sweet peas, halved diagonally

1 carrot, julienned

1 head cabbage, sliced into thin strips

10 ears baby corn, halved diagonally

1 bamboo shoot, cut into strips, or 3 ounces canned sliced bamboo shoots (drained)

4 cups (about 6 ounces) bean sprouts, blanched in boiling water for 30 seconds

1 tablespoon cornstarch mixed with 1 tablespoon cold water

Chili paste, for serving

In a small bowl, combine 1 cup of the water, 2 tablespoons of the soy sauce, the hoisin sauce, and the vinegar.

In a large bowl, combine 1 tablespoon of the soy sauce, the wine, and 1½ teaspoons of the water. Add the tofu and toss to coat; let it marinate while you cook the noodles.

Cook the noodles according to the package directions (for fresh noodles, boil for about 3 minutes).

Drain the noodles and return them to the cooking pot. Add 1 teaspoon of the oil and the remaining 1 tablespoon of soy sauce and toss to coat.

Heat the remaining 1⅔ tablespoons of the oil in a wok or skillet over high heat. Add the garlic and mushrooms, and cook, stirring occasionally, for 2 minutes.

Add the sweet peas, carrot, cabbage, corn, bamboo shoots, and bean sprouts, and cook, stirring, for 2 minutes.

Add the marinated tofu and the sauce mixture. Reduce the heat to low, cover, and simmer until the vegetables are crisp-tender, about 3 minutes.

Add the cornstarch mixture to the skillet and simmer, stirring, until the sauce thickens.

Add the vegetables and sauce to the noodles and toss gently to mix.

Drizzle with a bit of vinegar, if desired, or serve vinegar on the side. Top with chili paste to taste.

KEITH LIM AND KAREN DUREG, HOME COOKS IN HONOLULU, HAWAII

Jai (Monks' Stew or Buddha's Delight)

TOTAL COOK TIME: 3 HOURS 30 MINUTES • SERVES 4 TO 5

Jai—also called lo han jai, monks' stew, or Buddha's delight—is a Chinese vegetarian dish traditionally eaten by Buddhist monks. It is commonly seen on Chinese restaurant menus as a great meat-free option. It's especially popular on the first day of the Lunar New Year. Tradition has it that one should eat a vegetarian diet to start the year off pure. Furthermore, many of the ingredients used in this dish symbolize good luck, and it is thought to bring luck to those who eat it. This version includes dried mushrooms, dates, lily buds, and other ingredients that are soaked in water to rehydrate. The soaking liquid is then used as the basis of the sauce, which is seasoned with soy sauce, garlic, ginger, and turmeric. This vegetarian stew is full of nutrition and flavor.

½ ounce dried chestnuts or ½ (5-ounce) can water chestnuts

1 ounce dried red dates (jujubes)

1 ounce dried shiitake mushrooms

1 ounce dried wood ear mushrooms

3 ounces dried bean curd sticks (bean threads)

½ ounce dried lily flower buds

½ ounce dried black moss

2 ounces dried mung bean vermicelli noodles

2 tablespoons vegetable oil

½ teaspoon minced garlic

½ teaspoon minced fresh ginger

½ teaspoon minced fresh turmeric

2 ounces fermented bean curd (red or white), cut into ½-inch cubes

¼ cup canned white ginkgo nuts, drained

½ (5-ounce) can shredded bamboo shoots

5 ounces (fresh or canned) fried wheat gluten

1 cup fresh snow peas

1 cup sliced carrot

1½ cups sliced napa cabbage

1 tablespoon soy sauce

Rinse the chestnuts, dates, shiitake mushrooms, wood ear mushrooms, bean curd sticks, lily flower buds, and black moss. Put each into separate bowls and cover with water. Let them soak for at least 3 hours. Drain, reserving the soaking water (the soaking water for all can be combined). Cut the ingredients into bite-size pieces.

Soak the mung bean noodles in warm water for about 15 minutes and then drain (discard the soaking water).

In a wok, heat the oil over medium-high heat. Add the garlic, ginger, and turmeric, and cook, stirring, until they begin to brown, 30 seconds to 1 minute.

Add about 2 cups of the reserved soaking liquid and bring to a boil.

Add the fermented bean curd and the rehydrated chestnuts, dates, mushrooms, bean curd sticks, lily flower buds, and black moss, and cook, stirring frequently, until the mushrooms soften, about 5 minutes.

Stir in the ginkgo nuts, bamboo shoots, and wheat gluten. Then add the snow peas, carrot, cabbage, and soy sauce, and cook, stirring occasionally, until the vegetables are crisp-tender, adding more of the soaking liquid if needed to prevent the pan from going dry.

Add the mung bean noodles and cook for a few minutes to soften them and heat them through; they should soak up most of the liquid.

Serve hot.

NOTES
• If you can't find these ingredients at your regular grocery store, you can find them at an Asian grocery store or online.

• You can substitute 5 fresh shiitake and wood ear mushrooms for the dried mushrooms. Fresh mushrooms don't need to be soaked.

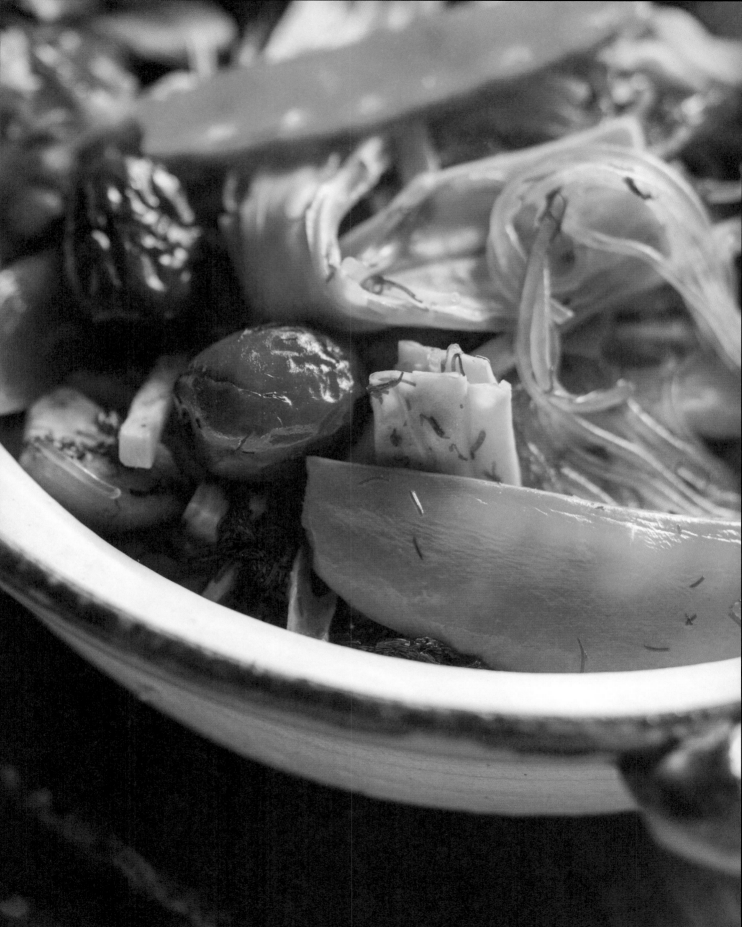

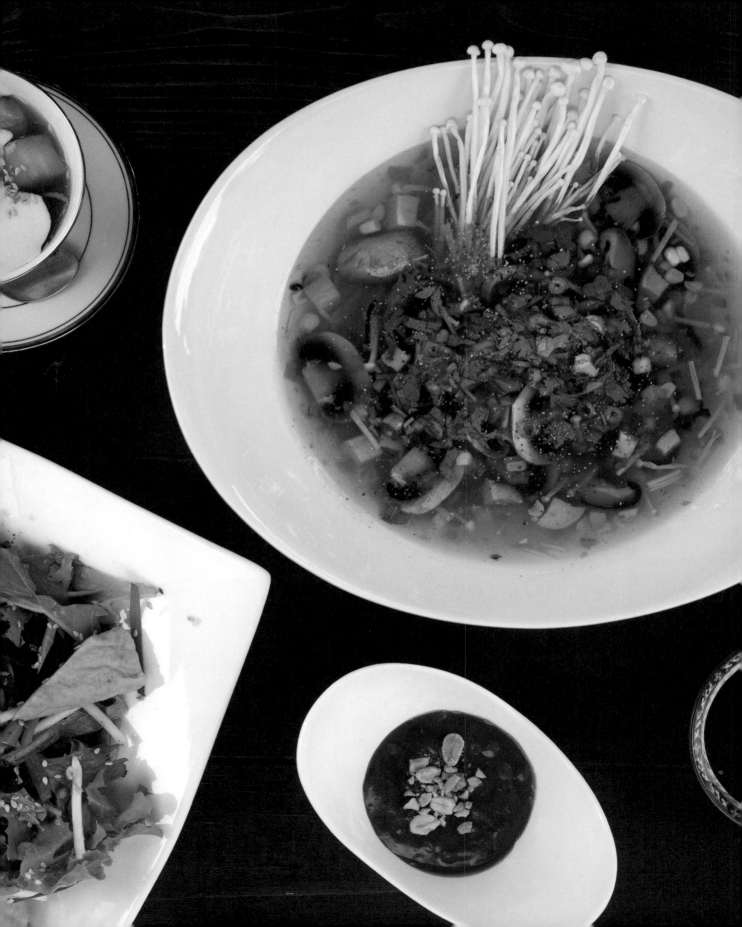

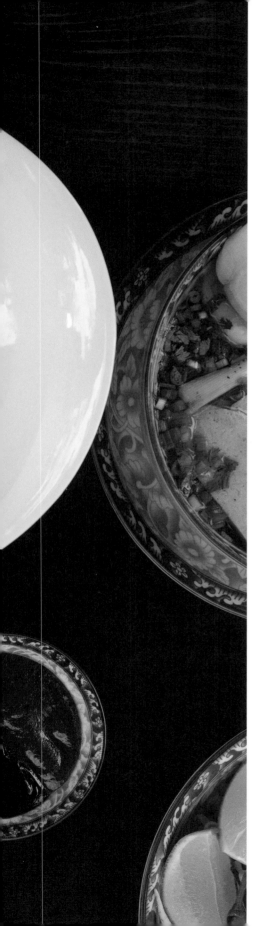

Mushroom Medley Soup

TOTAL COOK TIME: 1 HOUR 10 MINUTES • SERVES 6

Born in Saigon, Vinh "Kathy" Nguyen came to the United States in the 1980s. She started as a radio host, then became a radio cooking show host, and then a host on Vietnamese TV.

10 cups water

1 king mushroom, diced small

1 jicama, quartered

1 medium daikon, cut into 8 pieces

1 head cabbage, quartered

1 white onion, quartered

1 carrot, peeled and quartered

1 ounce rock sugar

1½ teaspoons salt

2 tablespoons mushroom bouillon powder

1 tablespoon dried black mushroom, soaked in warm water 20 minutes to soften, finely chopped

6 ounces fresh corn

4 fresh shiitake mushrooms, thinly sliced

4 white button mushrooms, thinly sliced

4 ounces enoki mushrooms

3 tablespoons tapioca starch mixed with 5 tablespoons water

1 teaspoon sesame oil

Green onions, chopped, for garnish

Fresh cilantro, chopped, for garnish

Freshly ground black pepper, for garnish

In a large stockpot, bring the water to a boil. Add the king mushroom, jicama, daikon, cabbage, onion, and 3 of the carrot quarters, and cook over medium heat for 1 hour. Remove the vegetables and strain the broth, discarding the solids.

Add the sugar, salt, and mushroom bouillon powder to the broth, and bring to a boil.

Finely chop the remaining quarter carrot and add it to the broth along with the black mushrooms and corn, and simmer for 5 minutes.

Add the shiitake, button, and enoki mushrooms, and cook for 3 minutes to soften. Remove from the heat and stir in the tapioca mixture and sesame oil.

Serve hot, garnished with green onion, cilantro, and pepper.

Stuffed Mustard Green Rolls With Peanut Sauce

TOTAL COOK TIME: 10 MINUTES • MAKES 10 ROLLS

FOR THE MUSTARD GREEN ROLLS:

1 tablespoon vegetable oil

1 shallot, thinly sliced

1 yellow or red bell pepper, thinly sliced

10 mustard green leaves, stemmed and cut into 8-by-3-inch rectangles

¼ fresh pineapple, cut into 3-by-1-inch strips

1 ripe avocado, sliced into 3-by-1-inch strips

1 package mustard sprouts

1 carrot, shredded

1 bunch Chinese chives

FOR THE PEANUT SAUCE:

1 tablespoon vegetable oil

1 shallot, sliced

3 tablespoons peanut butter or 2 tablespoons bean paste

3 tablespoons hoisin sauce

¼ cup water

½ teaspoon salt

2 teaspoons sugar

2 tablespoons chopped roasted peanuts, for garnish

To make the mustard green rolls, in a small skillet, heat the vegetable oil over medium heat. Add the shallot and pepper and cook, stirring, until lightly browned, about 3 minutes.

Remove the pan from the heat and let cool.

Lay a mustard leaf on your work surface and top it with some of the shallot mixture, and then add some of the pineapple, avocado, sprouts, and carrot. Roll the leaf up to contain them. Use a chive to tie the leaf up around the filling. Repeat with the remaining leaves and filling.

To make the peanut sauce, in a small pan, heat the oil over medium heat and add the shallot. Cook, stirring, until the shallot begins to brown, about 3 minutes. Reduce the heat to low and add the peanut butter and hoisin sauce and cook for 1 minute.

Raise the heat to medium and add the water, salt, and sugar.

Bring to a boil and then remove from the heat. Set aside to cool.

Transfer the sauce to a serving bowl and garnish with the peanuts.

Serve the mustard green rolls with the peanut sauce for dipping.

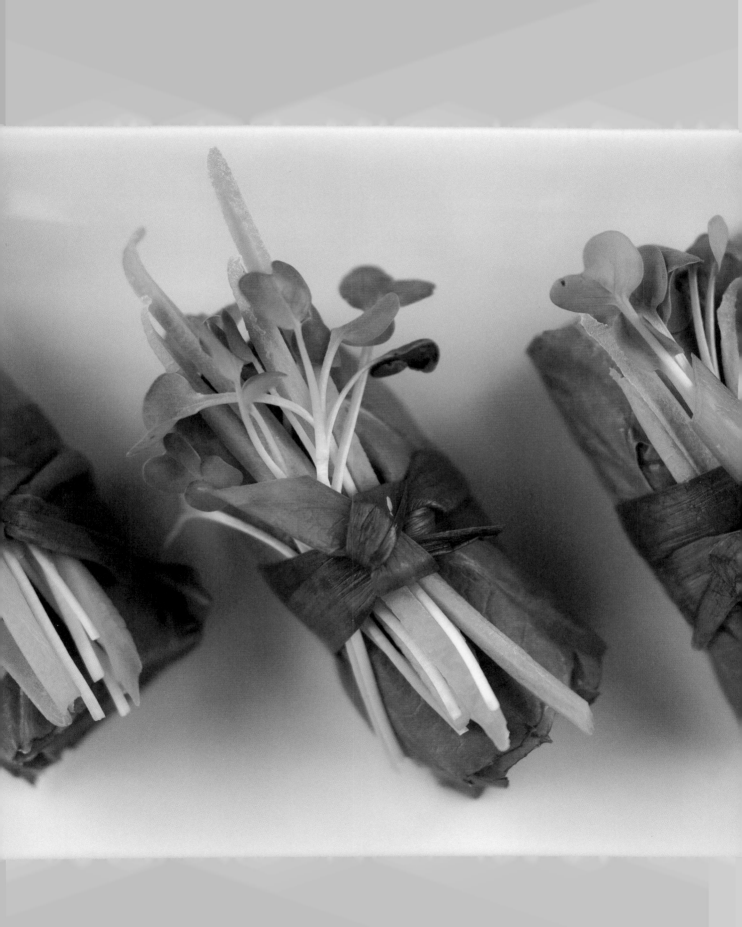

Sweet Full-Color Yams With Coconut Sauce

TOTAL COOK TIME: 30 MINUTES • SERVES 4

FOR THE YAMS:

8 ounces cassava, peeled and cut into ½-inch cubes

1 purple yam, peeled and cut into ½-inch cubes

1 yellow yam, peeled and cut into ½-inch cubes

6 tablespoons tapioca starch, divided

8 ounces rock sugar

2 liters water

1 teaspoon vanilla extract

FOR THE COCONUT SAUCE:

1 (13-ounce) can unsweetened coconut milk

1 cup water

1 tablespoon sugar

½ teaspoon salt

2 tablespoons tapioca starch mixed with 3 tablespoons water

1 tablespoon toasted sesame seeds, for garnish

Bring a large pot of water to a boil over high heat. Add the cassava and boil for 8 to 10 minutes. Drain and transfer it to a bowl.

Bring another pot of water to a boil, add the purple yam, and boil for 8 to 10 minutes. Drain and transfer the yam to a separate bowl from the cassava.

Boil the yellow yam the same way, drain, and transfer it to its own bowl.

Sprinkle 2 tablespoons of the tapioca starch over each (cassava, purple yam, and yellow yam). Toss to mix.

In a medium pot, combine the rock sugar and 2 liters of water. Bring to a boil over high heat and cook, stirring, until the sugar dissolves.

Reduce the heat to medium and add the cassava and purple and yellow yams, and cook, stirring gently with a wooden spoon, until the mixture thickens.

Remove from the heat and stir in the vanilla.

To make the coconut sauce, in a small saucepan, combine the coconut milk, water, sugar, and salt, and heat over medium heat.

Slowly add the tapioca mixture to the pot while stirring constantly. When it comes to a boil, remove it from the heat.

Serve the yams in small bowls, drizzled with the coconut sauce and garnished with toasted sesame seeds.

Fried Tofu Salad

TOTAL COOK TIME: 5 MINUTES • SERVES 2

FOR THE DRESSING:

1½ tablespoons white vinegar

1 tablespoon sugar

2 tablespoons water

1½ tablespoons soy sauce

1 teaspoon sesame oil

¼ teaspoon freshly ground black
  pepper

FOR THE SALAD:

4 ounces fried tofu

4 ounces mixed lettuce leaves

2 ounces bean sprouts

10 Chinese chives, cut into 2-inch
  lengths

2 ounces shredded carrot

1 tablespoon toasted sesame seeds,
  for garnish

To make the dressing, in a small bowl, combine all the ingredients and
whisk together.

To make the salad, in a large bowl, combine the tofu, lettuce, bean sprouts,
chives, and carrot, and toss to mix.

Add the dressing to the salad and toss to coat.

Serve garnished with the sesame seeds.

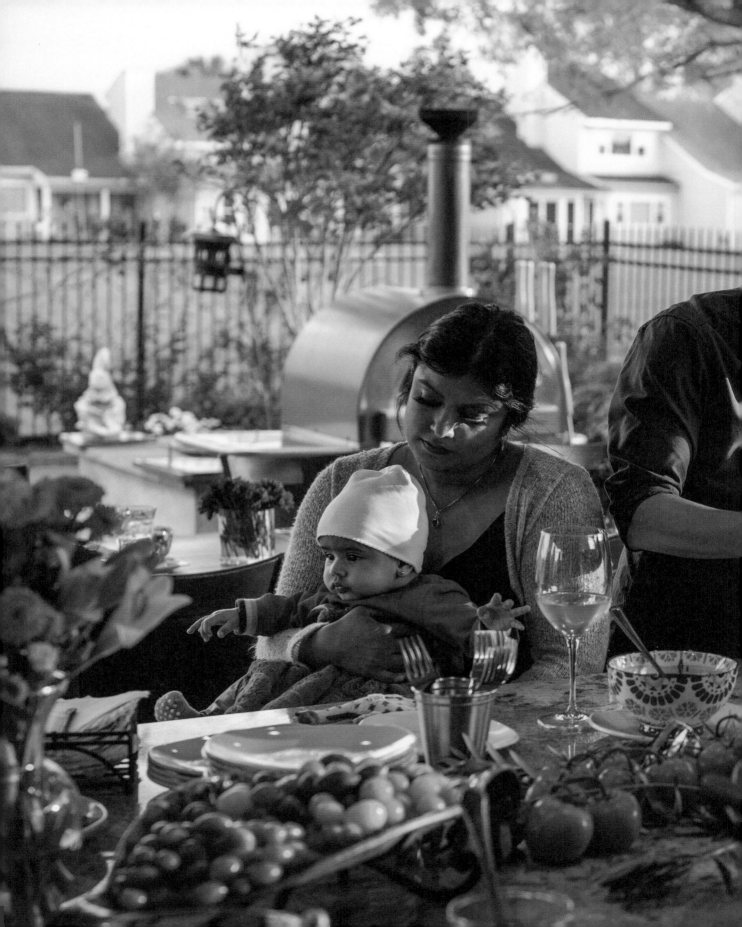

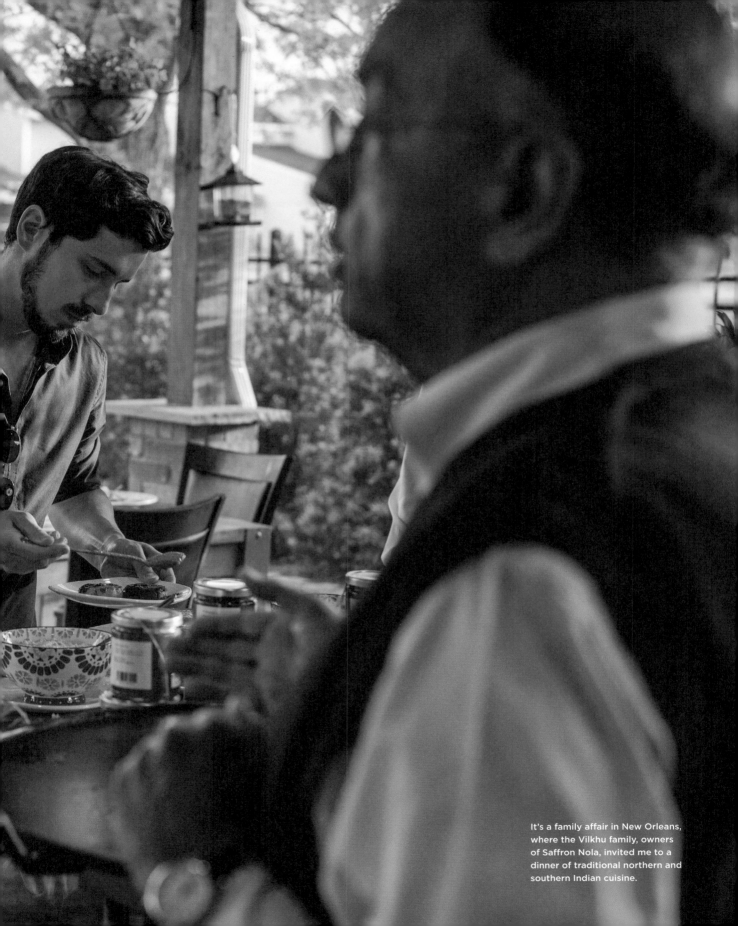

It's a family affair in New Orleans, where the Vilkhu family, owners of Saffron Nola, invited me to a dinner of traditional northern and southern Indian cuisine.

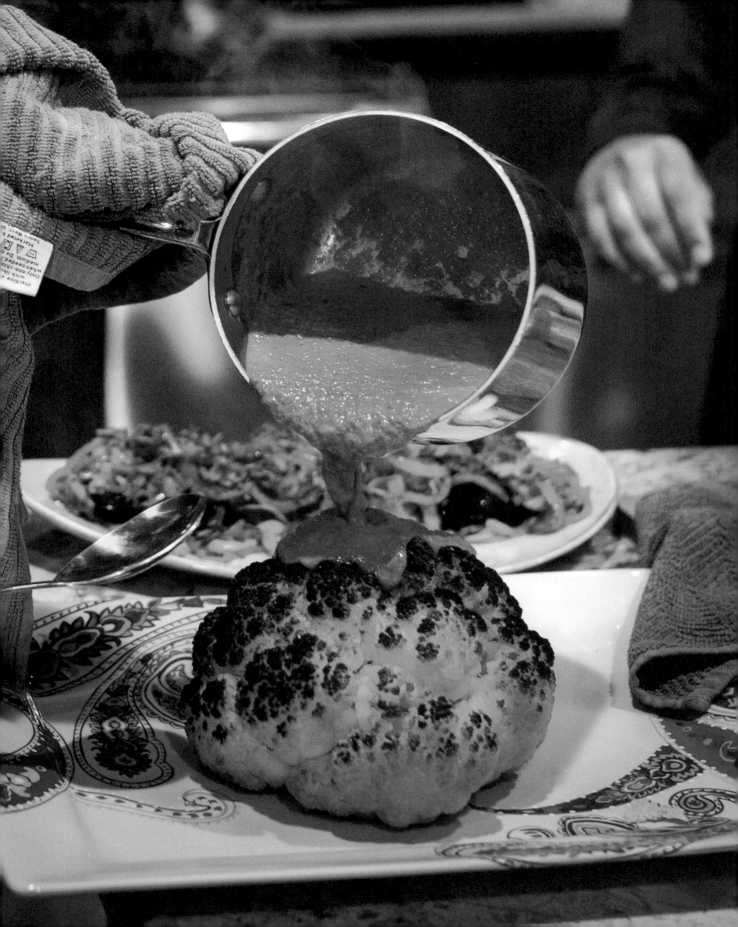

Whole Cauliflower With Makhani Sauce

TOTAL COOK TIME: 45 MINUTES • SERVES 4 TO 6

Saffron Nola is a Vilkhu family business that incorporates local New Orleans ingredients and flavors into traditional Indian cuisine. It received a James Beard nomination for Best New Restaurant in 2018.

FOR THE CAULIFLOWER:

2 teaspoons salt

½ teaspoon ground turmeric

½ teaspoon red chili powder

1 head cauliflower

FOR THE MAKHANI SAUCE:

2 tablespoons oil

1 dried red chili

1 onion, diced

1 teaspoon ginger paste

1 teaspoon garlic paste

2 teaspoons ground coriander

½ teaspoon ground cumin

½ teaspoon ground turmeric

1 cup tomato puree

¾ teaspoon salt

½ cup cashew paste

1 tablespoon dried fenugreek leaves

2 tablespoons chopped cilantro, for garnish

To blanch the cauliflower, bring a large pot of water to a boil. Add the salt, turmeric, and chili powder, followed by the whole cauliflower. Cover the pot and cook for about 8 minutes, flipping the cauliflower if needed, until it is tender. Remove cauliflower from the pot and cool in an ice bath.

To make the makhani sauce, heat the oil in a skillet over medium-high heat. Add the dried chili and onion and cook, stirring occasionally, until the onion is golden brown, about 7 minutes.

Add the ginger paste and garlic paste and cook for 2 more minutes. Add the coriander, cumin, and turmeric and cook for 2 more minutes.

Add the tomato puree and salt, and cook, stirring occasionally, until the sauce thickens, about 5 minutes. Stir in the cashew paste and fenugreek leaves and remove from the heat. If using an immersion blender, puree until smooth. If you are using a countertop blender, set aside to cool. Once the sauce is cool, transfer it to the blender and puree until smooth.

Preheat the oven to 400°F.

Place the blanched cauliflower in a baking dish and pour half the pureed sauce over the top.

Bake for 20 minutes.

While the cauliflower is in the oven, heat the remaining sauce in a saucepan.

Put the heated sauce in a serving bowl and add the cauliflower to the bowl after removing it from the oven. Serve hot, garnished with cilantro.

Uttapam (Savory Lentil Pancakes)

TOTAL COOK TIME: 1 HOUR + 16 HOURS SOAKING AND RESTING • SERVES 4

FOR THE BATTER:

1½ cups basmati rice

½ cup urad dal

2 tablespoons chana dal (split chickpea lentils)

½ teaspoon fenugreek seeds

½ teaspoon salt

1 teaspoon oil

FOR THE TOPPINGS:

½ cup diced onion

½ cup diced tomatoes

½ cup chopped cilantro

1 or 2 green chilis (such as jalapeños), chopped

Coconut Chutney (page 181), for serving

To make the batter, rinse the rice, urad dal, chana dal, and fenugreek seeds in cold running water. Cover them with cold water and soak overnight.

Drain most of the water, and using a high-speed blender, blend the soaked ingredients with enough water to make a thick, smooth, pourable batter; the rice will make the batter slightly grainy, which is okay, but make sure to process it until the grains are very small.

Add the salt and set the batter aside in a warm place to ferment overnight, or until the batter rises.

To cook the uttapam, return the batter to a pourable consistency by adding additional water a little at a time—up to 1 cup—stirring after each addition until you reach desired consistency, adding more only if needed.

Heat the oil in a flat-bottomed skillet over medium-high heat. Pour or ladle about ½ cup of the batter into the skillet, and then tilt and turn the skillet to spread the batter out a bit to a circle about 6 inches in diameter.

Reduce the heat to medium and scatter half the toppings over the batter. Add a little oil around the edges if needed to prevent sticking, and cook over medium heat for about 2 minutes, until the top looks dry and has lots of little holes all over. Using a thin spatula, carefully flip the uttapam over and then cook it 1 to 2 minutes more, until the underside is cooked.

Repeat with the rest of the batter and toppings.

Transfer to a serving plate and serve with the coconut chutney.

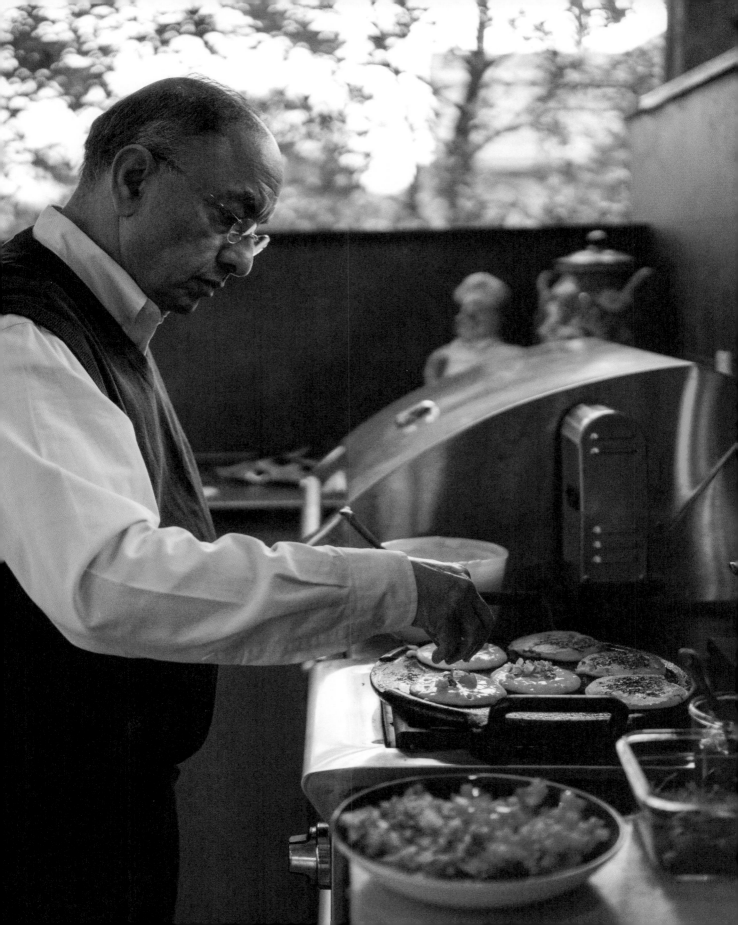

Aloo Tikki (Crispy Potato Patties)

TOTAL COOK TIME: 30 MINUTES • MAKES 12 PATTIES

These crunchy potato patties are a popular North Indian street food and are easy and delicious to make at home. They are sometimes stuffed with chana dal or served with curry on the side.

2 pounds small, thin-skinned potatoes (such as Yukon Gold)

2 ounces cornstarch

Salt

2 tablespoons oil, plus additional for frying

1 teaspoon cumin seeds

1 cup fresh or frozen peas

1 tablespoon ground coriander

1 teaspoon ground red chili

Mint Chutney (page 180), for serving

Cover the potatoes in cold water in a saucepan and bring to a boil. Cook until tender, about 15 minutes. Drain the potatoes and let cool. When they're cool enough to handle, peel the potatoes (the peels should slip off easily), discard the peels, and grate the peeled potatoes on the large holes of a box grater.

Put the grated potato in a large mixing bowl and stir in the cornstarch and salt. Mix well and then divide into 12 equal portions, rolling each into a ball.

Heat the 2 tablespoons of oil in a pan over medium-high heat. Add the cumin seeds and cook, stirring, until the seeds begin to crackle, about 30 seconds. Add the peas, coriander, and red chili, and cook, stirring occasionally, until the peas are tender, about 2 minutes. Transfer the pea mixture to a bowl and let cool. Mash the peas well.

Flatten each potato ball into a disk and place a spoonful of the pea filling on top, dividing the filling equally between the 12 potato balls. Press the potato patty around the filling to enclose it, forming it back into a ball. Flatten the filled ball to a disk about ¾ inch thick.

In a large skillet, add enough oil to cover the bottom in a thin layer and heat over medium-high heat. Add the patties and cook until the bottoms are crisp and golden brown, 2 to 3 minutes. Flip the patties over and cook until the second side is golden brown and crisp, 2 to 3 minutes more. For extra crispness, flip them over again and fry for another minute or so on each side.

Transfer the cooked patties to a plate lined with paper towels to drain.

Serve hot with mint chutney.

Poori (Indian Fried Bread)

TOTAL COOK TIME: 20 MINUTES • MAKES 8 POORI

These puffy, crisp, fried bread rounds are quick and easy to make. Serve them alongside Mint Chutney (page 180) or Tomato and Ginger Chutney (page 180).

1 cup whole wheat flour, plus additional as needed

1 teaspoon semolina flour

Pinch of salt

½ cup water

1 teaspoon oil, divided, plus additional for frying

In a medium bowl, combine the whole wheat flour, semolina flour, and salt. Add the water and ½ teaspoon of oil, and mix until it comes together in a soft but not sticky dough. If the dough is too stiff, add a bit more water, 1 tablespoon at a time. If the dough is too sticky, add more whole wheat flour, 1 tablespoon at a time.

Drizzle the remaining ½ teaspoon of oil onto the dough and knead lightly with your hands.

Place the dough in a large bowl and cover with a clean dishtowel. Set aside to rise for 5 to 10 minutes.

Divide the dough into eight parts and roll them into balls.

On a well-floured board using a well-floured rolling pin, roll the balls out into thin disks. They should be about 6 inches across and the thickness of a corn tortilla.

Fill a high-sided pot or wok with about 3 inches of oil and heat over medium-high heat until the oil is very hot and begins to shimmer (you can drop a small ball of dough into the oil to test it—if it sizzles and immediately floats to the top, then the oil is hot enough).

Slide one poori into the oil and cook it until it puffs up and the bottom turns golden brown, about 1½ to 2 minutes. Flip it over and cook for about 30 seconds more, until the second side is golden brown. Remove it from the oil and drain it on a plate lined with paper towels. Repeat with the remaining poori.

Serve hot.

Chutney Three Ways

Tomato and Ginger Chutney

TOTAL COOK TIME: 15 MINUTES • MAKES ABOUT 3 CUPS

¼ cup vegetable oil

4 dried red chilis, chopped

1 teaspoon mustard seeds

12 curry leaves

½ cup peeled and julienned fresh
  ginger

1 teaspoon salt

1 teaspoon Kashmiri chili powder

4 cups tomato puree

¼ cup malt vinegar

Heat the oil in a medium saucepan over medium-high heat. Add the chilis, mustard seeds, and curry leaves, and cook, stirring, until the seeds begin to pop, 30 to 60 seconds. Add the ginger and salt, and cook, stirring occasionally, for 2 minutes more.

Stir in the chili powder and tomato puree and reduce the heat to medium. Cook until the mixture thickens, about 10 minutes.

Add the vinegar and cook for 2 more minutes.

Mint Chutney

TOTAL COOK TIME: 15 MINUTES • MAKES ABOUT 1 CUP

1 cup mint leaves

1 cup cilantro leaves

1 green chili pepper (such as
  jalapeño)

1 garlic clove

½ cup pureed mango

2 tablespoons freshly squeezed
  lemon juice

½ teaspoon salt

Combine all the ingredients in a blender and process until smooth. Taste and adjust the seasoning as needed.

Serve immediately or refrigerate, covered, for up to five days.

Coconut Chutney

TOTAL COOK TIME: 1 HOUR 15 MINUTES • MAKES ABOUT 1½ CUPS

¼ cup chana dal (split chickpea
   lentils)

2 cups water

2 teaspoons vegetable oil

1 dried red chili

1 teaspoon mustard seeds

10 curry leaves

1 cup grated coconut

1 cup cilantro

1 tablespoon minced fresh ginger

1 tablespoon lemon juice

In a medium bowl, combine the chana dal and water and let stand for at least 1 hour.

Heat the oil in a skillet and add the red chili and mustard seeds. Cook until the mustard seeds begin to pop, about 30 to 60 seconds, and then add the curry leaves.

Drain the chana dal and add it to the skillet. Cook, stirring occasionally, until the chana dal is browned and cooked through, 10 to 12 minutes.

In a blender, combine the coconut with the cilantro, ginger, lemon juice, and chana dal mixture from the skillet. Process to a smooth paste.

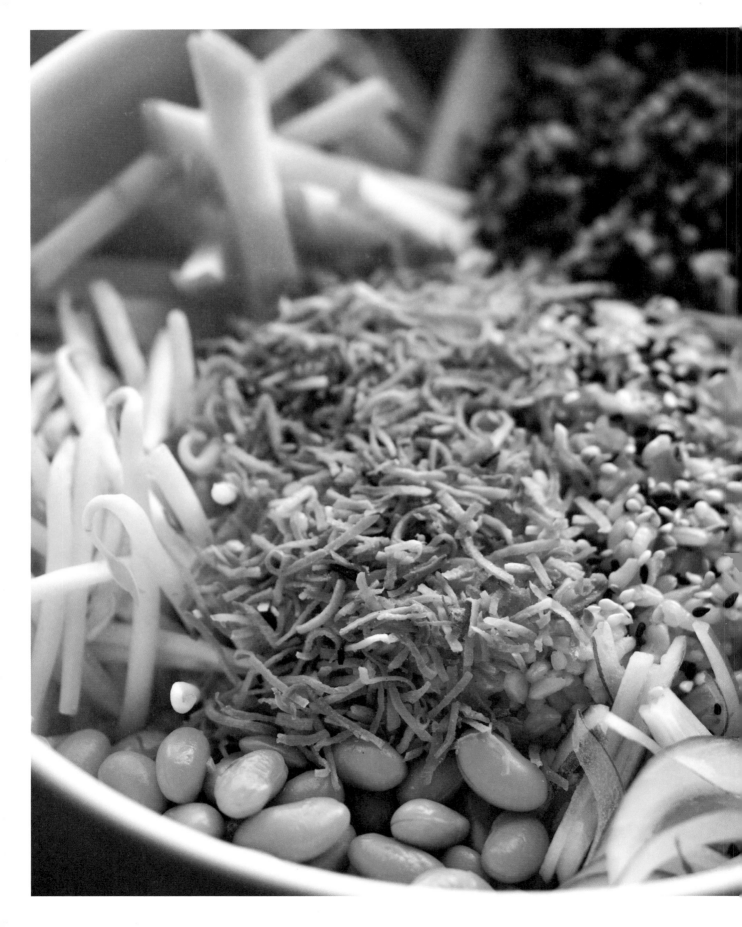

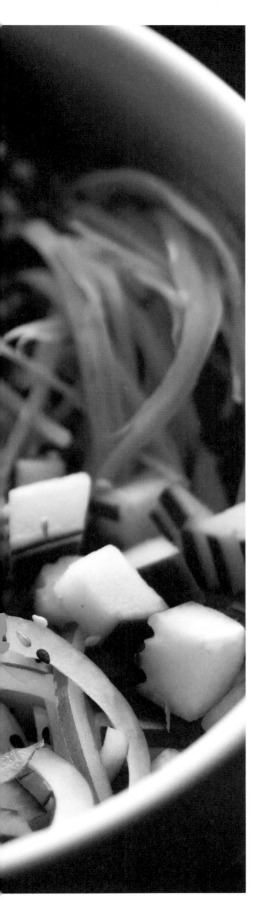

Khao Yum
(Rainbow Rice Salad)

TOTAL COOK TIME: 45 MINUTES • SERVES 4

Nat Ruengsamutr immigrated to the United States in her 20s and started Bulan Thai Vegetarian Kitchen in 2006 with three other women in the Silver Lake neighborhood of Los Angeles. They saw the need for authentic Thai vegetarian cooking in the area, and each brought something special to the table.

FOR THE DRESSING:

3 tablespoons soy sauce

1 tablespoon palm sugar or brown sugar

6 tablespoons freshly squeezed lime juice

1 tablespoon finely minced lemongrass

1 tablespoon finely grated galangal

1 Thai chili, grated or finely minced (optional)

FOR THE SALAD:

2 cups cooked brown rice

¼ cup steamed diced squash or pumpkin

¼ cup diced cucumber

¼ cup diced red onion

½ cup diced green apple

½ cup bean sprouts

½ cup shredded carrots

¼ cup edamame

¼ cup quinoa

¼ cup shredded coconut, lightly toasted

2 teaspoons sesame seeds, lightly toasted, for garnish

To make the dressing, in a small bowl, whisk together the soy sauce and palm sugar. Add the lime juice, lemongrass, galangal, and chili, if using.

To assemble the salad, place the rice in a bowl and then add the squash, cucumber, red onion, green apple, bean sprouts, carrots, edamame, quinoa, and toasted coconut in separate mounds around or on top of the rice.

At the table, add the dressing to the salad, toss to combine, and then garnish with the toasted sesame seeds.

NOTE
• Toast the shredded coconut and sesame seeds separately in a skillet over medium-high heat until just lightly browned and aromatic.

Honey-Marinated Tomatoes

TOTAL COOK TIME: 3 HOURS • SERVES 4

1 pound cherry tomatoes, peeled

½ cup honey

1 teaspoon olive oil (optional)

Put the peeled tomatoes in a 32-ounce jar.

Add the honey to the tomatoes, along with the olive oil, if using.

Cover and refrigerate for at least 3 hours before serving.

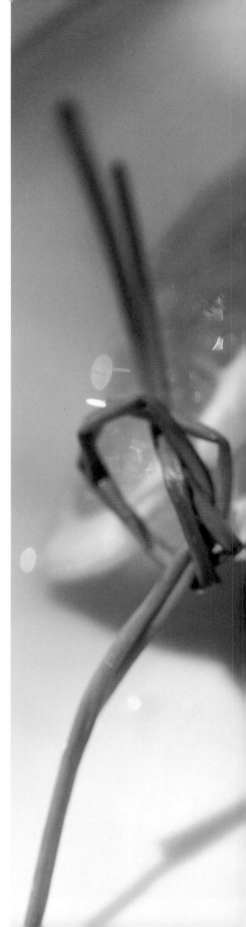

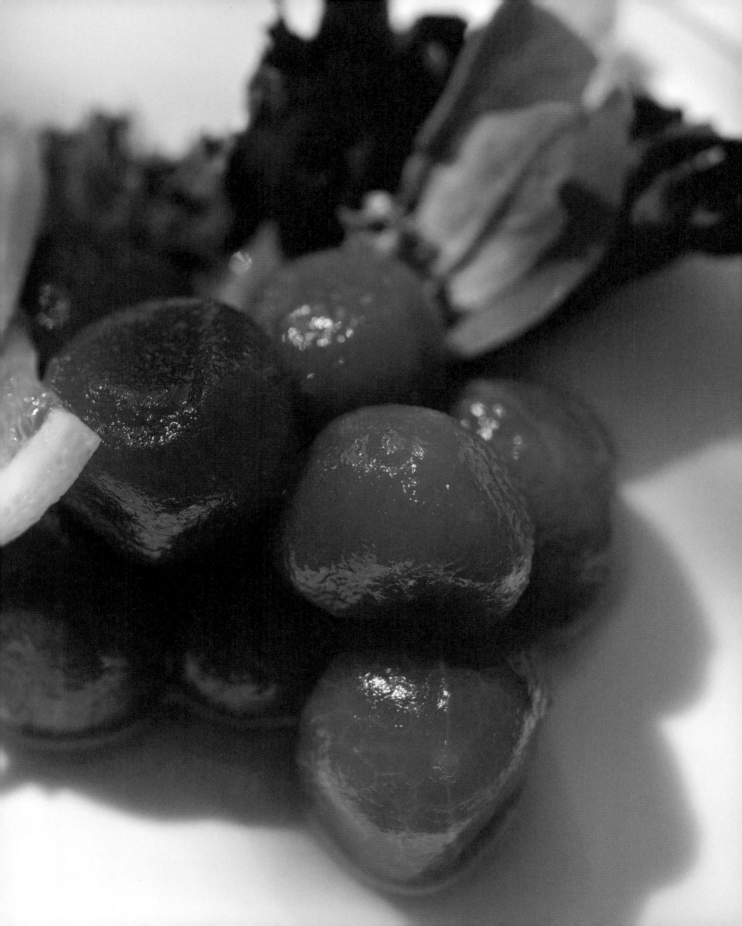

Cha Soba Noodle Salad

TOTAL COOK TIME: 10 MINUTES • SERVES 4

4 ounces cha soba noodles (green tea noodles)

2 ounces rice vinegar

2 ounces soy sauce

1 tablespoon agave syrup

2 ounces avocado oil

1 tablespoon sriracha

4 ounces mushrooms (use any kind such as shimeji, maitake, shiitake, enoki, or a combination), sliced, for garnish

Sesame seeds, for garnish

Cook the noodles al dente, according to the package directions.

In a medium bowl, combine the vinegar, soy sauce, agave syrup, avocado oil, and sriracha and mix well. Add the noodles and toss to coat.

Serve garnished with the mushrooms and sesame seeds

NOTE
• If cha soba noodles aren't available in your regular grocery store, look in nearby Asian markets.

Teriyaki Tofu and Onion Rounds

TOTAL COOK TIME: 20 MINUTES • SERVES 4

FOR THE TERIYAKI SAUCE:

2 tablespoons soy sauce

2 tablespoons water

2 tablespoons mirin

1 tablespoon sugar

FOR THE TOFU:

1 (16-ounce) package medium-firm tofu, cut into ½-inch-thick slabs

1 onion, sliced into ½-inch-thick rings

1 cup flour

Avocado oil

Shredded daikon, for garnish

Enoki mushrooms, for garnish

To make the teriyaki sauce, combine all the ingredients in a small saucepan and heat over medium heat until the sugar dissolves and the sauce thickens. Remove from the heat and set aside.

To make the tofu, use a round cookie cutter or biscuit cutter with a slightly smaller diameter than the onion rings to cut the tofu slabs into rounds. Place the tofu rounds inside the onion rings.

Sprinkle the flour over the onion and tofu on both sides.

Heat a large drizzle of oil in a skillet over medium-high heat. Add the onion-wrapped tofu to the pan and cook until browned on both sides, about 10 minutes total.

Serve the tofu drizzled with the teriyaki sauce and garnished with the shredded daikon and mushrooms.

NOTE
• If you don't have mirin, add a bit more water and sugar to the sauce.

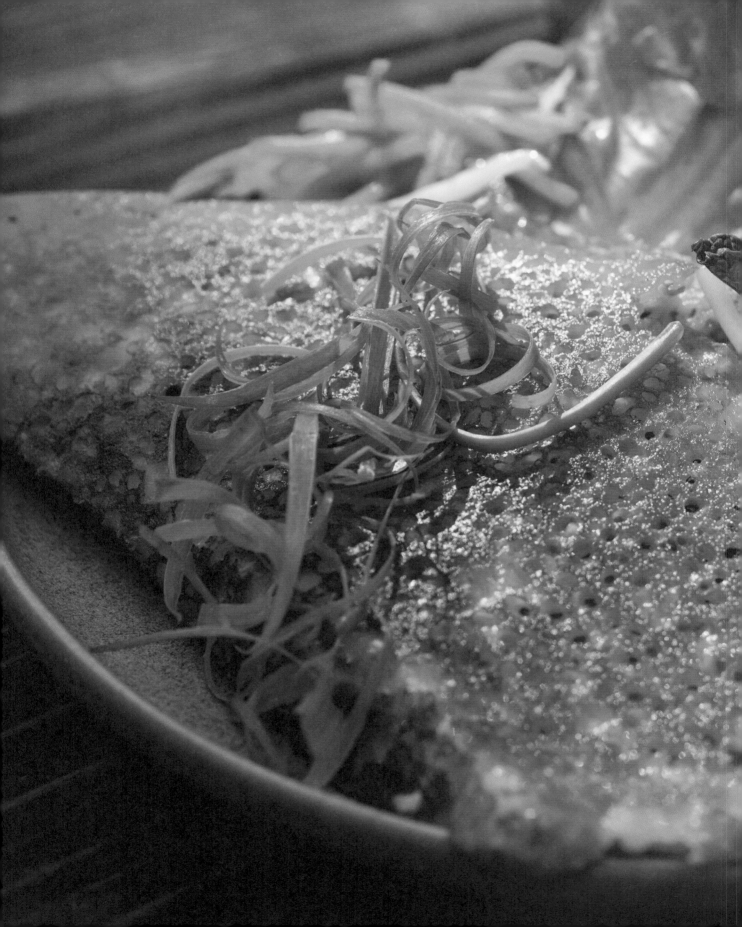

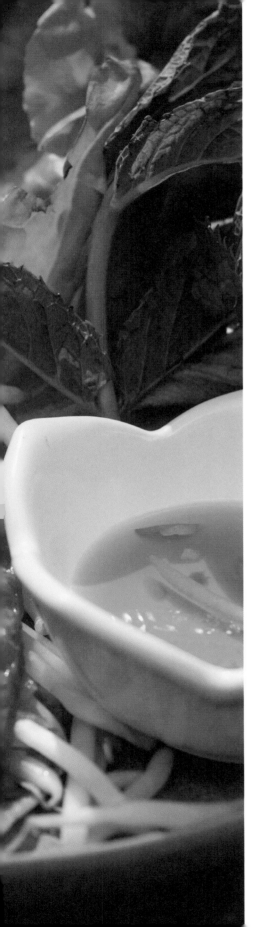

Bánh Xèo
(Savory Vietnamese Crepe)

TOTAL COOK TIME: 1 HOUR 15 MINUTES • MAKES 4 TO 6 CREPES

Henry Pineda serves Filipino soul food in his restaurant. His kamayan feasts, where the food is placed in the center of the table and diners eat communally without utensils, are praised for their excellence and as a unique experience people can't often get in the United States.

FOR THE CREPE BATTER:

1½ cups rice flour

¾ cup all-purpose flour

1½ cups unsweetened coconut milk

2 teaspoons ground turmeric

2½ cups water

1 teaspoon salt

1 tablespoon chopped green onion

FOR THE NƯỚC CHẤM DIPPING SAUCE:

2 tablespoons vegan fish sauce

3 tablespoons water

2 tablespoons sugar

1 tablespoon freshly squeezed lime juice

2 teaspoons minced garlic

1 teaspoon thinly sliced Thai chili

FOR THE FILLING:

1 tablespoon oil, plus more if needed

½ cup sliced onion

1 tablespoon minced garlic

8 ounces bean sprouts

FOR THE GARNISHES:

Romaine lettuce leaves

Fresh mint

Lime wedges

Thinly sliced cucumber

In a medium bowl, combine the rice flour, all-purpose flour, coconut milk, turmeric, water, and salt, and mix well. Let stand for 1 hour or refrigerate overnight. Just before cooking, stir the green onion into the batter.

To make the nước chấm dipping sauce, in a bowl, whisk all the ingredients together.

To make the filling, in a skillet over high heat, heat the oil. Add the onion and garlic and cook, stirring occasionally, until golden brown, about 10 minutes. Remove filling and set aside in a bowl.

Add about a quarter of the filling back to the pan, with more oil if needed, and with the skillet over medium-high heat, pour in about ½ to ¾ cup of the batter (enough batter to cover the bottom of the pan in a thin layer).

Reduce the heat to medium and add a handful of bean sprouts. Cover with a lid and cook for about 3 minutes, or until the bean sprouts are slightly cooked. Remove the lid and continue cooking until the edges of the crepe begin to crisp up and flake along the side of the pan.

Once the edges look crispy and flaky, fold the crepe in half and transfer it to a plate. Repeat with remaining batter and filling.

Serve with dipping sauce and garnishes.

Mung Beans With Coconut Cream and Leafy Green Vegetables

TOTAL COOK TIME: 45 MINUTES • SERVES 4

2 tablespoons olive oil

1 onion, diced

¼ cup minced garlic

1 tomato, quartered

1 cup dried mung beans, soaked overnight and drained

2 cups coconut cream

2 cups water, or more if needed

2 bunches bok choy, cut and chopped

2 ounces horseradish leaves

8 ounces spinach

¼ cup vegan fish sauce

1 tablespoon soy sauce

Salt

Freshly ground black pepper

In a stockpot, heat the oil over medium-high heat. Add the onion and garlic and cook, stirring frequently, until golden brown, about 8 minutes. Add the tomato and mung beans and continue to cook, stirring, for 2 to 4 minutes.

Reduce the heat to medium and add the coconut cream and 1 cup of water. Cook, stirring occasionally, for about 25 minutes, or until the mung beans are soft. Add more water if needed to keep the pot from drying out.

When the beans are soft, add the bok choy, horseradish leaves, spinach, fish sauce, and soy sauce. Cook until the vegetables are soft. Add the salt and pepper to taste.

Serve on its own or over rice.

Sinigang (Filipino Tamarind Vegetable Soup)

TOTAL COOK TIME: 45 MINUTES • SERVES 4 TO 6

Sinigang is a Filipino dish that gets a big dose of sour flavor from tamarind. This vegetable-forward recipe is hearty with tomatoes, okra, Chinese long beans, spinach, and eggplant. Sinigang was recently named the best vegetable soup in the world by TasteAtlas.

12 cups water

2 tomatoes, quartered

1 onion, diced

8 to 16 ounces tamarind paste, to taste

1 Filipino eggplant, sliced into ¼-inch medallions

4 ounces okra

2 ounces Chinese long beans, quartered

2 stalks bok choy, sliced

4 ounces spinach

¼ cup vegan fish sauce

Salt

In a stockpot, bring the water to a boil. Add the tomatoes, onion, and tamarind paste, and cook until the tomatoes are soft enough to smash.

Using a ladle inside the stockpot, smash the tomatoes to release their juices.

Add the eggplant, okra, and long beans. Continue to simmer until the vegetables soften, 5 to 10 minutes.

Add the bok choy, spinach, and fish sauce, and then remove the stockpot from the heat and let the flavors incorporate for about 15 minutes. Add salt to taste, and enjoy by itself or with a nice bowl of steamed rice.

Bibimbap (Korean Mixed Rice Bowl)

TOTAL COOK TIME: 50 MINUTES • SERVES 4

Bibimbap is one of Korea's favorite foods. There really is no wrong way to prepare this beloved dish. It always starts with a base of cooked rice. An assortment of vegetables and often meat and/or a fried egg are mixed in and drizzled with a spicy gochujang sauce. You can add different vegetables from those listed for variety.

FOR THE PURPLE RICE:

1 cup short grain white rice

1 cup pressed barley

¼ cup black rice

2 cups water

FOR THE VEGETABLE TOPPINGS:

4 teaspoons cooking oil, divided

4 ounces mushrooms (white, oyster, king oyster, or a mix), julienned

4 ounces carrot, peeled and julienned

1 cup spinach, julienned

4 ounces soybean sprouts

Salt

Freshly ground black pepper

2 red leaf lettuce leaves, julienned

4 sliced perilla leaves, julienned

1 small Persian cucumber, halved horizontally and sliced

4 ounces Korean radish, julienned

Strips of dried seaweed, for garnish

FOR THE GOCHUJANG SAUCE:

¼ cup gochujang (Korean fermented hot pepper paste)

1 tablespoon doenjang (Korean fermented soybean paste)

1 garlic clove, minced

1 tablespoon sesame oil, plus more for drizzling

2 teaspoons sugar

1 teaspoon toasted sesame seeds, plus more for garnish

To make the purple rice, rinse the white rice and barley together until the water runs clear.

In a medium saucepan, combine the white rice, barley, black rice, and water and bring to a boil. Reduce the heat to low, cover, and simmer for 30 minutes. Alternatively, you can use a rice cooker.

To make the vegetable topping, heat 1 teaspoon of the oil in a small skillet over medium-high heat. Add the mushrooms and cook, stirring occasionally, until softened, about 5 minutes. Transfer to a bowl.

Add another teaspoon of oil to the same skillet and heat over medium-high heat. Add the carrot and cook, stirring occasionally, until softened, about 5 minutes. Transfer to a bowl.

Add another teaspoon of oil to the skillet and heat over medium-high heat. Add the spinach and cook just until wilted, about 1 minute.

Add the remaining teaspoon of oil to the same skillet and heat over medium-high heat. Add the bean sprouts and cook, stirring occasionally, just until softened, about 1 minute. Transfer to a bowl.

To make the gochujang sauce, in a small bowl, combine all the ingredients and mix well.

To serve, place ½ to 1 cup of rice in a serving bowl. Add a layer of the lettuce and perilla leaves. Top that with a layer of the cooked vegetables, followed by the cucumber and radish, arranged on top so that each has in its own section.

Drizzle with some additional sesame seed oil and sprinkle the toasted sesame seeds on top. Garnish with the seaweed.

Serve with the gochujang sauce on the side to be added individually.

NOTE

• You can store the gochujang sauce in an airtight container in your refrigerator for up to a month.

Doenjang Jjigae
(Korean Stew With Zucchini, Tofu, and Mushrooms)

TOTAL COOK TIME: 20 MINUTES • SERVES 4

This stew is one of the most popular everyday Korean dishes. *Jjigae* means "stew" in Korean, and doenjang is a Korean fermented soybean paste (very similar to miso). This spicy, savory, and hearty stew is made with mushrooms, zucchini, and tofu. Perilla seeds look like smaller, rounder, and darker sesame seeds, and their flavor is reminiscent of fresh herbs like mint or basil. You can find perilla seed powder in Korean grocery stores, or you can use regular sesame seeds in its place.

1 tablespoon sesame oil

1 oyster mushroom, sliced diagonally into strips

2 shiitake mushrooms, sliced

2 button mushrooms, sliced

2 cups water

1 potato, diced small

1 onion, diced small

1 small zucchini, diced small

¼ cup doenjang (Korean fermented soybean paste)

1 tablespoon gochujang (Korean fermented hot pepper paste)

1 teaspoon minced garlic

2 tablespoons perilla seed powder

6 ounces firm tofu, cut into ½-inch cubes

1 red jalapeño, sliced

1 green onion, sliced, for garnish

In a medium saucepan or Korean hot pot over medium-high heat, heat the sesame oil. Add all the mushrooms and cook, stirring, for a minute or two.

Add the water, potato, onion, zucchini, doenjang, gochujang, garlic, and perilla seed powder, and bring to a boil. Cover and reduce the heat to medium-low. Simmer for 10 minutes.

Add the tofu and jalapeño, and simmer for another 5 minutes.

Serve hot and garnish with the green onion.

NOTE
• You can use dried mushrooms soaked in warm water for 30 minutes instead of fresh. Use the mushroom-soaking liquid in place of the water.

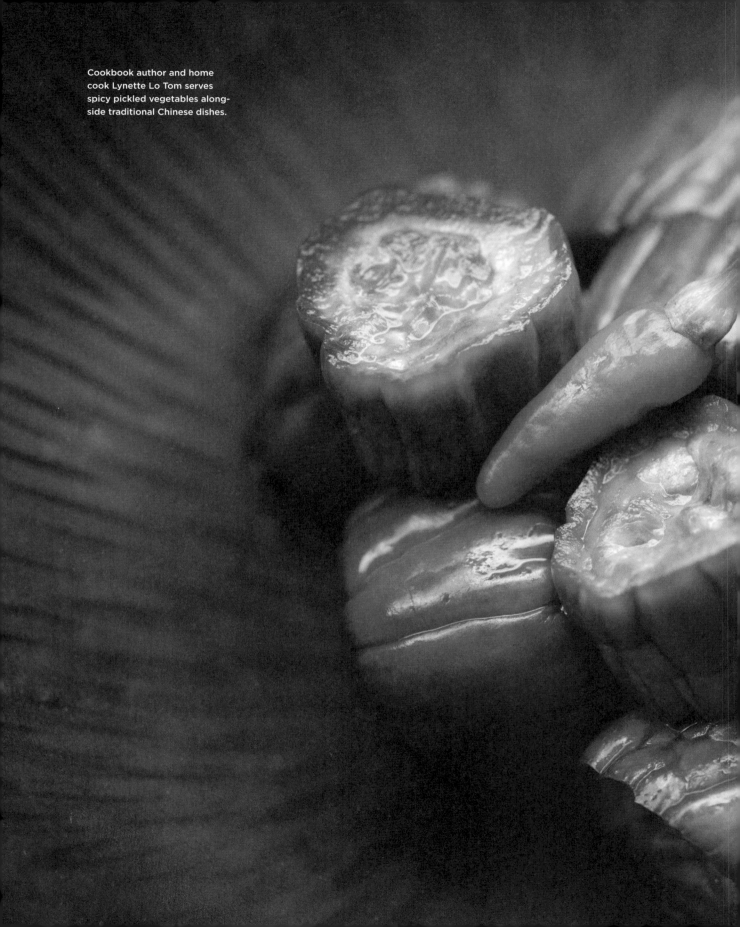

Cookbook author and home cook Lynette Lo Tom serves spicy pickled vegetables along-side traditional Chinese dishes.

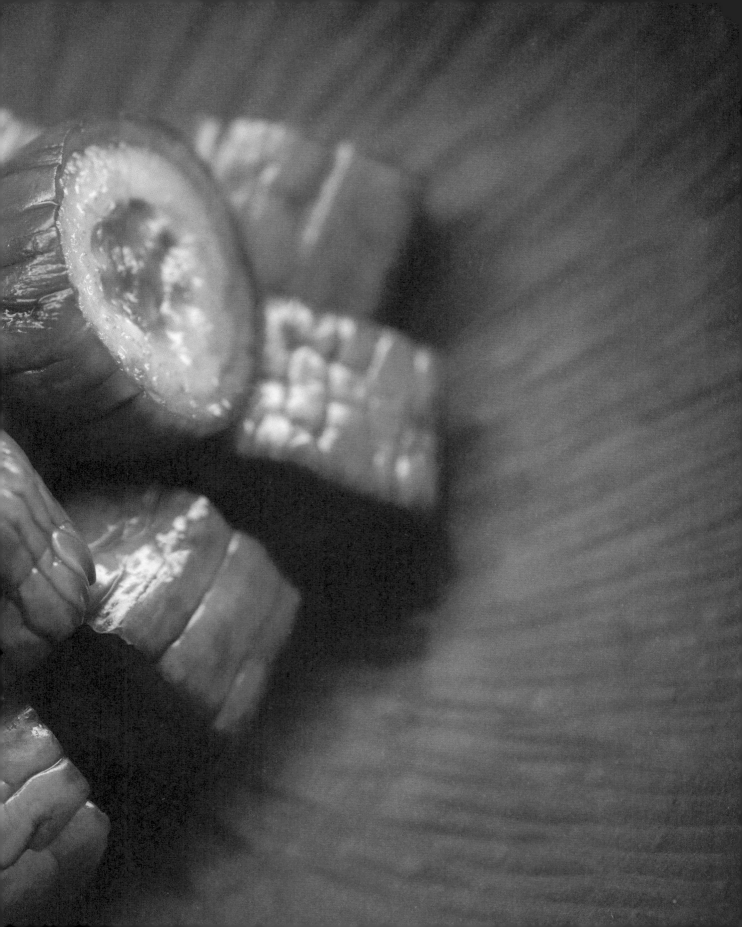

Cambodian Coconut Corn

TOTAL COOK TIME: 20 MINUTES • SERVES 3

Chad Phuong serves up Texas-meets-Cambodia barbecue every week at his pop-up in Long Beach, California. This simple but flavorful Cambodian corn dish is a crowd favorite.

2 cups fresh corn kernels

½ cup unsweetened coconut milk

⅓ cup sugar

½ teaspoon salt

¼ cup chives, chopped

Preheat the oven to 350°F.

Spread the corn kernels in a baking dish in an even layer and roast them in the oven for 10 minutes.

Meanwhile, in a small saucepan, bring the coconut milk to a boil.

Add the sugar and salt and reduce the heat to low. Simmer for 5 minutes.

Add the chives and simmer for 1 minute more.

Pour the coconut milk mixture over the corn kernels and return the dish to the oven to bake for about 5 minutes, until lightly brown on top.

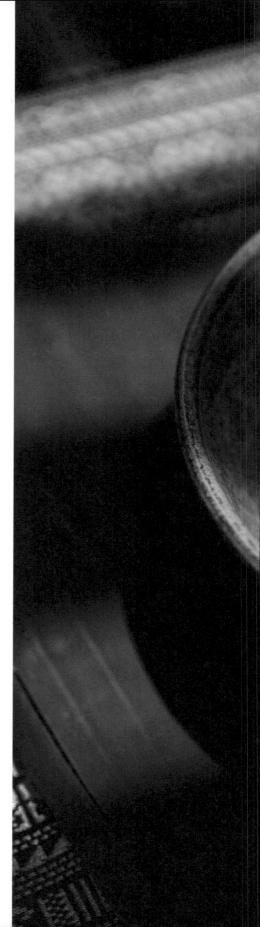

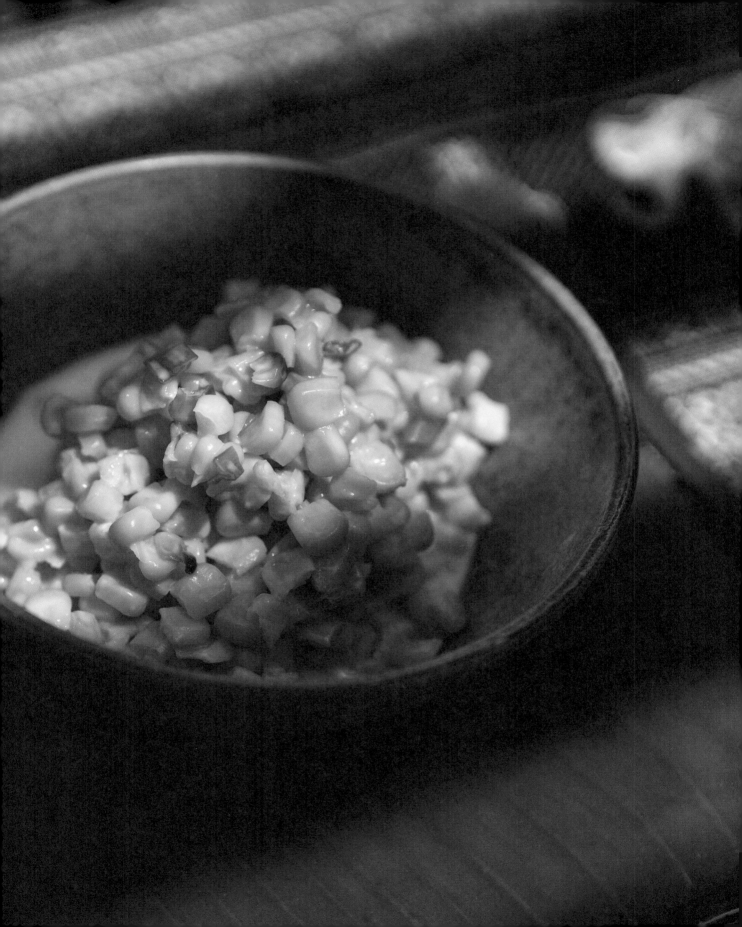

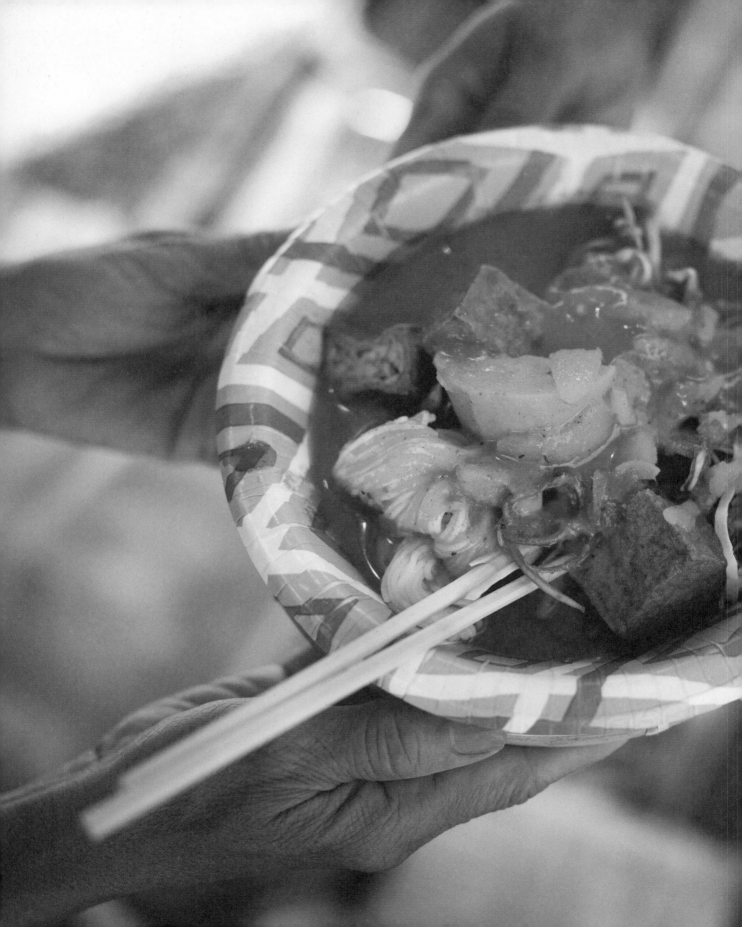

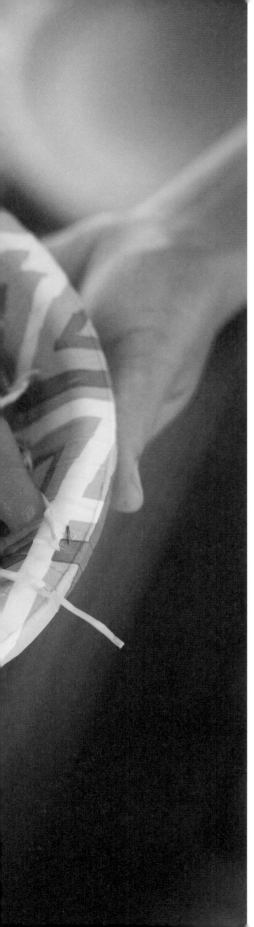

Red Cambodian Curry

TOTAL COOK TIME: 45 MINUTES • SERVES 4

This Cambodian curry uses a lemongrass paste made with red chili peppers that gives the dish a bright red color. Kroeung, the lemongrass paste, is an essential part of Khmer cooking. Although fresh is best, you can buy prepared kroeung in Asian markets and online if it's difficult to source some of these ingredients.

FOR THE RED KROEUNG PASTE:

6 large dried red chilis

2 lemongrass stalks, thinly sliced

4 garlic cloves, minced

2 inches galangal root, finely minced

4 shallots, chopped

2 makrut lime leaves, stemmed and julienned

1 tablespoon chopped ginger

1 tablespoon finely minced fresh turmeric

1 bird's eye chili

¼ teaspoon salt

FOR THE CURRY:

1½ tablespoons olive oil

3 to 5 tablespoons red kroeung paste, to taste

¾ cup unsweetened coconut milk, divided

½ large onion, roughly chopped

4 Chinese long beans, cut into 2-inch pieces

1 small eggplant, cut into 2-inch pieces

1 small white potato, peeled and cut into 2-inch pieces

1 small sweet potato, peeled and cut into 2-inch pieces

1 to 1½ tablespoons vegan fish sauce

1 tablespoon palm sugar

½ teaspoon sea salt

2 cups water

To make the kroeung (lemongrass paste), soak the red chilis in 1 cup or more hot water (enough to cover chilis) for 10 minutes. Drain, reserving ¾ cup of the soaking liquid.

In a blender or food processor, combine the rehydrated chilis and their reserved soaking liquid with the rest of the kroeung ingredients. Process to a smooth paste. Store the excess in the freezer for later use.

To make the curry, in a stockpot over medium heat, heat the oil. Add the red kroeung paste and cook, stirring, for 1 minute. Add ½ cup of the coconut milk and cook, stirring, for 2 minutes.

Add the onion, beans, eggplant, white potato, and sweet potato, and stir to combine.

Add the remaining ¼ cup of coconut milk, fish sauce, sugar, salt, and water. Increase the heat to bring the mixture to a boil, then decrease it to medium-low and simmer for 20 to 25 minutes, until the vegetables are soft.

Serve with French sourdough bread, rice, or noodles.

Mayak Gimbap (Korean Rice Rolls)

TOTAL COOK TIME: 20 MINUTES • MAKES 10 SMALL ROLLS

Every Korean meal comes with side dishes, whether it's two or 12, and these "side" dishes can even make a full meal with the addition of rice and soup. That explains why Krissy Song's company is named Zip Banchan ("house of sides") and why their food deliveries are in such high demand. Based in Los Angeles, they make 50 to 60 types of dishes a week and deliver all over the L.A. metro area.

Gimbap means "seaweed and rice," but it is so much more. Similar to Japanese sushi rolls (maki), gimbap is seasoned rice with fillings rolled up in seaweed. The main difference is that in the Korean version, the rice is seasoned with sesame oil instead of vinegar, and the fillings are not raw fish but anything and everything from tofu, meat, fish, pickled vegetables, eggs, and sometimes even cheese. These gimbap have a combination of cooked, pickled, and raw vegetables inside. It's the kind of classic Korean food Krissy Song makes at Zip Banchan: quick, healthy, and heavy on vegetables and flavor.

FOR THE GIMBAP:

4 cups hot cooked rice

¾ teaspoon salt, divided

2½ tablespoons toasted sesame oil, divided

1 large carrot, peeled and cut into matchsticks (about 1½ cups)

Vegetable oil

5 sheets gim (seaweed paper), roasted slightly, cut into quarters

5 strips yellow pickled radish (use precut danmuji)

Any type of vegetable of your choice (fresh or steamed)

FOR THE KOREAN MUSTARD SAUCE:

1 tablespoon Korean yellow mustard powder

1 tablespoon soy sauce

1 tablespoon sugar

1 tablespoon vinegar

1 tablespoon water

1 teaspoon sesame oil

1 teaspoon minced garlic

To make the gimbap, place the hot cooked rice in a large, shallow bowl. Gently mix in ½ teaspoon of the salt and 2 teaspoons of the sesame oil with a rice scoop or a wooden spoon.

Let the rice cool down enough so that it's no longer steaming. Cover and set aside.

In a medium bowl, combine the carrots with the remaining ¼ teaspoon of salt. Mix well and let it sweat for 5 to 10 minutes. Squeeze the excess water from the carrots.

Heat a skillet and add a few drops of vegetable oil. Add the carrots and cook, stirring occasionally, for about 1 minute.

Place a quarter sheet of gim on a bamboo mat with the shiny side down. Evenly spread about 2 spoonfuls of the cooked rice over the top of it, leaving about ¼ inch of the gim uncovered on one edge.

Place the carrots, pickled radish, and any other vegetables you are using in the center of the rice.

Use both hands to roll the mat (along with gim and rice) over the fillings, so that one edge of the rice and gim reaches the opposite edge.

Grab the mat with both hands and press it tightly as you continue rolling the gimbap. Push out the mat as you roll, so it doesn't get wrapped in the gimbap.

Remove the roll from the mat at the end and set it aside with the seam down to seal it nicely. Repeat with the remaining ingredients.

Brush remaining toasted sesame oil on the finished rolls and sprinkle some sesame seeds over top.

To make the Korean mustard sauce, in a bowl, combine all the ingredients and stir to mix well.

Serve the gimbap immediately with Korean mustard sauce for flavor!

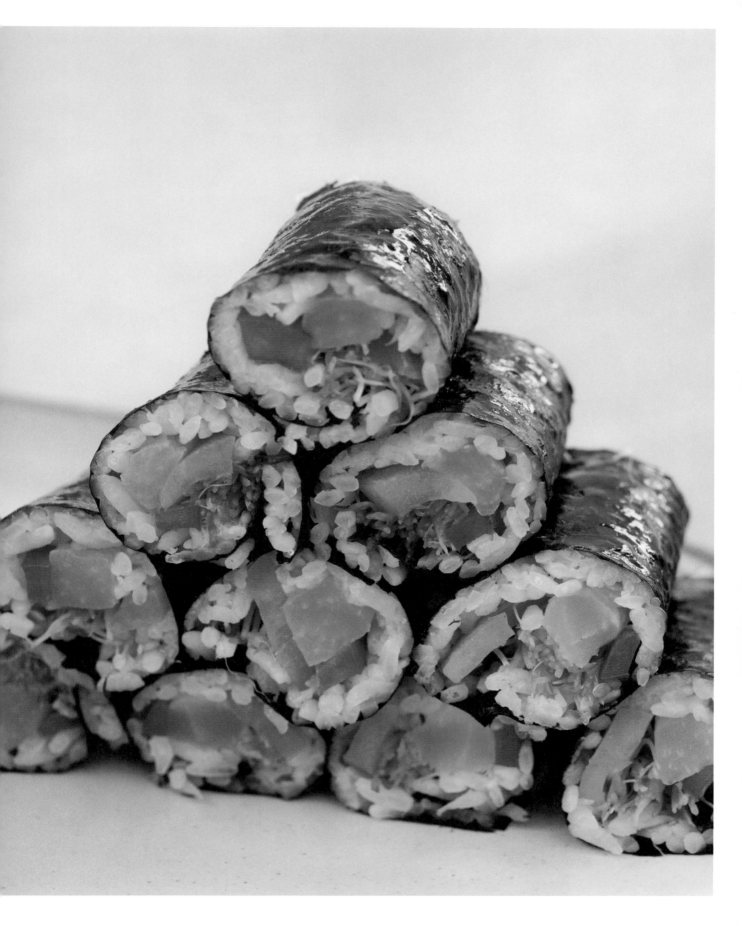

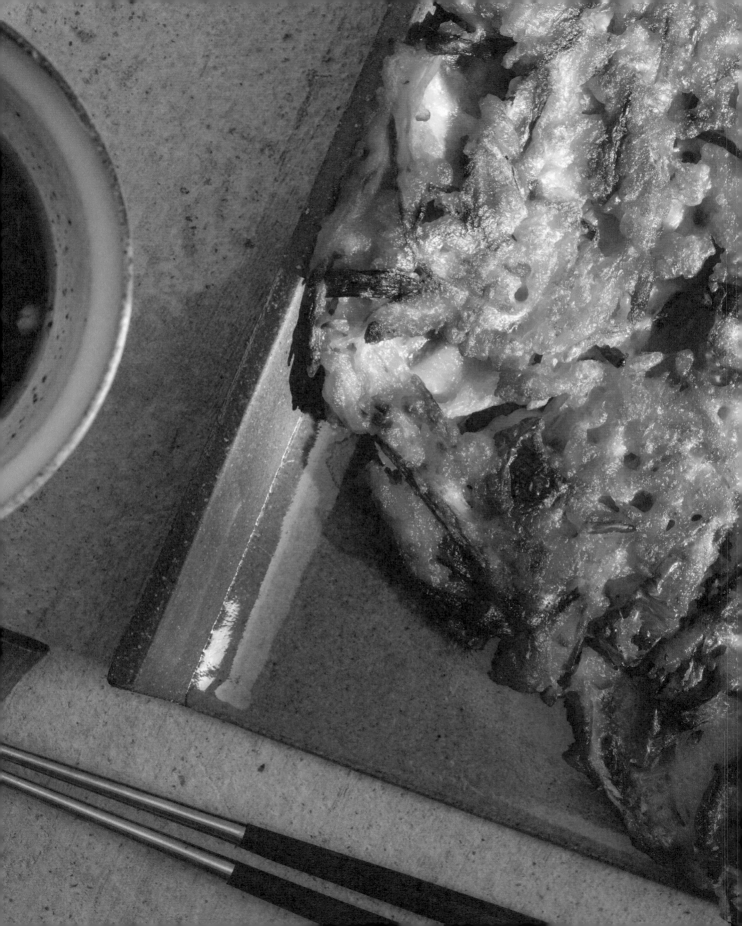

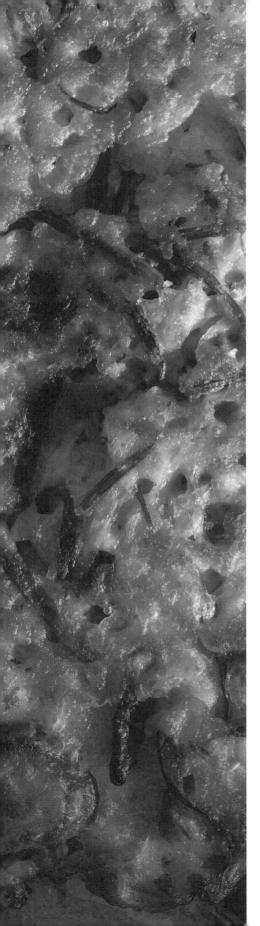

Korean Kimchi Pancake

TOTAL COOK TIME: 5 MINUTES • MAKES 2 PANCAKES

Kimchi pancakes are a popular Korean snack. They're quick to make, require only a few basic ingredients—the most important, of course, being a good kimchi—and are delicious. You could make one big pancake if you like, but making two in a smaller pan is a bit easier.

½ pound well-fermented napa cabbage kimchi, chopped into small pieces, plus 2 tablespoons of the kimchi brine

3 scallions, chopped

½ teaspoon sugar

½ cup all-purpose flour or all-purpose gluten-free flour

½ cup water

2 tablespoons oil, divided

In a medium bowl, combine the kimchi and kimchi brine, scallions, sugar, flour, and water, and mix well with a spoon.

In an 8-inch nonstick skillet over medium-high heat, heat 1 tablespoon of the oil until it shimmers, swirling the pan to coat the entire bottom.

Add half the batter to the pan, spreading it to the edges of the pan and smoothing it with a spatula or the back of a spoon into an even layer. Cook for 3 to 5 minutes, until the bottom is golden brown and beginning to crisp. Transfer to a plate.

Repeat with the remaining oil and batter to cook a second pancake.

Cut the pancakes into wedges and serve hot.

Miso Ramen

TOTAL COOK TIME: 1 HOUR 15 MINUTES • SERVES 4

Kim Huynh has owned restaurants for 30 years and learned vegan and vegetarian cooking from her Buddhist family. Co-owned with her son Viet Pham, Good Vibes Cafe is anchored in their Vietnamese background but flavored with ingredients and influences from all over the world.

FOR THE BROTH:

1 bulb garlic, halved

1 onion, peeled and halved

3 to 4 large, thick slices fresh ginger

2 carrots, peeled and halved

4 green onions, halved

6 cups cold water

4 cups mushroom stock

2 sheets kombu (dried kelp)

5 dried shiitake mushrooms

FOR THE SPICY MISO TARE:

½ cup yellow miso paste

2 tablespoons doubanjiang (hot bean paste)

½ cup sake

½ cup mirin

FOR THE NOODLES:

12 ounces dried ramen noodles or 18 ounces fresh ramen noodles

FOR THE TOPPINGS (OPTIONAL):

Sliced green onion

Corn

Kimchi

Nori sheets, cut into strips

Shichimi togarashi

Sliced bamboo shoots

To make the broth, in a large stockpot, combine the garlic, onion, ginger, carrots, green onions, water, and mushroom stock. Bring to a boil over high heat, then reduce the heat to medium-low and simmer for 30 to 45 minutes. Strain the broth, discarding the solids.

Return the broth to the pot and bring it back up to a simmer. Add the kombu and mushrooms, and remove the pot from the heat. Let it stand for 30 minutes and then remove and discard the kombu. Remove the mushrooms, slice them into strips, and reserve.

To make the spicy miso tare, in a bowl, stir together all the ingredients until well mixed.

To make the noodles, cook them according to the package directions and then drain.

To serve the soup, bring the broth back up to a hearty simmer. Place 2 tablespoons of the tare into the bottom of each of four large serving bowls. Add noodles to each bowl, dividing them evenly. Ladle the broth over the noodles, and then top with the reserved sliced shiitake mushrooms and any other toppings, if using.

Serve hot.

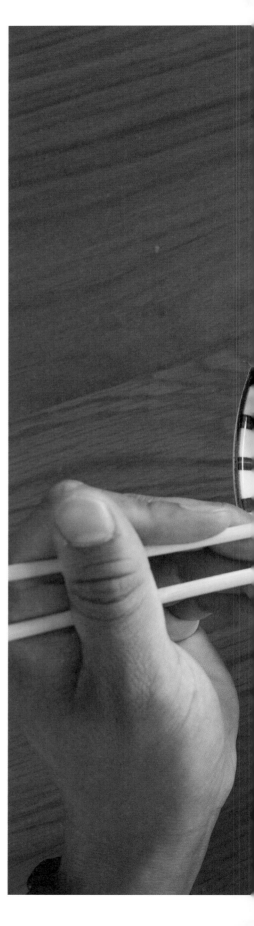

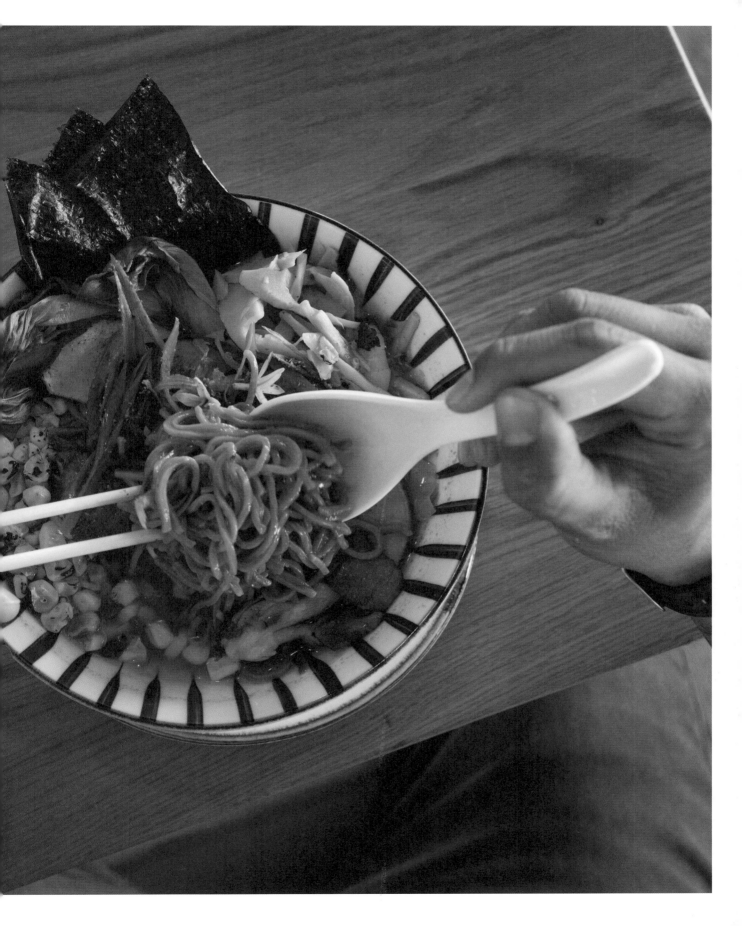

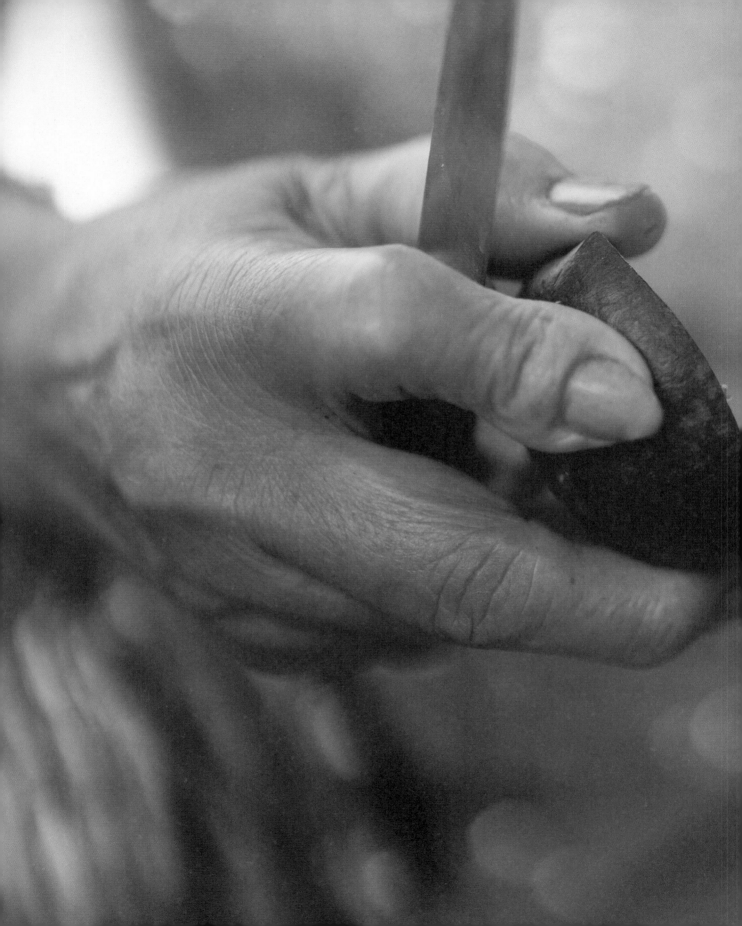

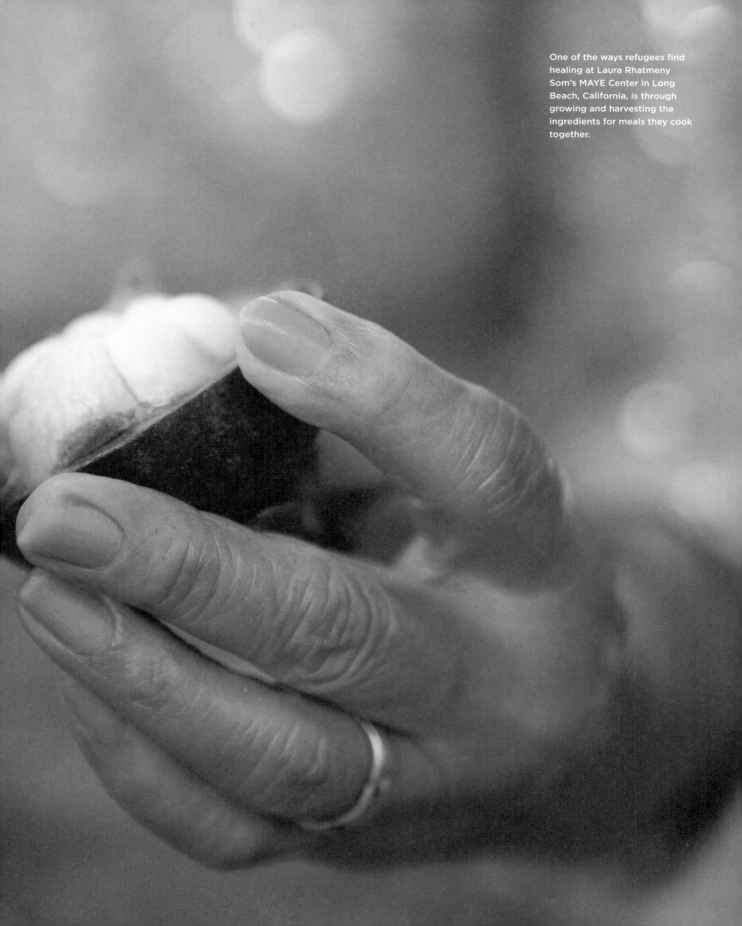

One of the ways refugees find healing at Laura Rhatmeny Som's MAYE Center in Long Beach, California, is through growing and harvesting the ingredients for meals they cook together.

Tao Bowl

TOTAL COOK TIME: 1 HOUR + 6 HOURS SOAKING • SERVES 4

This namesake dish from Anna Needham's restaurant is a crowd favorite for its beauty, balance, and simplicity. It hearkens back to the hippie era, when veggies and brown rice represented a radical return to self-care and living gently on this Earth. That movement is as strong today as it was in the 1960s, and Tao Natural Foods is proud to have served this no-frills, earnest meal for nearly 50 years. May it bring health, happiness, and a bit of mindfulness to your day.

2 cups short-grain brown rice, soaked for 6 hours and then drained

10 cups water, divided

2 cups dried black beans, soaked for 6 hours and then drained

¼ teaspoon salt

1 bay leaf

3 or 4 slices fresh, peeled ginger root, ¼ inch thick

6 cups chopped vegetables (use any combination of broccoli, red cabbage, celery, carrot, kale, cauliflower, etc.)

2 avocados, halved and sliced

1 cup sauerkraut

4 tablespoons tamari or soy sauce

½ cup toasted sesame oil

2 to 3 tablespoons sesame seeds

In a saucepan, combine the rice with 4 cups of the water and bring to a boil. Reduce the heat to low, cover, and simmer for 40 minutes, or until the rice has absorbed all the water and is tender.

In a separate large saucepan or a stockpot, combine the beans with the remaining 6 cups of water. Add the salt and bay leaf. Bring to a boil, then reduce the heat to low and simmer, uncovered, until the beans are tender, about 45 minutes. Drain off any excess liquid.

Prepare a pot to be fitted with a steamer by filling the pot with 1 inch of water. Add the ginger slices to the water and bring it to a boil. Put the vegetables into the steamer and add to the pot. Cover and steam over medium heat for about 15 minutes, until the vegetables are tender. Discard the ginger.

To each bowl, add 1 cup of rice, ½ cup of black beans, 1½ cups of steamed veggies, a quarter of the avocado slices, and ¼ cup of sauerkraut.

Garnish each bowl with 1 tablespoon of tamari, 2 tablespoons of sesame oil, and a generous sprinkle of sesame seeds.

Serve immediately.

The Sun

TOTAL COOK TIME: 1 HOUR • MAKES 8 SERVINGS

This bright, nourishing drink combines creamy, fresh cashew-date milk with a hearty dose of anti-inflammatory herbs that are rich in immune-supporting vitamin C. It's wildly delicious and deeply soothing. Enjoy it warm or iced. Many of these ingredients can be sourced from a local herbal shop or ordered online at taoherbery.com.

FOR THE HERBAL BLEND:

1 tablespoon ground turmeric

1 tablespoon ground ginger

⅛ teaspoon finely ground black pepper

¼ teaspoon ground amla root

¼ teaspoon camu camu fruit powder

¼ teaspoon magnesium (citrate) powder

¼ teaspoon ascorbic acid (vitamin C) powder

¼ teaspoon hawthorn berry powder

½ teaspoon vanilla powder

FOR THE CASHEW MILK:

Cashew-date milk

1½ cups raw, organic cashews, soaked in hot water, covered, for 10 minutes and then drained

3 pitted dates

8 teaspoons honey or sweetener of choice

5 cups filtered water

To make the herbal blend, combine all the ingredients in a lidded jar.

To make the cashew milk, in a blender, combine all the ingredients and blend on high speed for 2 minutes. Strain through fine cloth or a nut-milk bag, if desired. Store covered in the refrigerator for up to three days.

To make one serving, combine 10 ounces of the cashew-date milk with 1 heaping teaspoon of the herbal blend and mix well.

To make it a warm beverage, warm the cashew milk before mixing it with the herbal blend.

For an iced version, combine cold cashew milk with the herbal blend, mix well, and pour it over ice.

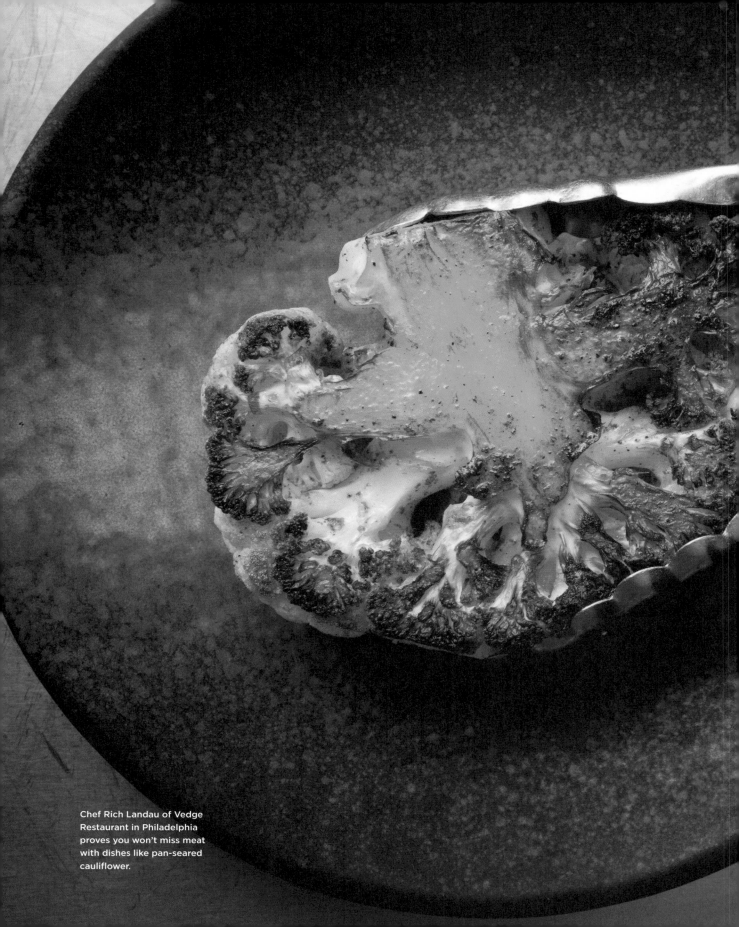

Chef Rich Landau of Vedge Restaurant in Philadelphia proves you won't miss meat with dishes like pan-seared cauliflower.

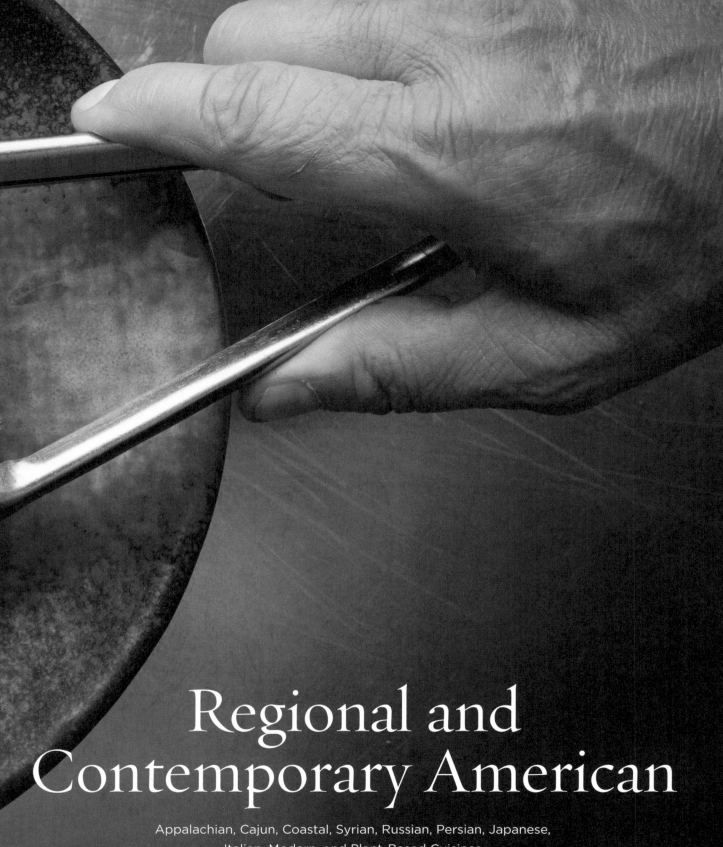

Regional and
Contemporary American

Appalachian, Cajun, Coastal, Syrian, Russian, Persian, Japanese,
Italian, Modern, and Plant-Based Cuisines

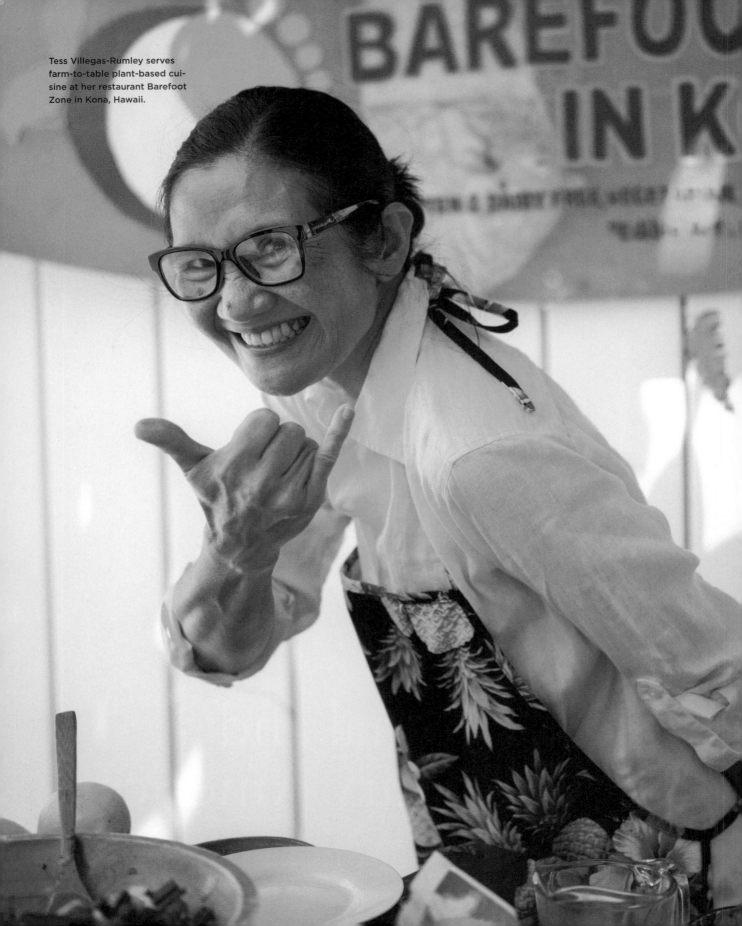

Tess Villegas-Rumley serves farm-to-table plant-based cuisine at her restaurant Barefoot Zone in Kona, Hawaii.

"I switched to a whole-food, plant-based diet to save my life."

~STEPHEN ROUELLE

M ost of this book explores the historical diets of four different demographic groups in America, revealing patterns of eating that could likely help the average American live another decade or so. This chapter is a bit different. Rather than focus on cultural foodways, we look at regional cooking and the food innovators of today who are focusing on the modern techniques and plant-based foodways. These chefs incorporate plant-based cooking into their craft or have dedicated their professional lives to developing delicious recipes that are accessible to the masses.

Our search for these innovators takes us to Rich Landau and Kate Jacoby, the husband-and-wife founders of Philadelphia's famous Vedge Restaurant. Philadelphia has a long history of vegetarianism. Ben Franklin was a vegetarian for a time and is credited with introducing tofu to the Colonies. In 1817, drawn by Philadelphia's reputation for tolerance, the Bible Christians (established by William Metcalfe) created the first vegetarian church and large-scale plant-based organization. Metcalfe later joined Sylvester Graham (Presbyterian minister and inventor of the Graham cracker) and William Andrus Alcott (an American educator and physician) to found the U.S. Vegetarian Society, which promoted plant-based eating across the nation.

Today, Rich and Kate continue to burnish Philadelphia's vegetarian reputation. In addition to elevating plant-based food to fine dining, Rich and Kate have also trained most of the city's best vegan chefs. Case in point: We also meet Vedge alum Rachel Klein of Philly's Miss Rachel's Pantry. She makes plant-based Seitan Brisket (page 221) so good it's indistinguishable from its meaty analog.

Outside a 400-year-old New England farm, we meet James Beard Award–winning chef James Wayman at what he calls the "Fire Beast." In this druid-like

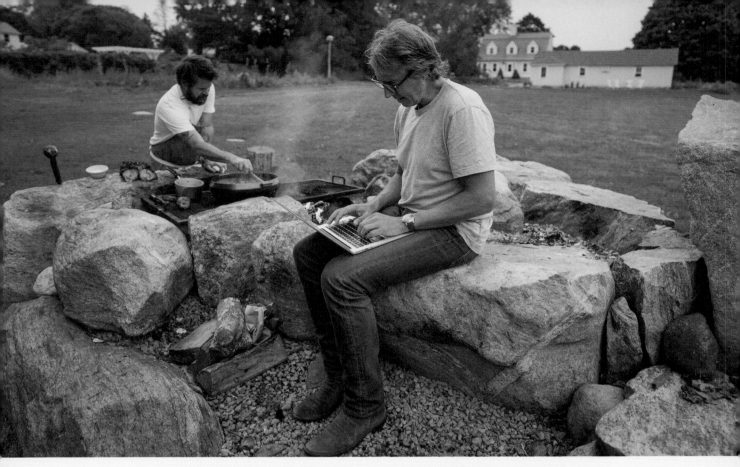

Above: Chef James Wayman uses an open fire to prepare dinner at Stone Acres Farm in Stonington, Connecticut. Opposite: Rachel Klein, chef and owner of Miss Rachel's Pantry, makes a delicious vegan version of matzo ball soup.

assemblage of boulders, he's fashioned a half dozen firepits, where he coaxes the most amazing flavors from the most pedestrian of vegetables. In one of the pits, he fires tomato halves slathered with sweet miso and sesame seed. Within a minute, the glaze browns and forms a crust. ("An orgasm in my mouth" is how David described his bite, tomato juice dripping down his chin.) Into another fire pit he chucks a Georgia candy roaster squash, leaving the flame to scorch the skin. Ten minutes later, he busts the blackened squash open, revealing sweet, golden flesh that could have easily stood alone as a meal.

In New Orleans, we spend two days in an Airbnb with chefs Blake Lofton, Chris DeBarr, and Mel Braden, who riff on Cajun recipes from 100-year-old cookbooks. Who knew that peanut butter and black-eyed peas made good bedfellows (see Black-Eyed Pea and Peanut Butter Hummus, page 269), or that a simple onion could be honey-baked into a satisfying side dish?

Moving across the country, in Central Texas, on a tumbleweed-blown street, we meet another plant-based Cajun chef, Camryn Clements. She shows us how to prepare mushrooms that are a dead ringer for crustaceans in her crawfishless Mushroom Étouffée (page 227).

Back in my hometown of Minneapolis, my good buddy and celebrity chef Andrew Zimmern spends an afternoon in his kitchen creating his version of Kimchi Jjigae, Korean kimchi stew (page 235). And at my favorite lunch haunt, Tao Natural Foods, chef Anna Needham shares the recipe for their Tao Bowl (page 208), a macrobiotic feast.

I spend a morning in Los Angeles with the chef at my favorite restaurant in America, Gjelina, in Venice Beach. Executive chef Juan Hernandez has pulled together a kitchen staff from his native Oaxaca, Mexico. They work in the tiny kitchen as if they were a single organism. Gjelina excels in vegetable dishes. Each day, Juan sends out trucks to collect fresh vegetables from local farms. He personally tastes each batch and then begins the creative work of enhancing flavor without losing a vegetable's integrity. The season dictates whether it's left raw, blanched, or charred. Then he adds a touch of acidity from preserved lemons, sweet pomegranates, or savory sauces to enhance natural flavors. I've tasted vegetables on five continents and can say that no one transforms vegetables into a meal better than Juan.

Back in Hawaii, chef Stephen Rouelle has transformed a former health crisis into a thriving business. Fifteen years ago, suffering from diabetes and weighing 450 pounds, he collapsed with deathly chest pains. "I switched to a whole-food, plant-based diet to save my life," he tells me. A trained chef, he began developing vegan

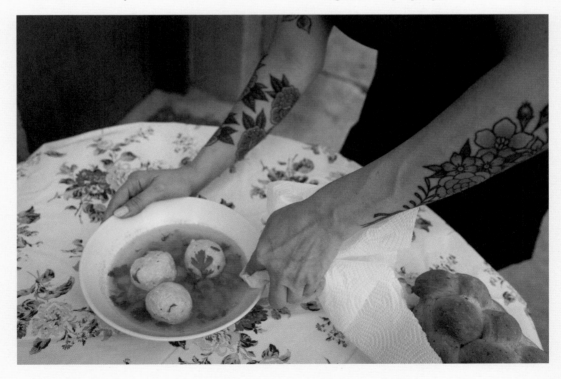

recipes. Now he's more than 200 pounds lighter, and his Under the Bodhi Tree restaurant is packed with customers who come for his Reuben's Garden sandwich (with pressed, marinated tofu that mimics roast beef) and his BLT made with coconut "bacon."

Think eating delicious plant-based food has to be expensive? Forager chef Alan Bergo and his health-advocate partner, Pilar Gerasimo, host us at their 400-acre Wisconsin farm. Alan has foraged a meal of Fave e Cicoria (Fava Bean Puree With Wild Chicory, page 245), stewed wild chicory cooked with garlic and hot pepper, served with a puree of fava beans. For dessert we eat chokecherry cake truffles made with wild honey and pine pollen. Total cost: $0. Everything he made was found right on the farm or nearby land.

Finally, my dad, who grew up on a dairy farm, seems to have an epiphany of his own. After joining us for two Blue Zones Kitchen cookbooks, he has learned a thing or two tasting plant-based dishes from as far as Okinawa, Japan, and as near as Louisiana. He decides to put his Blue Zones experience and knowledge to the test with his own recipe. He invites us to his Minnesota garden, where he harvests the ingredients for Tomato, Eggplant, and Sweet Potato Pasta Sauce (page 238). Then he serves us a vegan supper. (That's right. My meat-and-potatoes father has learned a thing or two. A vegan supper is a no-brainer to him these days.) It is the perfect ending to this one-of-a-kind cross-country road trip.

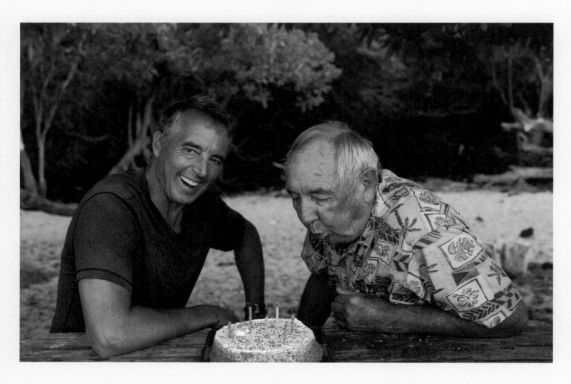

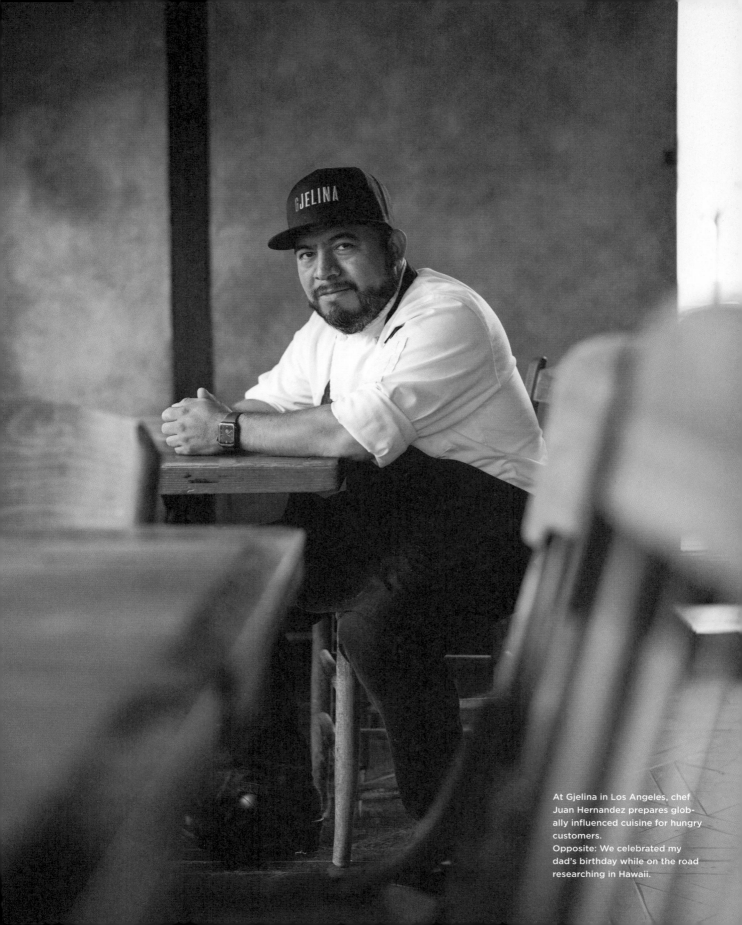

At Gjelina in Los Angeles, chef Juan Hernandez prepares globally influenced cuisine for hungry customers.
Opposite: We celebrated my dad's birthday while on the road researching in Hawaii.

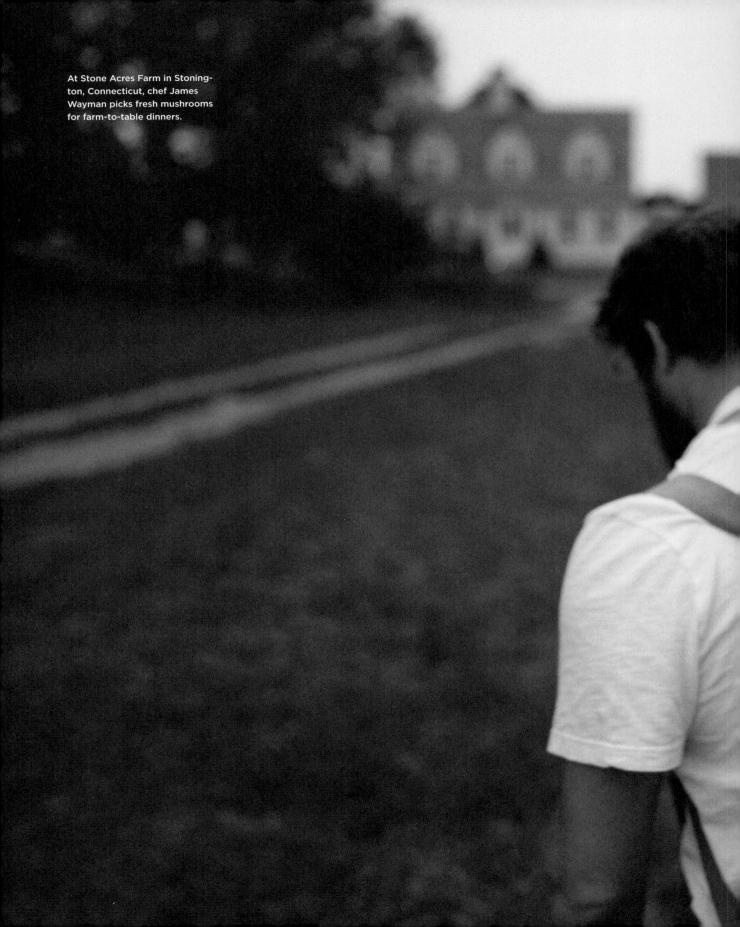

At Stone Acres Farm in Stonington, Connecticut, chef James Wayman picks fresh mushrooms for farm-to-table dinners.

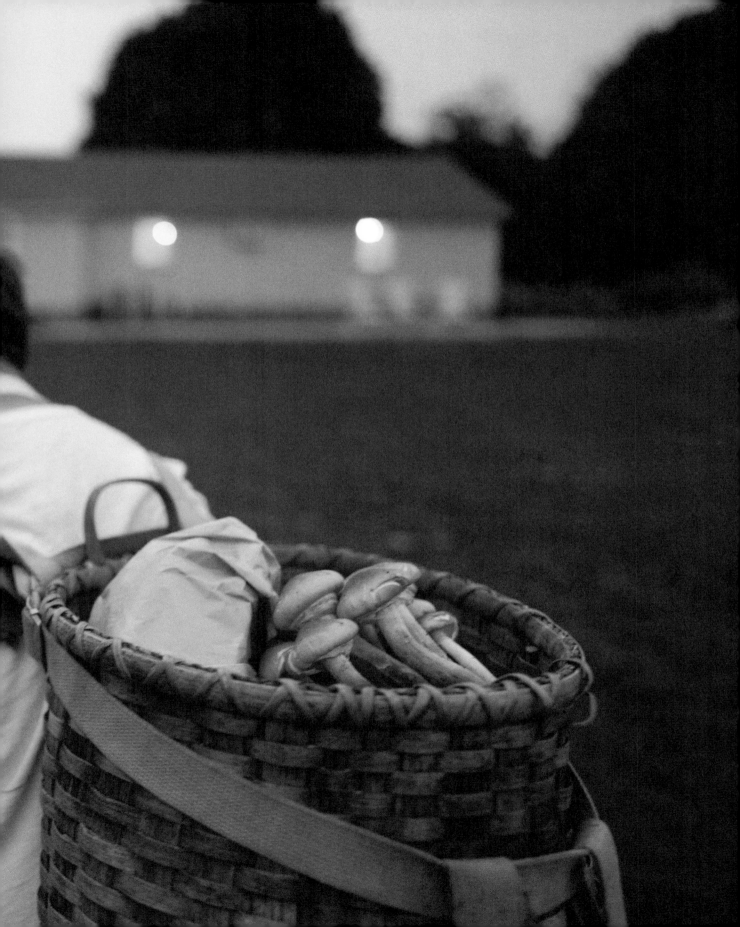

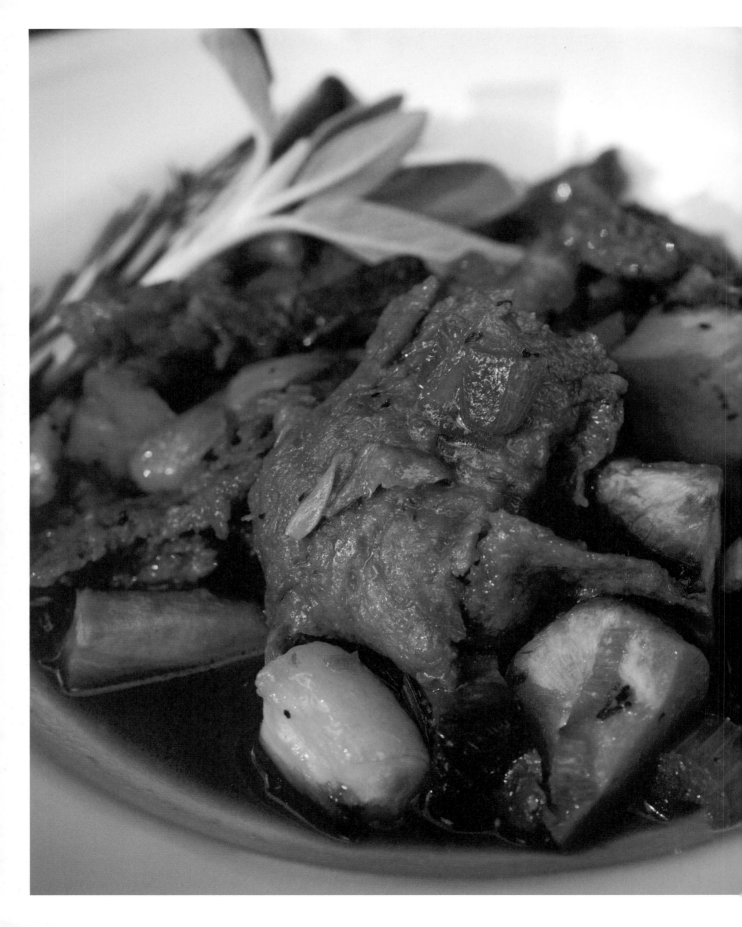

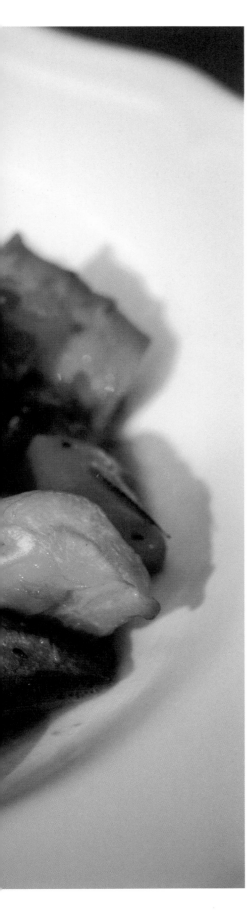

Seitan Brisket

TOTAL COOK TIME: 1 HOUR • SERVES 4

Seitan brisket is a warm and comforting dish with lots of autumn aromatics. It can be paired with roasted vegetables, ladled over polenta, or spooned over pasta. The jus, made with herbs and veggies in a rich tamari broth, is strained to make a thin gravy to cook the seitan in and is to be poured over the dish during plating or tableside.

FOR THE JUS:

1 cup chopped portobello, cremini, or shiitake mushrooms

¾ cup tamari

1 onion, diced

¼ cup minced garlic

¼ cup red wine or canned or boxed Roma tomatoes, blended

3 cups water

½ cup rough chopped carrot

½ cup rough chopped celery

¼ cup oil (use a neutral-flavored oil such as sunflower)

3 sprigs rosemary

3 sprigs thyme

1 tablespoon granulated onion

Salt

Freshly ground black pepper

FOR THE SEITAN:

2 cups 2-inch pieces seitan

1 teaspoon salt

2 tablespoons oil

1 carrot, chopped

1 teaspoon freshly ground black pepper

1 teaspoon granulated garlic

1 teaspoon granulated onion

1 teaspoon fresh thyme leaves

1 teaspoon olive oil

1 to 2 teaspoons agave or coconut nectar

To make the jus, in a stockpot over medium heat, combine all the ingredients and bring to a boil. Reduce the heat to a simmer and cook until the carrots, onion, and celery are tender, 6 to 8 minutes. Strain through a mesh sieve and set aside, reserving both the broth and the solids.

Preheat the oven to 350°F.

Season the seitan with salt and toss it in the oil along with the carrot, pepper, garlic, onion, and thyme. Arrange the seitan on a baking sheet and bake for 15 minutes.

Remove the seitan from the oven and raise the heat to 375°F.

Transfer the seitan and carrots to a roasting pan. Toss them with 1 cup of the jus. Cover the pan with foil, and heat it in the oven for 10 minutes.

Remove the foil and add ½ cup more jus. Return to the oven uncovered and cook for 15 more minutes.

Heat the olive oil in a skillet over medium-high heat. Add the seitan along with the agave, and cook until the outside of the seitan is caramelized, 3 to 4 minutes, flipping halfway through. Add more jus, 1 tablespoon at a time, to prevent the seitan from burning.

Transfer the seitan to a serving platter and pour the remaining jus over the top.

Syrian Brined Beets and Cauliflower

TOTAL COOK TIME: 25 MINUTES • MAKES 2 QUARTS

This garlicky pickle is perfect for meze. A squeeze of fresh lemon over the pickles just before serving will add zip to their flavor.

4 large beets, peeled and quartered

2 quarts spring water

1 cup red wine vinegar

¼ cup pickling salt

1 small head cauliflower, broken into florets

8 large garlic cloves, halved lengthwise

Place the beets in a stockpot with the water and cook over medium heat until they are tender (easily pierced with a skewer). Strain the cooking liquid into a bowl and set both the liquid and the beets aside.

Heat the reserved beet cooking liquid, vinegar, and salt in a large stainless steel (or other nonreactive) saucepan.

While the brine is heating, slice the beets and make a layer on the bottom of a hot, sanitized 2-quart canning jar. Add some of the cauliflower and some of the garlic. Add more beets, garlic, and cauliflower, and continue layering until the jar is full, ending with a layer of beets.

Once the pickling brine comes to a full rolling boil, pour it over the vegetable mixture. Seal tightly with a lid and set the jar aside to cool.

Once the jar has cooled, refrigerate it for at least 2 weeks before using.

The pickles will keep in the refrigerator for up to 6 months.

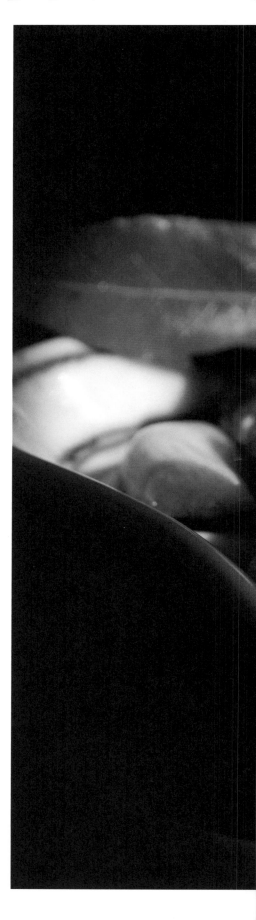

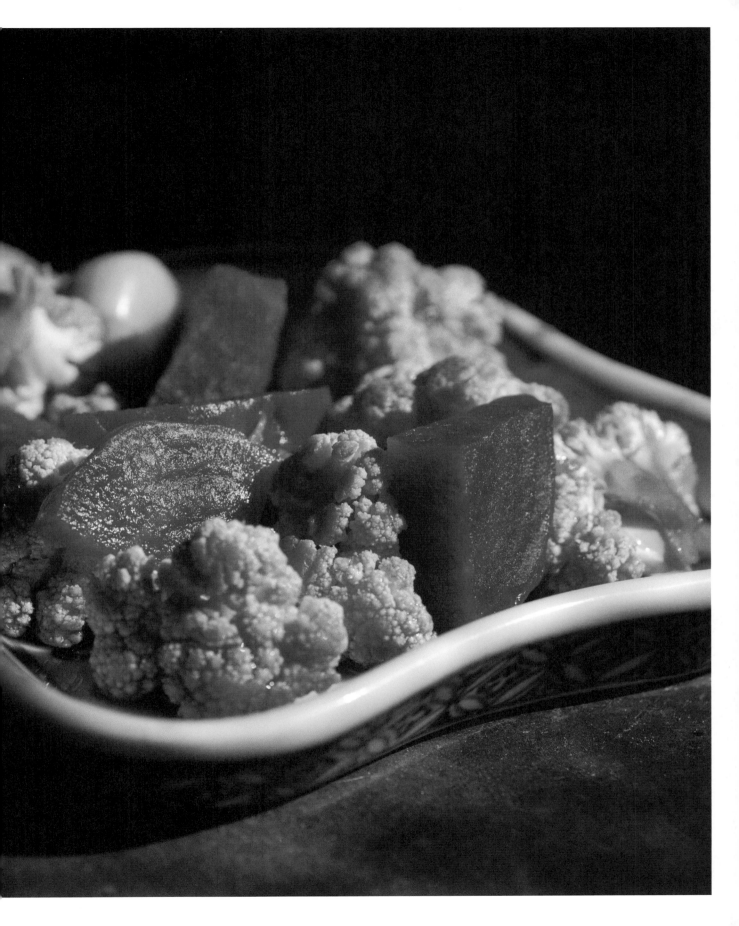

Old Chub–Braised Collard Greens

TOTAL COOK TIME: 45 MINUTES • SERVES 5

Chef Katina Hansen draws on her Greek heritage and local Appalachian traditions and ingredients in her cooking. Her popular café, Blue Ridge Bakery in Brevard, North Carolina, is a local gathering spot and was the first Blue Zones Project Approved restaurant in her town, which means it is part of the statewide movement to create cities and counties where people live better and longer lives. She also hosts Blue Zones Project cooking classes for free at the bakery to help people in her community learn how to cook delicious, healthy meals.

2 tablespoons olive oil

1 onion, diced

4 bunches collard greens, stemmed and chopped

1 (12-ounce) can Oskar Blues Old Chub beer (or other Scottish-style ale)

Pinch of cayenne

¼ cup molasses or brown sugar

1 teaspoon nutritional yeast

Salt

Freshly ground black pepper

In a wide-bottomed pot, heat the oil over high heat. Add the onion and cook, stirring occasionally, until the onion has caramelized, about 5 minutes.

Reduce the heat to medium-high heat and add half the collard greens and all the beer. Cook, stirring, until the collards wilt and then add the remaining collards.

Add the cayenne, molasses or brown sugar, nutritional yeast, salt, and pepper, and reduce the heat to low. Cover and let it cook for 30 minutes or until the greens are tender.

Chewy Apricot Cereal Bars

TOTAL COOK TIME: 1 HOUR 10 MINUTES • SERVES 5

¼ cup coconut oil

½ cup honey

¼ cup brown sugar

¼ teaspoon vanilla extract

1¼ cup toasted old-fashioned rolled oats

1 cup chopped toasted walnuts or pecans

¼ cup toasted flax seeds

2½ cups puffed rice cereal

½ cup diced dried apricots or other fruit

½ teaspoon salt

Grease a 9-inch square baking pan with butter or baking spray. Line the pan with parchment paper.

In a small saucepan over medium heat, combine the coconut oil, honey, and brown sugar. Cook, stirring to fully dissolve the sugar, about 4 minutes.

Remove the pan from the heat and mix in the vanilla.

In a large bowl, combine the remaining ingredients and stir to mix.

Add the coconut-oil-and-honey mixture and stir to mix well.

Press the mixture into the prepared baking pan. Lay a piece of parchment on top and press the mixture into an even layer.

Refrigerate for at least 1 hour to set.

To serve, cut into bars and let them come to room temperature.

The bars will keep in an airtight container at room temperature for up to a week.

NOTE
• To toast the oats, nuts, and seeds, spread them in a single layer on a baking sheet and bake in a 350°F oven for about 5 minutes.

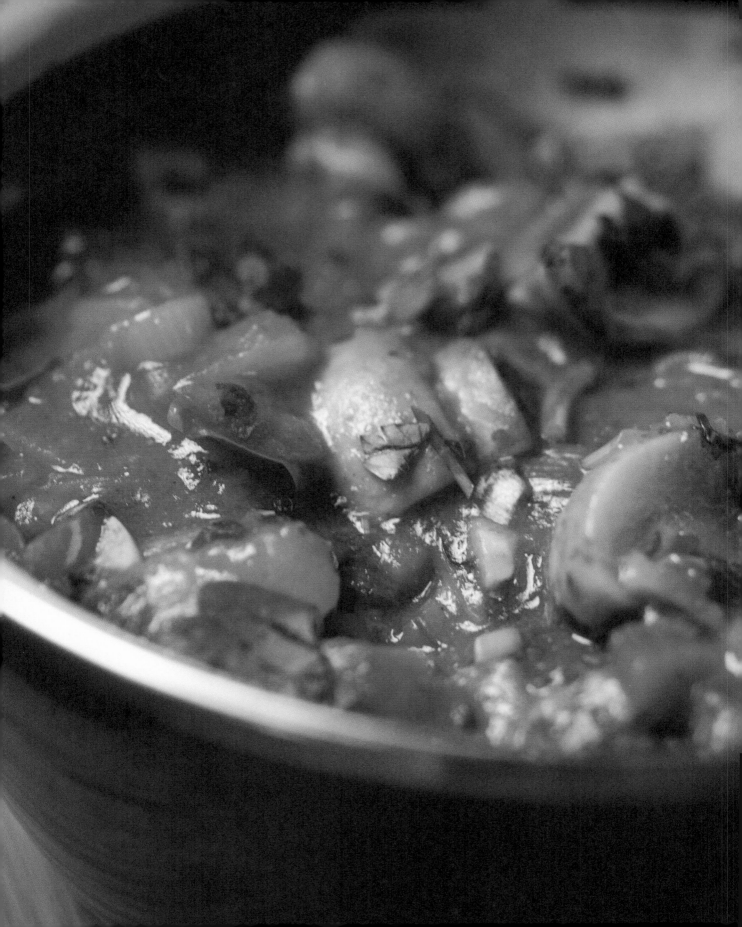

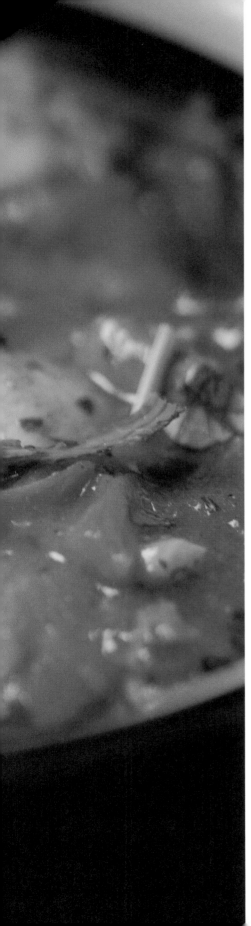

Mushroom Étouffée

TOTAL COOK TIME: 25 MINUTES • SERVES 4

Étouffée is a classic Creole cooking technique. The word literally translates to "smothered," and in this recipe the seasoned mushrooms are smothered in a sauce made with the "holy trinity" (onion, bell pepper, and celery), tomatoes, and seasonings. It's rich and flavorful—*and* plant-based.

FOR THE SAUCE:

¼ cup vegan butter

1 yellow onion, chopped

1 large stalk celery, chopped

1 green bell pepper, diced

¼ cup whole wheat flour

3 garlic cloves, minced

3 to 4 cups vegetable broth

½ cup tomato sauce

1 tablespoon sherry, dry white wine, or apple cider

1 tomato, diced

2 bay leaves

Salt

Freshly ground black pepper

1 bunch green onions, chopped, plus additional for garnish

¼ cup finely chopped parsley, plus additional for garnish

FOR THE MUSHROOM "CRAWFISH":

1½ pounds white mushrooms, stemmed and quartered

1½ teaspoons salt

¾ teaspoon celery seed

¾ teaspoon paprika

¾ teaspoon garlic powder

¾ teaspoon cayenne

Freshly ground black pepper

Zest and juice of 1 lemon

To make the sauce, in a large saucepan, melt the vegan butter over medium-high heat. Add the onion, celery, and bell pepper, and cook, stirring occasionally, until the vegetables are tender, about 10 minutes.

Add the flour and cook, stirring, until the flour begins to brown and gives off a nutty aroma, 3 to 4 minutes. Add the garlic and cook, stirring, 1 more minute.

Add the broth, tomato sauce, sherry, tomato, bay leaves, and salt and pepper to taste, and bring to a simmer.

To make the mushroom "crawfish," combine all the ingredients in a large bowl. Let stand for at least 5 minutes.

Add the seasoned mushrooms to the sauce and simmer for 3 minutes. Stir in the green onion and parsley. Taste and adjust seasonings as needed.

Serve hot over cooked brown rice. Garnish with green onions and parsley.

Cajun Cornbread

TOTAL COOK TIME: 25 MINUTES • SERVES 4

Aquafaba is the starchy liquid in a can of chickpeas. It works really well as an egg substitute and keeps this cornbread plant-based, allergy-friendly, and light.

1 cup cornmeal

1 cup whole wheat flour

1½ tablespoons baking powder

1 teaspoon salt

¼ cups raw cane sugar

½ cup aquafaba (liquid from 15-ounce can of chickpeas)

1½ cups nondairy milk

2 tablespoons oil

Preheat the oven to 400°F with a cast-iron skillet in the oven.

Whisk together the cornmeal, flour, baking powder, salt, and sugar. Add the aquafaba and milk and stir to mix well.

Remove the skillet from the oven, add the oil, and spread it all over the inside of the pan.

Transfer the batter to the greased skillet and spread it into an even layer. Bake for 20 to 25 minutes, until the edges begin to pull away from the sides of the skillet.

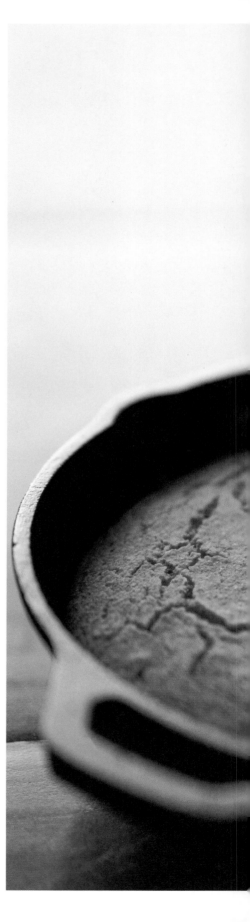

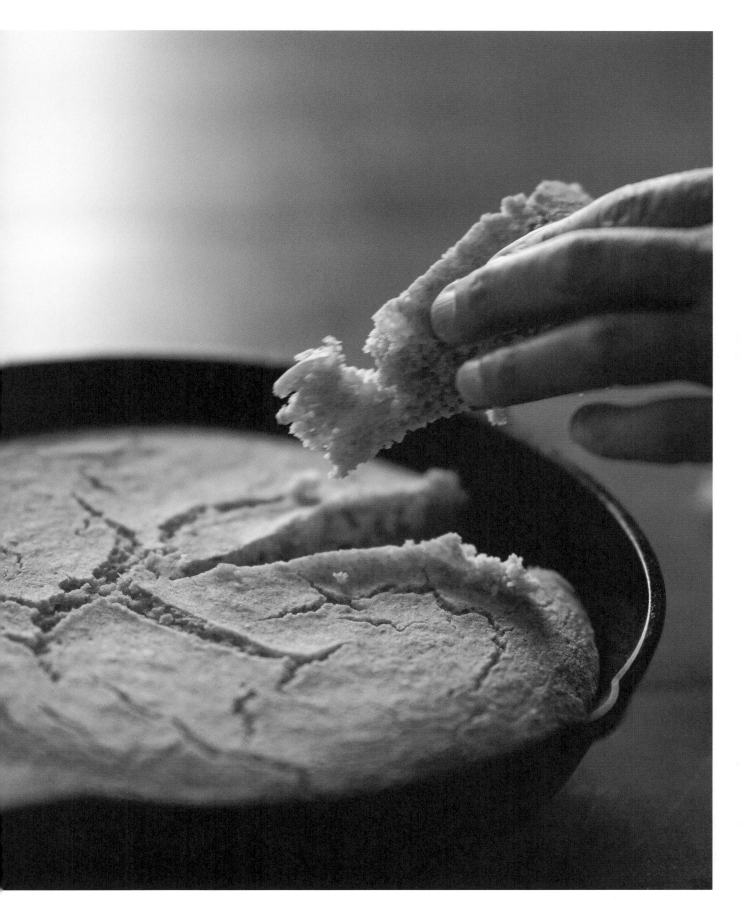

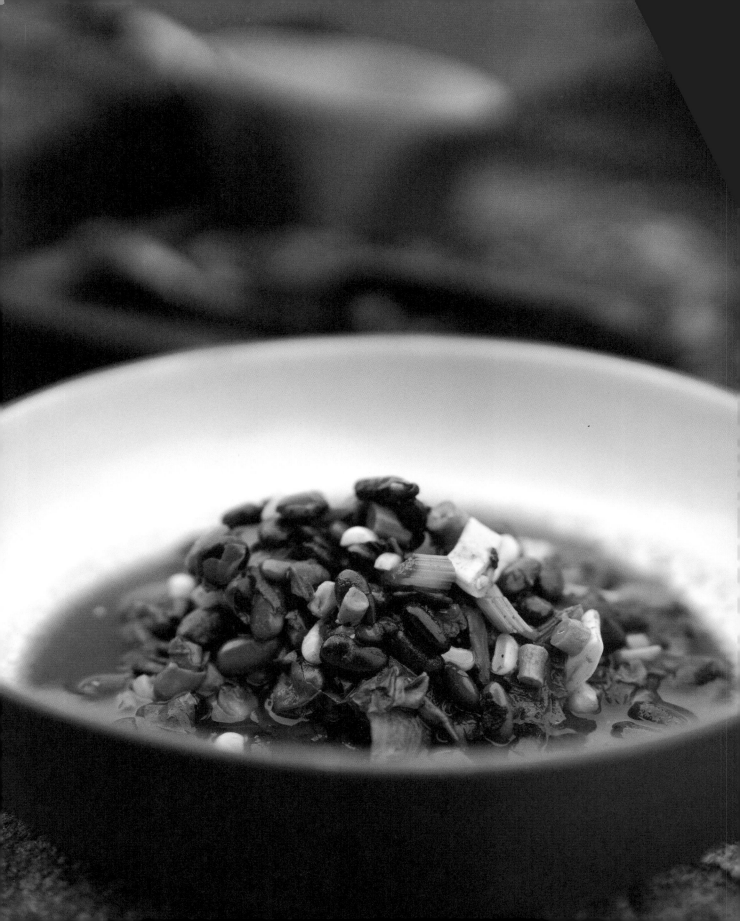

Beans and Greens and Beans

TOTAL COOK TIME: 1 HOUR 15 MINUTES • SERVES 4

2 cups dried Beefy Resilient bush beans or other dried beans (not soaked)

3 quarts water

2 tomatoes, whole

2 large or 3 small garlic cloves, skin on

1 red habanero pepper

1 ear sweet corn

2 sprigs fresh thyme

1 bay leaf

¾ cup finely chopped green and wax beans

2 cups greens such as Swiss chard or kale, julienned

Salt

Extra-virgin olive oil for serving

Heat a barbecue or grill to medium heat (preferably using hardwood) or use the stove.

In a stockpot, combine the dried beans and water and set on the grill or stovetop. Bring to a very slow simmer and cook until the beans are almost fully cooked, about 30 minutes.

Meanwhile, place the tomatoes, garlic cloves, and habanero pepper right onto the coals; or if using the stove, set them in a dry cast-iron skillet over medium heat (be sure to do this in a well-ventilated area). Cook until the vegetables are well charred on the outside. Transfer them to a plate to cool briefly.

When the tomatoes are cool enough to handle, chop them, leaving a bit of the char, and add them to the beans.

Remove and discard the burnt skin of the garlic, then mince the cloves. Add them to the beans.

Gently bruise the habanero pepper with the back of a knife, but be careful not to break the skin (unless you like a lot of spice in your beans). Add the pepper to the beans.

Cut the corn kernels from the cob, reserving both the cob and the kernels. Break the cob in half and add the halves to the beans along with the thyme and bay leaf. Continue to cook gently until the beans are tender, 15 to 30 minutes more. Taste the broth and add salt if needed, keeping in mind that the beans will soak up the salt, so you may need to add a little more when the cooking is finished.

When the beans are tender, add the corn kernels, the fresh beans, and the greens, and cook, stirring, just until the beans soften a bit and the greens wilt but the vegetables are still vibrant, 3 to 5 minutes.

Serve in bowls with a drizzle of extra-virgin olive oil.

NOTE
• When cooking dried beans, the cooking time and water ratios will differ greatly depending on the type of beans you use and how old they are. These instructions are approximate, and you may need to add more water or cook them longer.

Fall Harvest Panzanella

TOTAL COOK TIME: 1 HOUR • SERVES 4

Chef James Wayman likes to make this over a wood fire, as the fire adds a whole other layer of flavor. This salad is a perfect use of late summer and early fall produce—summer tomatoes, herbs, and zucchini, and fall squash and apples for heartier flavors.

¼ cup golden raisins

¼ cup champagne vinegar

1 ripe heirloom tomato

⅛ cup capers, rinsed

1 large garlic clove, minced

Pinch of cayenne

Salt

½ cup plus 2 tablespoons extra-virgin olive oil

1 small butternut squash

1 large or two small crisp apples

1 medium zucchini

1 small sprig fresh rosemary, chopped with stem removed

8 ounces shiitake mushrooms

2 cups sourdough bread, cut into 2-inch cubes

1 sweet bell pepper, cut into 1-inch squares

½ cup chopped fresh basil

Build a wood fire in your barbecue, making a 3-inch-deep bed of coals.

In a small saucepan, combine the raisins and vinegar. Once the coals have a nice, even flame, place the saucepan on the grill and bring to a simmer. Remove the dressing from the heat and let cool.

Using long tongs, place the tomato directly on the coals. Cook until the outside is nicely charred. Remove the tomato from the coals and chop. Add the tomato to the dressing in the saucepan, along with the capers, garlic, cayenne, salt, and 4 tablespoons of olive oil.

Keeping the coals at a nice and even flame, place the whole butternut squash on the grill, just a couple of inches from the coals. Cook, turning every 10 minutes or so, until the squash is tender enough to be pierced with a knife, about 30 minutes. Remove from the heat and let cool.

While the squash is cooking, put the apple and zucchini directly on the coals. Cook, turning every minute or so, until the outside is charred. Remove from the coals and set aside to cool.

In a small cast-iron skillet on the grill, heat the remaining oil with the rosemary. When the pan is hot, add the mushrooms and cook for about 5 minutes, mostly undisturbed, until the mushrooms are nicely browned. Remove from the heat.

Place the bread cubes directly on the grill and cook, turning occasionally, until they are nicely browned, 3 to 5 minutes. Remove from the heat and place in a large salad bowl.

Gently scrape the charred skin off the butternut squash, apples, and zucchini. Remove the seeds and cut the apple and squash into 1-inch pieces. Add them to the bowl with the bread.

Quarter the mushrooms and add them to the bowl along with the raw bell pepper. Salt to taste and add the basil and the raisin-tomato dressing just before serving. Toss well to combine.

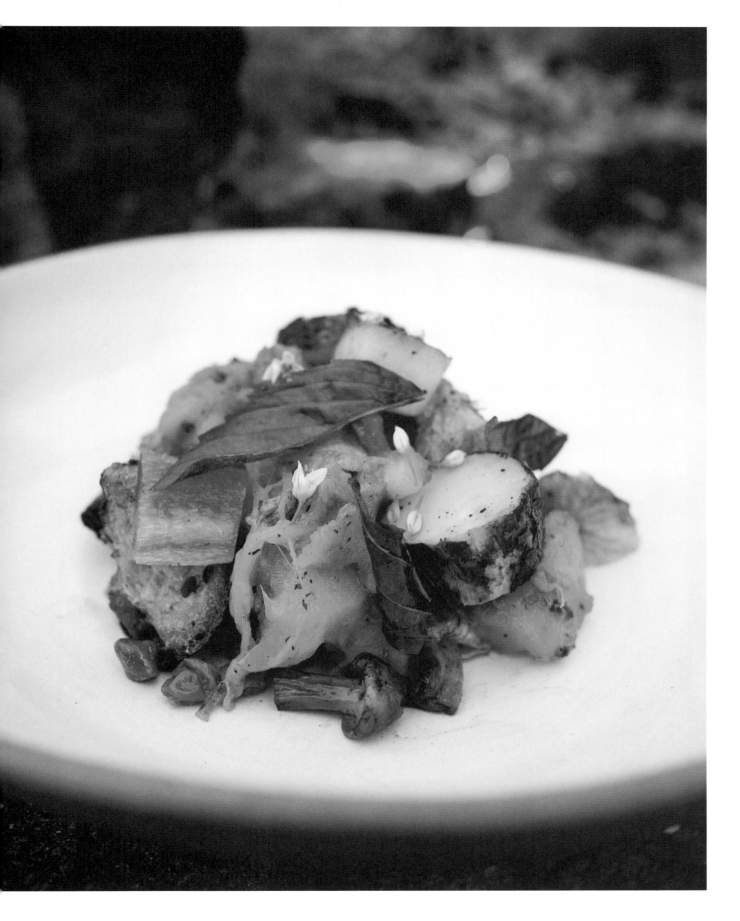

Red Lentil and Butter Bean Ful

TOTAL COOK TIME: 25 MINUTES • SERVES 8

1 tablespoon sunflower oil

1 cup diced onions

½ cup diced red bell pepper

2 teaspoons chopped garlic

1½ tablespoons ground cumin

1 teaspoon ground coriander

1 teaspoon smoked paprika

1 teaspoon ground turmeric

1½ tablespoons Moroccan tagine spice, dry harissa spice, or za'atar

1½ teaspoons salt

1 teaspoon freshly ground black pepper

2 cups diced Roma or beefsteak tomatoes

4 cups dry red lentils, rinsed

1 teaspoon tomato paste

10 cups vegetable stock

4 cups canned butter beans, drained

2 tablespoons olive oil

2 teaspoons lemon juice

In a skillet over medium-high heat, heat the sunflower oil. Add the onion, bell pepper, and garlic, and cook, stirring occasionally, until softened, 3 to 5 minutes.

Add the cumin, coriander, paprika, turmeric, tagine spice, salt, and pepper along with the tomatoes. Cook, stirring occasionally, for 5 minutes.

Add the lentils, tomato paste, and stock. Reduce the heat to medium-low and cook, stirring frequently, until the lentils break down, 12 to 15 minutes.

Stir in the butter beans, olive oil, and lemon juice, and remove from the heat.

Serve hot.

Kimchi Jjigae (Korean Kimchi Stew)

TOTAL COOK TIME: 1 HOUR • SERVES 2 TO 4

Emmy- and James Beard Award–winning chef and TV personality Andrew Zimmern has spent much of his professional career promoting understanding and culture through food. His influential *Bizarre Foods* franchise on the Travel Channel and his MSNBC series *What's Eating America*, among his many other projects, have explored authentic food experiences and discoveries with a wide audience.

FOR THE STOCK:

⅓ cup sliced daikon

4-by-5-inch piece dried Korean kelp (or Japanese kombu)

3 green onions

4 garlic cloves, smashed

4 cups vegetable stock

FOR THE STEW:

1 pound kimchi, cut into bite-size pieces

½ pound shiitake mushrooms, trimmed, stems discarded

1 medium onion, sliced

¼ cup kimchi brine

5 scallions

1 teaspoon salt

2 teaspoons sugar

2 teaspoons gochugaru (Korean hot pepper flakes)

1 teaspoon toasted sesame oil

1 tablespoon gochujang (Korean fermented hot pepper paste)

2 cups stock

½ pound Korean radish or daikon, cubed

1 package soft or medium silken tofu, sliced into ½-inch-thick bite-size pieces

16 ounces glass or bean thread noodles, prepared according to package directions

To make the stock, put all the ingredients in a saucepan. Boil for 25 minutes over medium-high heat.

Reduce the heat to low and simmer for another 5 minutes.

Strain the stock, discarding the contents of the strainer. This makes slightly more than 2 cups of stock.

To make the stew, place the kimchi, mushrooms, onion, and brine in a shallow braising pot with a lid.

Chop 4 of the scallions and add them to the pot with the salt, sugar, gochugaru, oil, gochujang, and stock.

Cover and cook for 10 minutes over medium-high heat.

Stir in the radish with a spoon. Lay the tofu over the top in an attractive line. Cover and cook for another 10 minutes over medium heat.

Add the noodles to the pot (nudge them under the tofu). Season with salt if needed.

Thinly slice the remaining scallion and add as a garnish. Remove the stew from the heat and serve right away with rice.

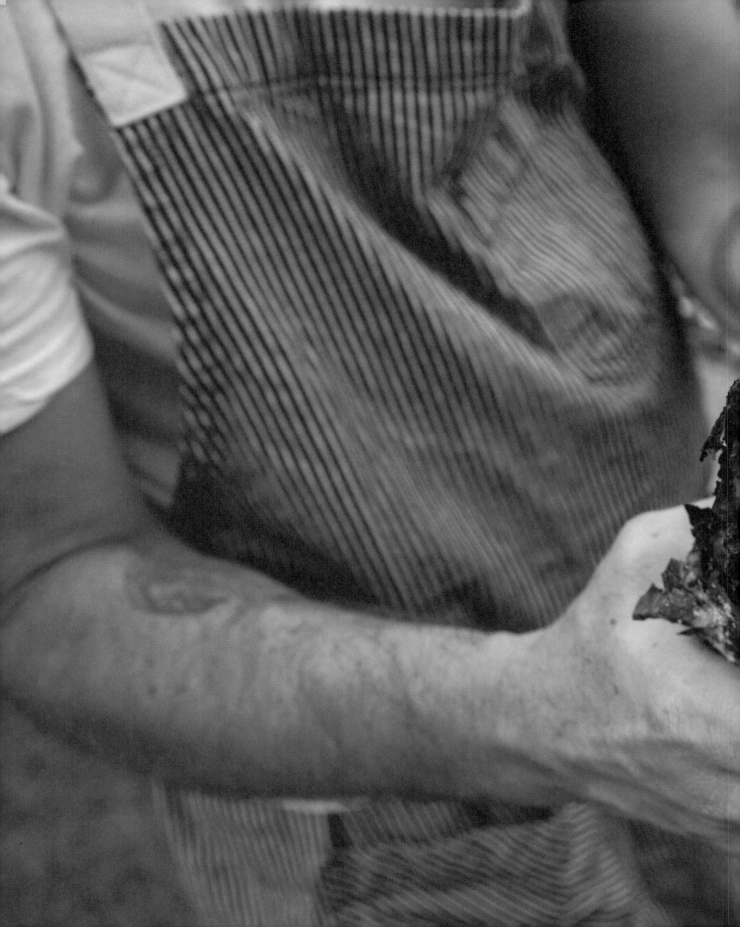

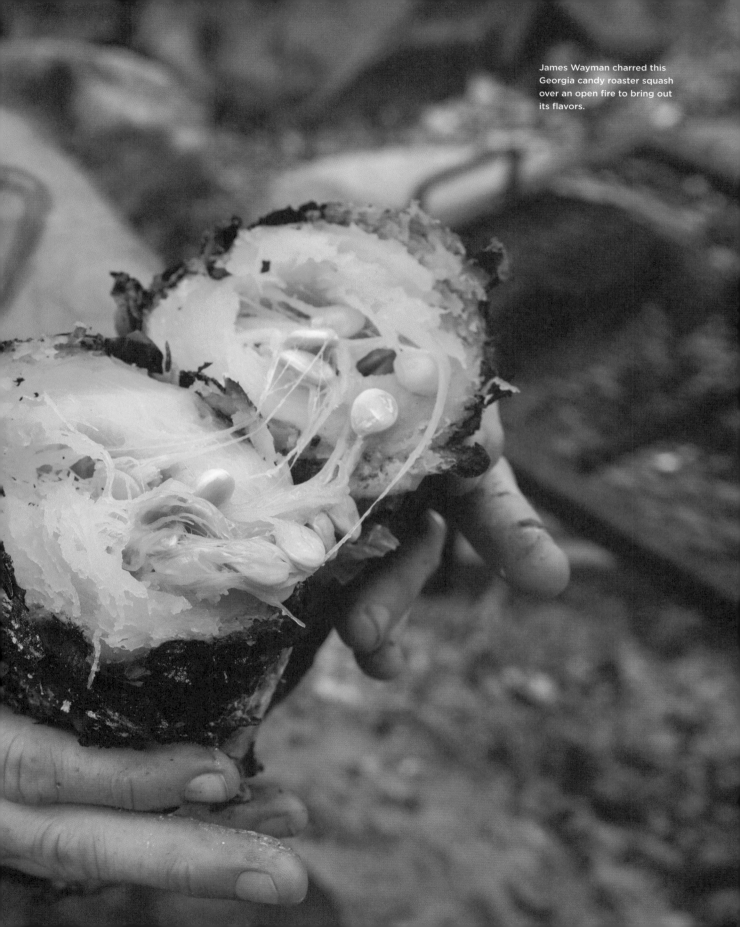

James Wayman charred this Georgia candy roaster squash over an open fire to bring out its flavors.

ROGER BUETTNER, DAN BUETTNER'S FATHER

Tomato, Eggplant, and Sweet Potato Pasta Sauce

TOTAL COOK TIME: 40 MINUTES • SERVES 6 TO 8

This quick pasta sauce is full of flavor. It's especially good made with home-canned garden tomatoes, but if you don't have them, use canned tomato puree. Serve it over pasta and garnish with chopped macadamia nuts.

¼ cup olive oil

1½ cups chopped onion

3 garlic cloves, minced

½ cup chopped bell pepper (red or green)

1½ cups peeled and chopped eggplant

1½ teaspoons dried basil

1½ teaspoons dried parsley

1½ teaspoons dried oregano

½ teaspoon dried rosemary

½ teaspoon dried thyme

2 quarts home-canned tomatoes pureed with their juice or 2 (28-ounce) cans tomato puree

½ cooked sweet potato, peeled and mashed

1 teaspoon salt

In a stockpot, heat the oil over medium-high heat. Add the onion, garlic, pepper, and eggplant, and cook, stirring occasionally, until the vegetables are soft, 8 to 10 minutes.

Add the basil, parsley, oregano, rosemary, thyme, and pureed tomatoes. Simmer for 30 minutes.

Add the sweet potato and salt, and cook, stirring, until heated through. Taste and adjust the seasoning as needed.

NOTE
• In place of the listed herbs, you can substitute 1½ tablespoons of Italian seasoning.

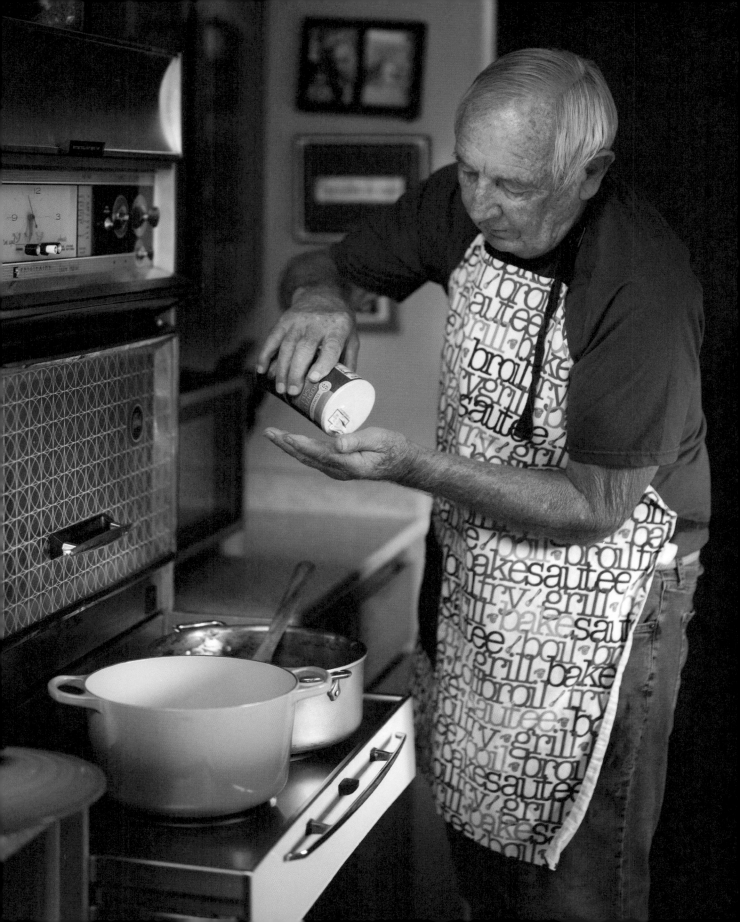

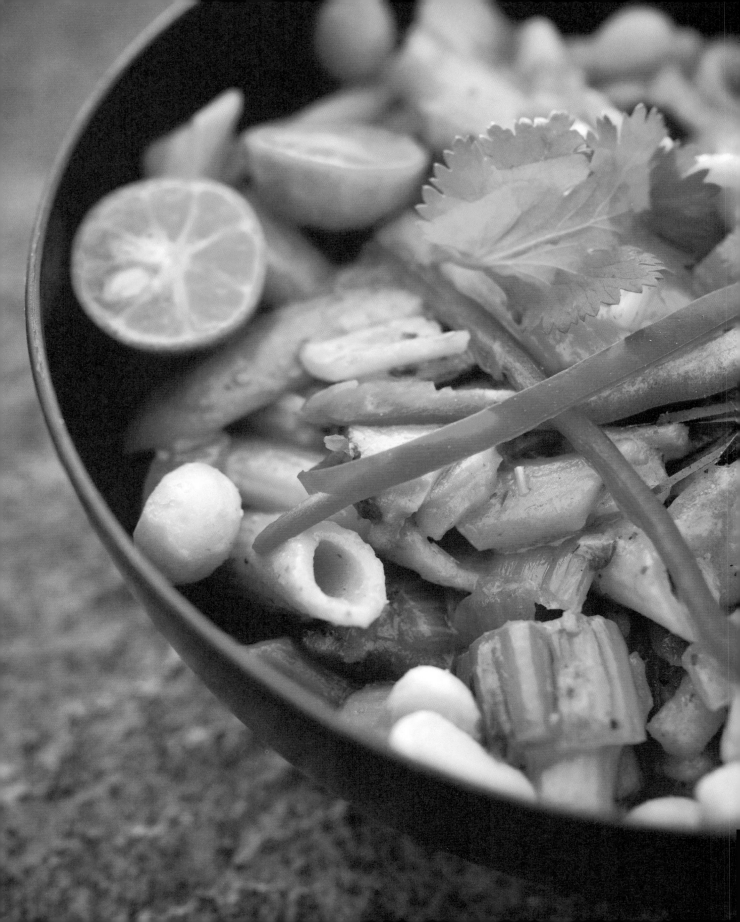

Nakhon Noodles (left)

TOTAL COOK TIME: 20 MINUTES • SERVES 4

8 to 10 ounces uncooked gluten-free noodles

2 tablespoons oil

¼ cup Island Thai Green Curry Paste (below)

1 cup minced onion

1 pound mushrooms (use king oyster mushrooms or any Asian mushrooms)

2 cups sliced bok choy

¼ cup tamari or soy sauce

2 cups unsweetened coconut milk

1 cup shredded carrots

½ cup macadamia nuts, chopped, for garnish

1 fresh lime, quartered, for garnish

Cook the noodles according to the package directions. Drain.

Heat the oil in a wok or skillet over medium-high heat. Add the curry paste and cook, stirring, for 1 minute. Add the onion and cook, stirring, until it softens, 4 to 5 minutes.

Add the mushrooms and bok choy and cook, stirring occasionally, until tender, about 4 minutes more.

Add the tamari and coconut milk and bring to a boil. Cook for a few minutes, until the sauce begins to thicken, and then add the shredded carrots. Cook for a few minutes more, until all the vegetables are tender, and then add the cooked noodles. Cook, tossing to coat the noodles with the sauce, until everything is heated through.

Serve hot in bowls, garnished with the macadamia nuts and lime wedges.

NOTE
• This dish is also great garnished with fresh cilantro sprigs and sriracha if you like.

Island Thai Green Curry Paste

TOTAL COOK TIME: 5 MINUTES • MAKES ABOUT ½ CUP

This spicy and beautifully green curry paste comes from Nakhon Ratchasima in central Thailand. It's delicious as a base for curries, like Nakhon Noodles (above).

2 makrut lime leaves

6 tablespoons chopped cilantro

2 stalks lemongrass

1 tablespoon minced fresh ginger

2 garlic cloves

2 tablespoons lime juice

2 hot red chili peppers (ideally, Hawaiian peppers)

¼ cup coconut oil

If you are using a high-speed blender, put all the ingredients in the blender and process to a smooth paste.

If you are using a mortar and pestle, start with the lime leaves and grind to a paste. Add the remaining ingredients, one at a time, and grind to a paste after each addition.

Transfer the paste to a jar or other container and store in the refrigerator until ready to use (within 2 weeks for best flavor).

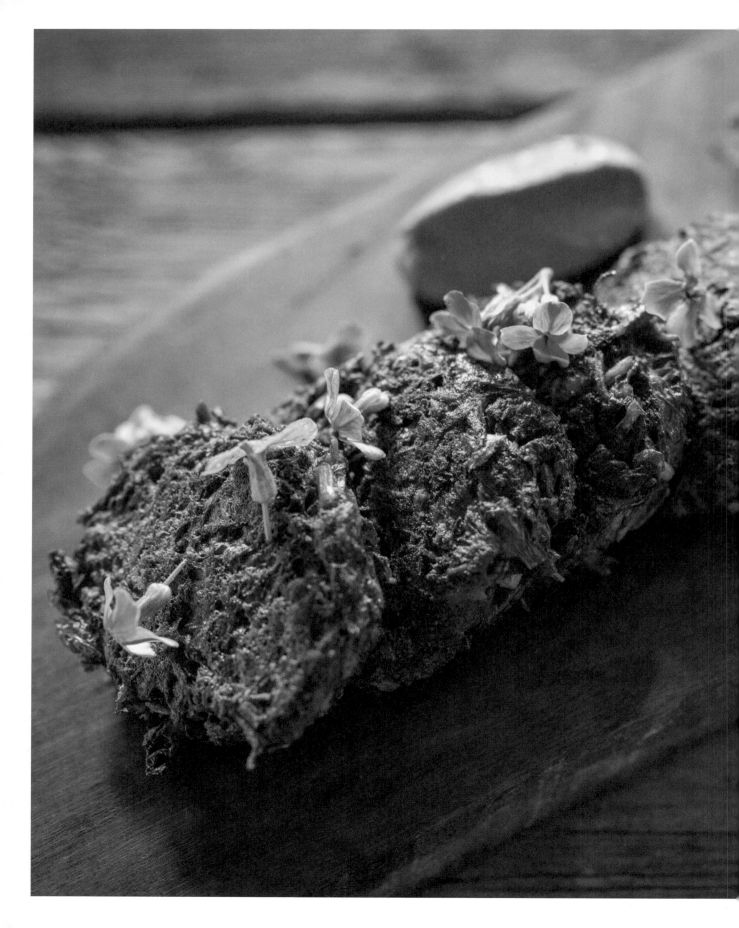

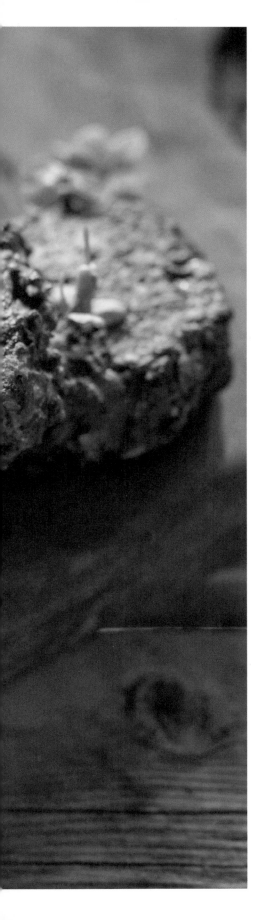

Wild Greens and Bean Cakes

TOTAL COOK TIME: 1 HOUR 10 MINUTES • SERVES 4

9 ounces wild greens, or a mix of spinach, parsley, and kale

2 ounces cooked white beans

1 cup chopped fresh herbs (cilantro, dill, parsley, and/or chives)

¼ teaspoon salt, plus more to taste

Freshly ground black pepper (about 4 or 5 cracks of the pepper mill)

½ teaspoon ground cumin (optional)

3 to 4 tablespoons alternative flour such as wild rice, chickpea, or buckwheat

Cooking oil

Wildflowers, for garnish

Spicy Thai-style sauce, sriracha aioli, or another condiment of your choice, for serving

Lemon wedges, for serving

Heat a large saucepan of lightly salted water to a simmer. Drop in the greens and cook until just tender, 3 to 4 minutes. Drain in a colander and let cool. Squeeze out any remaining water, and then chop the greens to an even consistency and eliminate any visibly long or uneven stems.

In a bowl, mash the cooked beans to a paste. Add the greens along with the herbs, salt, pepper, cumin, if using, and flour, and mix well. Let stand for 15 minutes.

Form the mixture into small, 2-inch-thick patties.

Coat the bottom of a skillet with cooking oil and heat over medium-high heat. Add the patties and cook them until nicely browned on both sides, about 10 minutes. Transfer the cakes to a plate lined with paper towels to remove excess oil.

Garnish the cakes with wildflowers, if using, and serve with your desired sauce and lemon wedges on the side.

NOTE
• This recipe is best made with wild greens like amaranth, nettle, or lamb's-quarters.

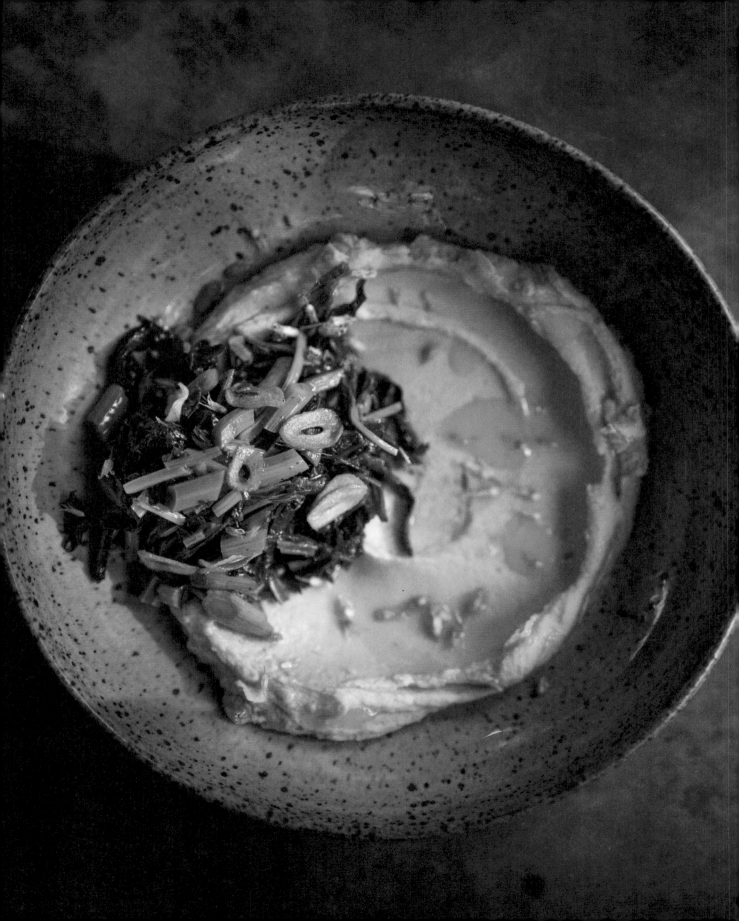

Fave e Cicoria
(Fava Bean Puree With Wild Chicory)

TOTAL COOK TIME: 1 HOUR 10 MINUTES • SERVES 4

This is a classic dish from the Puglia region of Italy, served as an appetizer or a side. True to much Southern Italian cuisine, the recipe relies on wild plants that can be foraged and a simple starch. It's a famous example of *cucina povera,* or "poverty cuisine." Wild chicory (*Cichorium intybus*) or dandelions are the traditional greens used here, but any bitter greens like kale, mustard, or radicchio make a nice counterpart to the silky fava bean puree.

FOR THE PUREE:

8 ounces dried, shelled fava beans

1 bay leaf

½ small yellow onion

3 cups water

Salt

2 tablespoons extra-virgin olive oil or another high-quality oil such as acorn or sunflower, plus extra for serving

FOR THE GREENS:

4 ounces fresh bitter wild greens, such as dandelions or garlic mustard, cut into 1-inch pieces

2 tablespoons cooking oil

1 large garlic clove, thinly sliced

1 small hot chili, preferably Calabrian or cherry bomb pepper, sliced

Salt

Good rustic bread, such as sourdough, for serving

Lemon wedges, for serving

To make the puree, in a stockpot, combine the fava beans, bay leaf, and onion with the water and bring to a simmer over high heat. Reduce the heat to medium-low, cover, and simmer for about 1 hour, until the beans are tender.

Remove the onion and bay leaf from the beans and discard, then drain the beans well and transfer them to a food processor. Puree the beans and season with salt to taste.

With the motor running, drizzle in the oil and process until the mixture is thick, fluffy, and smooth.

To make the greens, bring a large saucepan of lightly salted water to a simmer. Add the greens and cook, stirring occasionally, until tender, 3 to 4 minutes. Drain.

Meanwhile, in a skillet, heat the cooking oil over medium heat. Add the garlic and cook, stirring, for 30 seconds. Add the chili and cook for 1 minute more.

Add the cooked, drained greens to the skillet and cook, stirring, until heated through. Season to taste with salt.

To serve, spoon the fava bean puree into a shallow serving dish and put the greens on one side. Drizzle with olive oil and serve with crusty bread and lemon wedges.

NOTE
• Check your local Middle Eastern or Asian market for dried, shelled fava beans, or order them online.

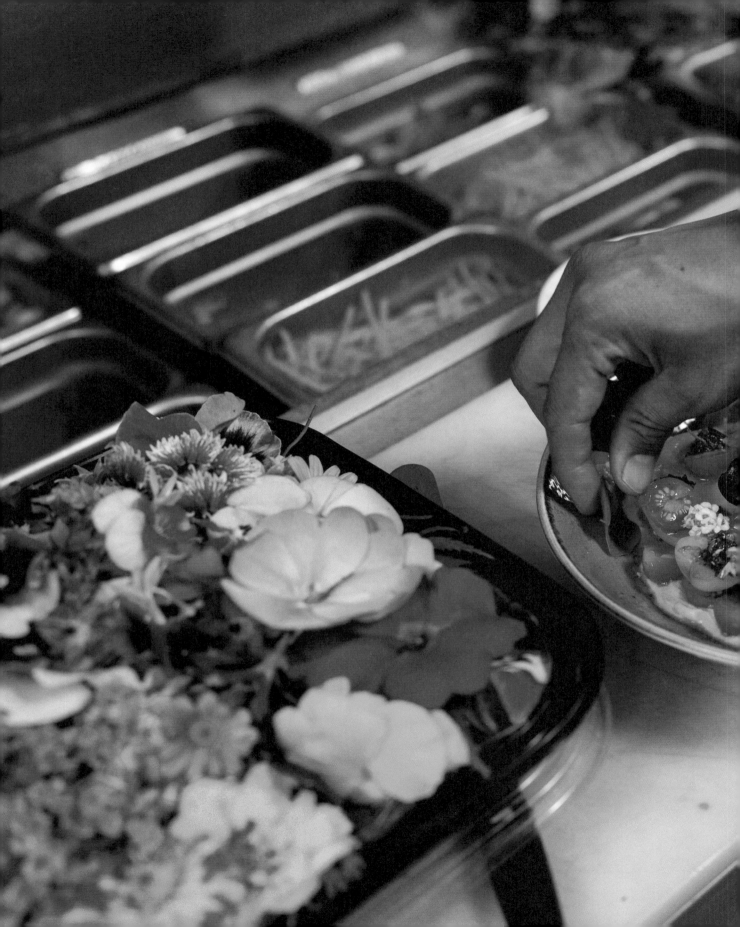

Borani Esfenaj (Lamb's-Quarter Dip)

TOTAL COOK TIME: 5 MINUTES • SERVES 8

This variation of a traditional Persian dip uses lamb's-quarter, a wild edible green, instead of spinach. American Black-feet were growing lamb's-quarters as long ago as the 16th century. They contain more iron and protein than spinach or cabbage and more B vitamins than many green and cruciferous vegetables. Lamb's-quarters are currently having a superfood moment, since they're highly nutritious and easy to grow. If you can't find them, you can substitute baby spinach leaves.

10 ounces tender clusters of lamb's-quarters

2 tablespoons extra-virgin olive oil

1 large garlic clove, minced

½ teaspoon ground cumin

⅛ to ¼ teaspoon crushed red pepper, plus additional as needed

¼ cup freshly cracked black or English walnuts, coarsely chopped

1 cup yogurt (such as CocoYo vegan coconut yogurt)

1½ ounces cilantro leaves and tender stems, or a mix of cilantro and fresh dill, or fresh mint, chopped

Juice of 1 small lemon

1 teaspoon lemon zest

Kosher salt

Freshly ground black pepper

¼ teaspoon sumac, for garnish

A few wild flowers (such as yellow mustard flowers), for garnish

Place the lamb's-quarters in a steamer basket over a pot of simmering water and steam until tender, 1 to 2 minutes. Remove from the heat and let them cool. Once they're cool enough to handle, chop them and place them in a bowl.

In a small pan, heat the oil with the garlic on medium until the garlic starts to brown around the edges and is aromatic. Add the cumin to the pan, turn off the heat, and swirl to allow the garlic to continue cooking with the residual heat. Stir in the red pepper, being careful not to let the garlic burn.

Pour the seasoned oil onto the lamb's-quarters, then add the walnuts (reserve a few for garnish), yogurt, cilantro, lemon juice, and zest. Add salt and pepper to taste. Mix well, taste, and adjust the seasoning as needed. Cover and chill before serving.

Serve cold, garnished with sumac and flowers, and with pita chips or bread for dipping.

Coconut Ceviche

TOTAL COOK TIME: 5 MINUTES • SERVES 4

FOR THE AGUACHILE SAUCE:

1 serrano chili, stemmed

6 tablespoons key lime juice

6 tablespoons Meyer lemon juice

6 tablespoons mandarin orange juice

Pinch of salt

FOR THE CEVICHE:

1 cup shredded coconut (unsweetened)

½ cup sliced mango

½ cup sliced cucumber

¼ cup pickled red onion

¼ cup diced heirloom tomato

2 tablespoons chopped cilantro

2 tablespoons sliced spring onion

Borage flowers, for garnish

To make the aguachile sauce, in a blender or food processor, combine all the ingredients and process until smooth.

To make the ceviche, put the coconut, mango, cucumber, pickled onion, tomato, cilantro, and spring onion in a medium bowl. Add ¼ cup of the aguachile sauce and toss to mix.

Serve garnished with borage flowers, if desired.

NOTE
• The extra aguachile sauce will keep in the refrigerator for up to a week. You can add olive oil to it to make a citrus vinaigrette for salads.

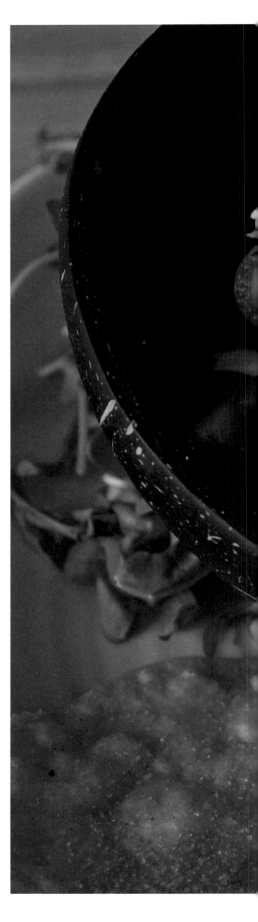

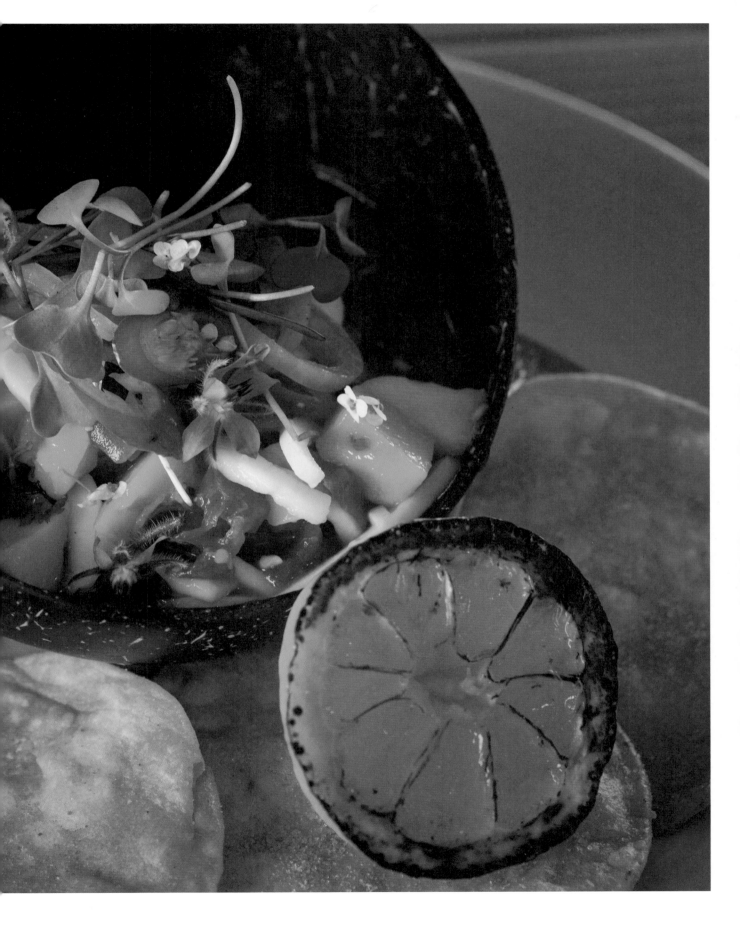

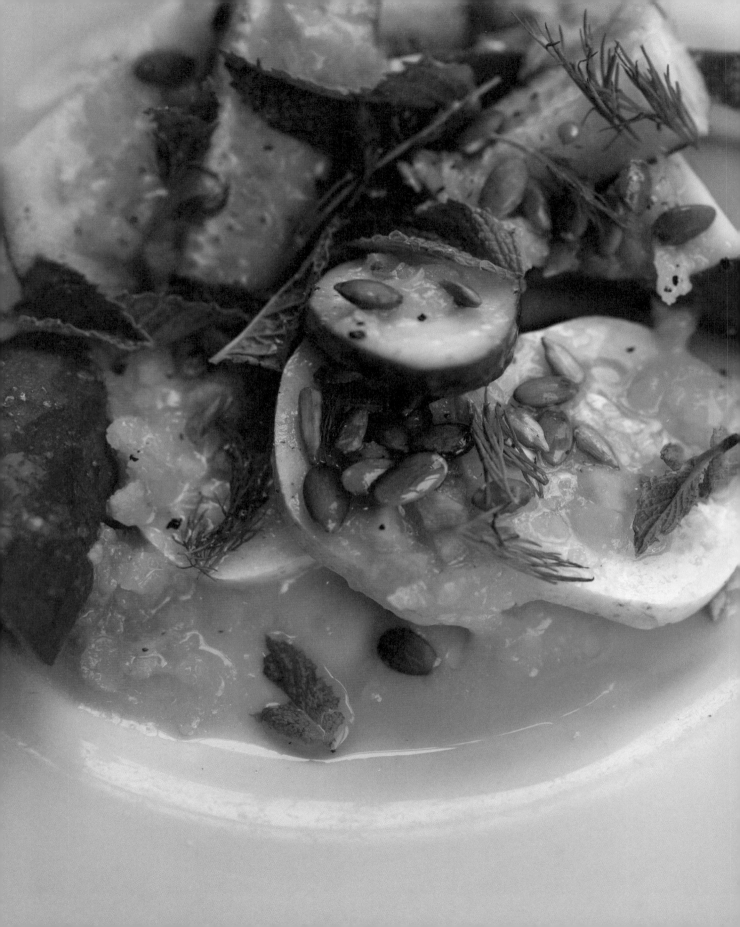

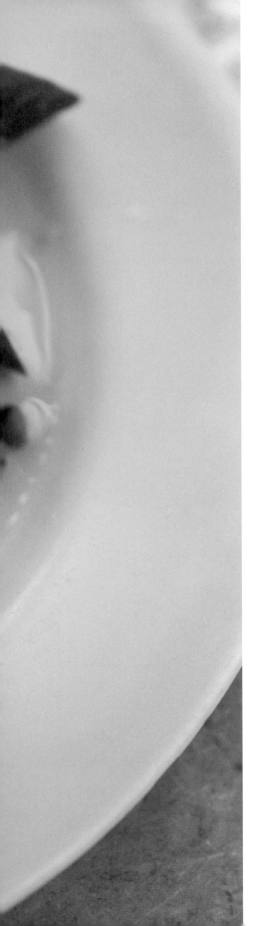

Heirloom Cucumber Salad With Preserved Lemon Vinaigrette

TOTAL COOK TIME: 5 MINUTES • SERVES 4

FOR THE SALAD:

2 lemon cucumbers, cut into bite-size pieces

1 Persian cucumber, cut into bite-size pieces

1 Armenian cucumber, cut into bite-size pieces

1 Japanese cucumber, cut into bite-size pieces

1 teaspoon Maldon sea salt

2 tablespoons toasted pepitas

2 tablespoons toasted sunflower seeds

1 tablespoon chopped fresh dill

1 tablespoon chopped fresh mint

FOR THE VINAIGRETTE:

⅓ cup preserved lemon rind

⅓ cup preserved orange rind

½ cup white wine vinegar

1 tablespoon honey

1 cup extra-virgin olive oil

To make the salad, arrange all the cucumbers on a plate or in a bowl and season with the salt.

To make the vinaigrette, in a food processor or blender, combine the preserved lemon, preserved orange, and vinegar. Process until the citrus rinds are finely chopped but still chunky. Transfer the mixture to a small bowl and stir in the honey and olive oil. Whisk to combine.

Drizzle the dressing over the top of the cucumbers and top with the pepitas, sunflower seeds, dill, and mint.

Seared Japanese Eggplant With Red Onion Agrodolce and Tahini Sauce

TOTAL COOK TIME: 10 MINUTES • SERVES 4

¼ cup extra-virgin olive oil, plus more for garnish

1 pound Japanese eggplant, halved lengthwise

Pinch of salt

½ cup Red Onion Agrodolce (page 253), plus more for garnish

6 cherry tomatoes, halved

1 tablespoon chopped parsley

1 tablespoon chopped fresh mint

Tahini Sauce (page 253)

1 teaspoon Maldon sea salt, for finishing

In a large skillet, heat the olive oil over medium heat. Add the eggplant, cut sides down, along with the salt. Cook until the bottom of the eggplant is golden brown, about 3 minutes. Flip the eggplant over and cook until the eggplant is soft, about 4 minutes more.

In a mixing bowl, toss together the red onion agrodolce, tomatoes, parsley, and mint.

Transfer the eggplant to a plate and drizzle the tahini sauce over the top. Garnish with the agrodolce, a drizzle of olive oil, and the sea salt.

Red Onion Agrodolce

TOTAL COOK TIME: 20 MINUTES • MAKES ABOUT 1 CUP

1 tablespoon extra-virgin olive oil

1 cup sliced red onion

1 clove garlic, sliced

2 sprigs fresh thyme

1 bay leaf

2 tablespoons sugar

¼ cup freshly squeezed orange juice

¼ cup red wine vinegar

¼ cup water

¼ teaspoon salt

In a medium saucepan over medium heat, combine the olive oil, red onion, garlic, thyme, and bay leaf. Cook for 5 minutes, stirring constantly, to keep the onion from browning.

Add the sugar and continue to cook, stirring, until the sugar dissolves, about 2 more minutes. Stir in the orange juice, vinegar, water, and salt, and let simmer for 10 minutes.

Remove from the heat and let cool. Store in an airtight container until ready to use; it will keep for up to a week in the refrigerator.

Tahini Sauce

TOTAL COOK TIME: 2 MINUTES • MAKES ABOUT ½ CUP

¼ cup tahini

¼ cup water

1 tablespoon white wine vinegar

¼ teaspoon salt

1 garlic clove, grated

In a small bowl, add all the ingredients and whisk until well combined.

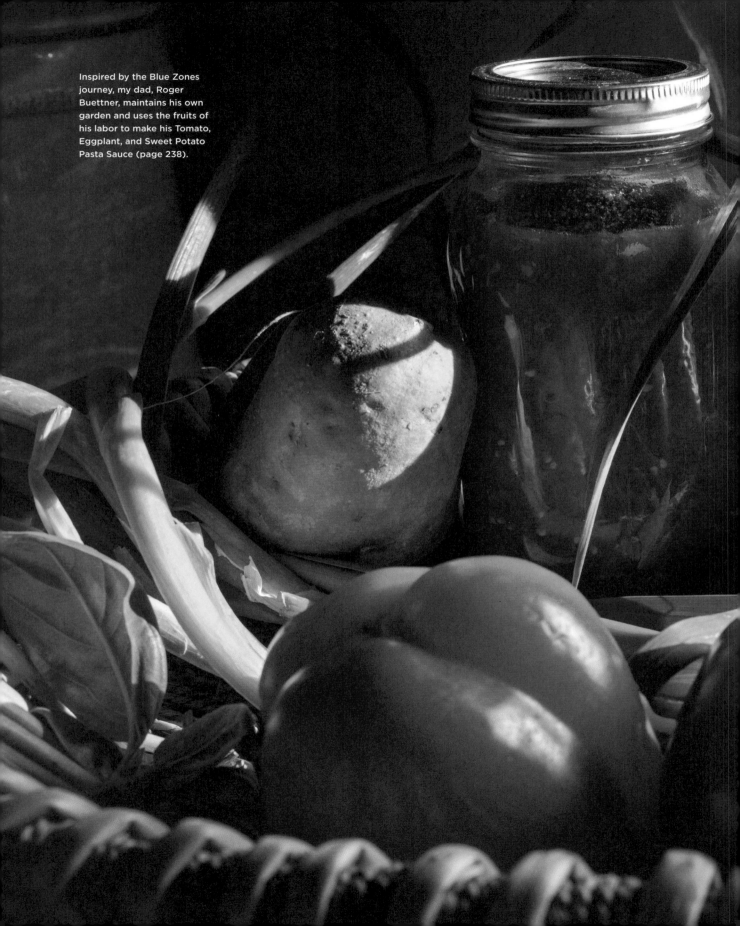

Inspired by the Blue Zones journey, my dad, Roger Buettner, maintains his own garden and uses the fruits of his labor to make his Tomato, Eggplant, and Sweet Potato Pasta Sauce (page 238).

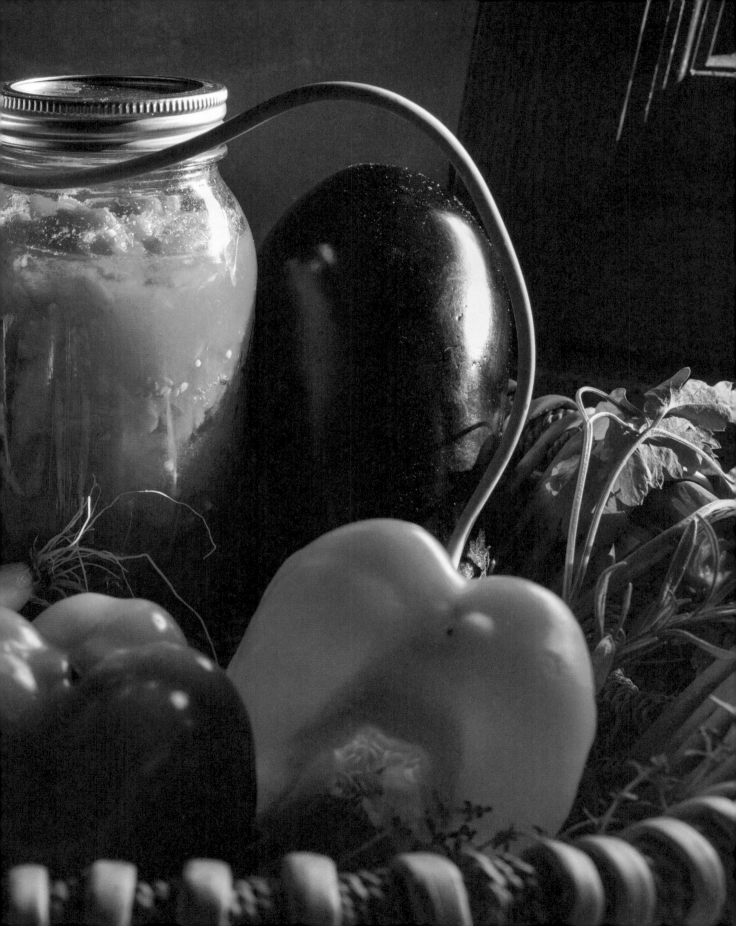

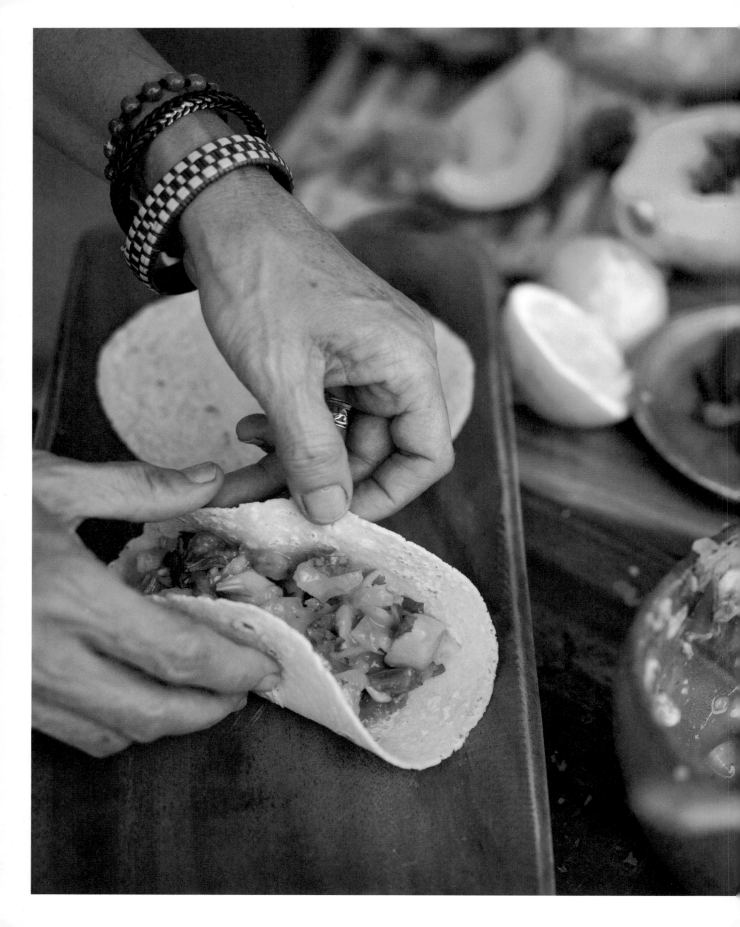

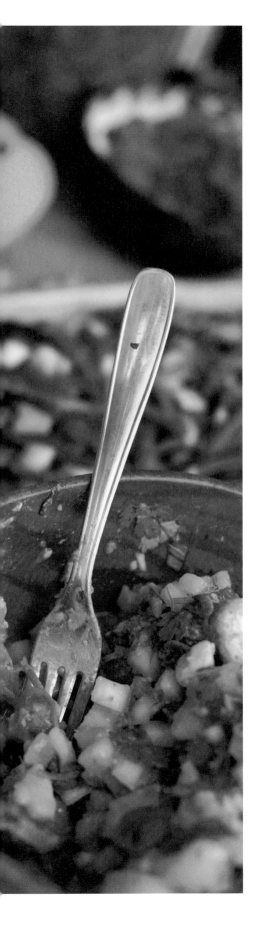

Hawaiian Fresh Fruit Tacos

TOTAL COOK TIME: 5 MINUTES • MAKES 12 TACOS

At her restaurant Barefoot Zone, Tess Villegas-Rumley serves fresh, plant-based foods meant to nourish the body and the spirit. Barefoot Zone is a Blue Zones Project Approved restaurant on the Big Island in Hawaii, which means they are part of the statewide movement to create cities and counties and islands where people live better and longer lives.

Tess's fresh fruit taco recipe is loaded with tropical fruit and irresistible flavor contrasts from onions, chili peppers, and lemon juice. The moringa flakes sprinkled on top are full of minerals, amino acids, and vitamins.

1 cup diced fresh pineapple

1 cup diced fresh mango

1 cup diced white onion

¼ cup chopped green onions

1 cup diced (peeled and seeded) tomatoes

1 cup chopped cilantro

Sea salt

¼ cup freshly squeezed lemon juice

3 pieces fresh Hawaiian chili pepper

12 soft corn tortillas

2 cups diced avocado

Moringa flakes, for garnish (optional)

Hot sauce (optional)

In a large bowl, combine the pineapple, mango, white onion, green onion, tomatoes, cilantro, salt, lemon juice, and chili pepper. Toss to mix well.

Heat the tortillas either in a crepe maker for about 30 seconds or on a baking sheet in a 400°F oven for a minute or two.

Fill the tortillas with the fruit filling and add the avocado, dividing equally.

Sprinkle moringa flakes over the fruit and add hot sauce, if using.

NOTE
• Dried cilantro can be substituted for the moringa flakes.

Hawaiian Fern Salad

TOTAL COOK TIME: 20 MINUTES • SERVES 4

1 pound young fiddlehead ferns, cut into 2-inch pieces

Juice of 1 lemon

1 slightly underripe mango

1 white onion, diced

3 tomatoes, peeled, seeded, and diced

¼ cup finely diced fresh ginger

½ cup Lilikoi Dressing or Pineapple Vinaigrette (page 259)

Sea salt

Moringa flakes, for garnish

Fill a large bowl with ice water for an ice bath.

Bring a large saucepan of water to a boil and then drop in the ferns. Cook, stirring, for 15 to 20 seconds. Then use a slotted spoon to remove the ferns and plunge them into the ice bath to stop the cooking process. Drain well.

Place the ferns in a large salad bowl. Squeeze lemon juice on top and toss to coat.

Add the mango, onion, tomatoes, ginger, dressing, and salt, and toss to mix.

Sprinkle the moringa flakes over the salad. Serve immediately.

NOTES

• You can substitute asparagus for the ferns.

• Dried cilantro can be substituted for the moringa flakes.

Lilikoi Dressing
or Pineapple Vinaigrette

TOTAL COOK TIME: 5 MINUTES • MAKES ½ CUP

Lilikoi, or Hawaiian passion fruit, is abundant in Hawaii, though it is actually native to South America and was brought to the islands only in the 1920s. It's a tart-sweet fruit that makes a flavorful salad dressing. Use it to dress leafy green salads or as a marinade for meat or fish. If you can't find lilikoi, swap in pineapple juice for an equally tropical dressing. This recipe offers both options.

¼ cup lilikoi juice with seeds (for lilikoi dressing) or pineapple juice (for pineapple vinaigrette)

¼ cup avocado oil (or olive oil or another oil)

1 tablespoon honey

Sea salt

Freshly ground black pepper

To make lilikoi dressing, combine the lilikoi juice, oil, honey, salt, and pepper in a blender and blend to combine well.

To make pineapple vinaigrette, combine the pineapple juice, oil, honey, salt, and pepper in a jar and shake to mix well.

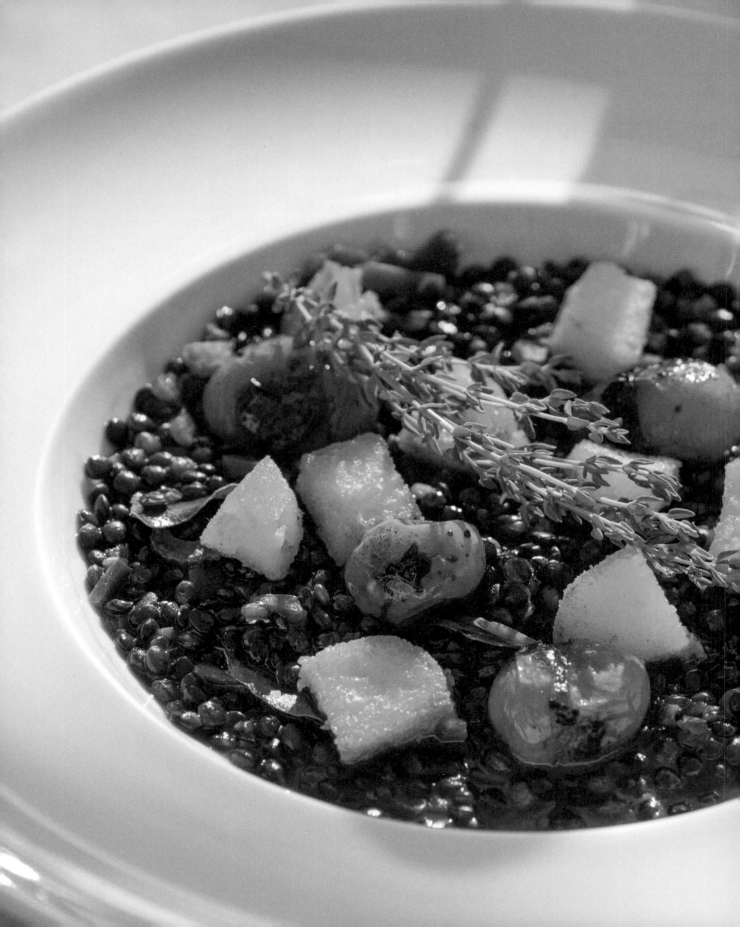

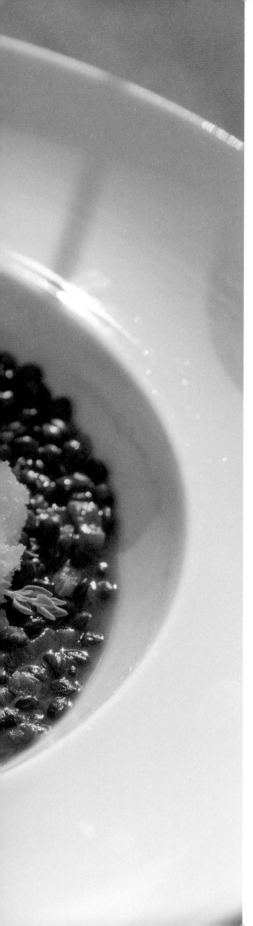

Umbria Black Beluga Lentil and Polenta Soup

TOTAL COOK TIME: 30 MINUTES • SERVES 4

2 tablespoons extra-virgin olive oil

½ onion, diced

2 carrots, peeled and diced

2 celery stalks, diced

⅔ cup black beluga lentils

4 cups vegetable broth or water

Sea salt

½ cup quick-cooking polenta

In a Dutch oven or stockpot over medium-low heat, heat the oil until it shimmers. Add the onion, carrots, and celery, and cook, stirring occasionally, until the vegetables are soft, about 12 minutes.

Add the lentils and continue to cook, stirring to coat them with the oil. Add the broth and bring to a boil. Reduce the heat to low and simmer for about 15 minutes, stirring occasionally, until the lentils are tender.

Add the salt to taste and some additional water if the liquid has evaporated too much; it should still be soupy.

Bring the mixture back up to a low boil and then whisk in the polenta. Reduce the heat to low again and simmer until the polenta is tender, about 2 minutes.

Taste and adjust the seasoning as needed, and add additional water if needed for consistency.

Chickpea Soup

TOTAL COOK TIME: 2 HOURS 30 MINUTES • SERVES 4

1 pound dried chickpeas, soaked and drained

2 tablespoons extra-virgin olive oil

½ onion, diced

2 carrots, peeled and diced

2 celery stalks, diced

4 cups vegetable broth

1 teaspoon chopped fresh rosemary leaves

Salt

Freshly ground black pepper

4 ounces Parmigiano-Reggiano (optional)

In a Dutch oven or stockpot, combine the chickpeas and enough water to cover them by about 2 inches. Bring to a boil over medium-high heat. Reduce the heat to low, cover, and simmer until the chickpeas are tender, about 2 hours. Drain.

In a Dutch oven or stockpot, heat the oil over medium-high heat. Add the onion, carrots, and celery, and cook, stirring occasionally, until the vegetables are soft, about 12 minutes.

Stir in the broth, chickpeas, rosemary, and salt and pepper to taste. Bring to a boil over medium-high heat. Reduce the heat to low and simmer for 15 minutes.

Serve hot. Garnish with grated cheese, if using.

16 Bean Soup

TOTAL COOK TIME: 10 HOURS, INCLUDING SOAKING TIME • SERVES 4

1 pound mixed dried beans (any combination of split peas, lentils, chickpeas, pinto beans, navy beans, cannellini beans, black beans, kidney beans, black-eyed peas, or lima beans)

2 tablespoons extra-virgin olive oil

½ cup sliced scallions

1 onion, diced

2 carrots, diced

4 cups vegetable broth

1 cup tomato puree (preferably San Marzano tomatoes)

1 bay leaf

1 teaspoon fresh thyme leaves

2 tablespoons chopped fresh basil

1 tablespoon chopped fresh oregano

Salt

Put the beans in a large bowl, Dutch oven, or stockpot and cover with water by at least 2 inches. Soak the beans overnight, then drain.

In a Dutch oven or stockpot, cover the beans with 2 inches of water and bring to a boil over medium-high heat. Reduce the heat to low and simmer until the beans are tender, 1 to 2 hours (depending on the combination of beans). Drain.

In a Dutch oven or stockpot, heat the oil over medium-high heat until it shimmers. Add the onion and carrots and cook, stirring occasionally, until soft, about 5 minutes.

Add the beans, broth, tomato puree, and bay leaf, and bring to a boil. Reduce the heat to low and simmer for 15 minutes.

Stir in the thyme, basil, and oregano. Season with salt to taste.

Serve hot.

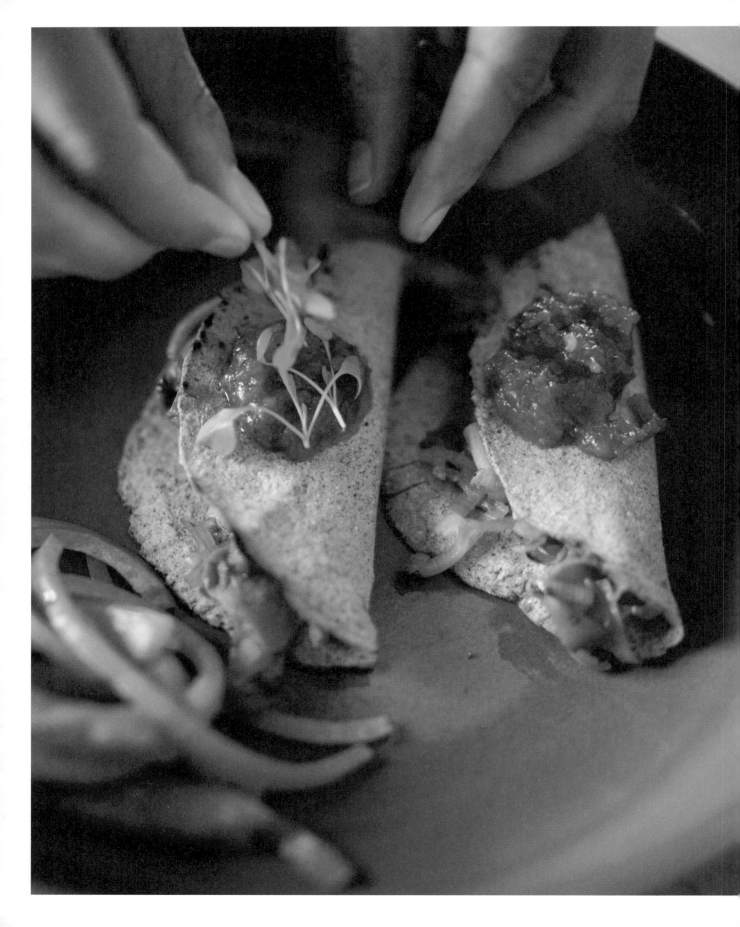

Mushroom Birria Tacos (left)

TOTAL COOK TIME: 1 HOUR 30 MINUTES • MAKES 6 TACOS

Traditional Mexican birria tacos are made with a savory stew and tortillas. Hao Tran's version replaces the meat with mushrooms and is flavored with sake and smoked shoyu for an Asian twist. You can find smoked shoyu in Asian markets.

½ cup unfiltered sake

2 teaspoons smoked shoyu

3 cups chopped cremini, button, shiitake, or portobello mushrooms

1 teaspoon sesame oil

1 teaspoon minced ginger

1 teaspoon minced garlic

½ cup chopped leek (white part only)

6 tortillas (corn or flour)

2 to 4 tablespoons vegetable oil

¼ cup chopped cilantro, for garnish

1 cup salsa or pico de gallo, for garnish

1 lime, cut into wedges, for serving

In a medium bowl, combine the sake and shoyu. Add the mushrooms and toss to coat. Let the mushrooms marinate for at least 1 hour.

Heat a skillet over medium heat and add the sesame oil, ginger, garlic, and leek. Cook, stirring, until aromatic, about 30 seconds.

Add the marinated mushrooms along with the marinating liquid. Cook, stirring occasionally, until the mushrooms soften, about 10 minutes. Using a slotted spoon, transfer the mushrooms from the skillet to a bowl, reserving the cooking liquid.

Place a couple of spoonfuls of the mushroom filling onto one half of each tortilla and fold the other half of the tortilla over the filling.

Heat 2 tablespoons of the vegetable oil in a heavy-bottomed skillet over medium-high heat.

Dip a filled taco in the reserved cooking liquid, then add it to the skillet and fry until it's crispy on both sides. Repeat with the remaining tacos, adding more oil as needed.

Serve immediately, garnished with cilantro, salsa, and a wedge of lime.

Carob Walnut Energy Balls

TOTAL COOK TIME: 10 MINUTES • SERVES 8 TO 10

1 cup old-fashioned oats (or about ¾ cup oat flour)

2 tablespoons carob powder

⅓ cup chopped walnuts

Pinch of sea salt

2 to 3 tablespoons coconut oil, melted

Scant 3 tablespoons honey

2 teaspoons vanilla extract

Optional toppings: unsweetened coconut chips or shredded coconut, chia seeds, or sunflower seeds

In a large bowl, combine the oats, carob powder, walnuts, and salt, and mix well.

Add the melted coconut oil, honey, and vanilla, and stir to combine.

Lightly oil your hands and scoop up about ¼ cup of the mixture at a time, rolling each scoop into a ball. If the mixture feels too dry and doesn't hold together well, add a few more teaspoons of coconut oil and honey to bind it.

Gently roll the balls over the toppings to coat them as desired.

Cover and refrigerate until ready to serve.

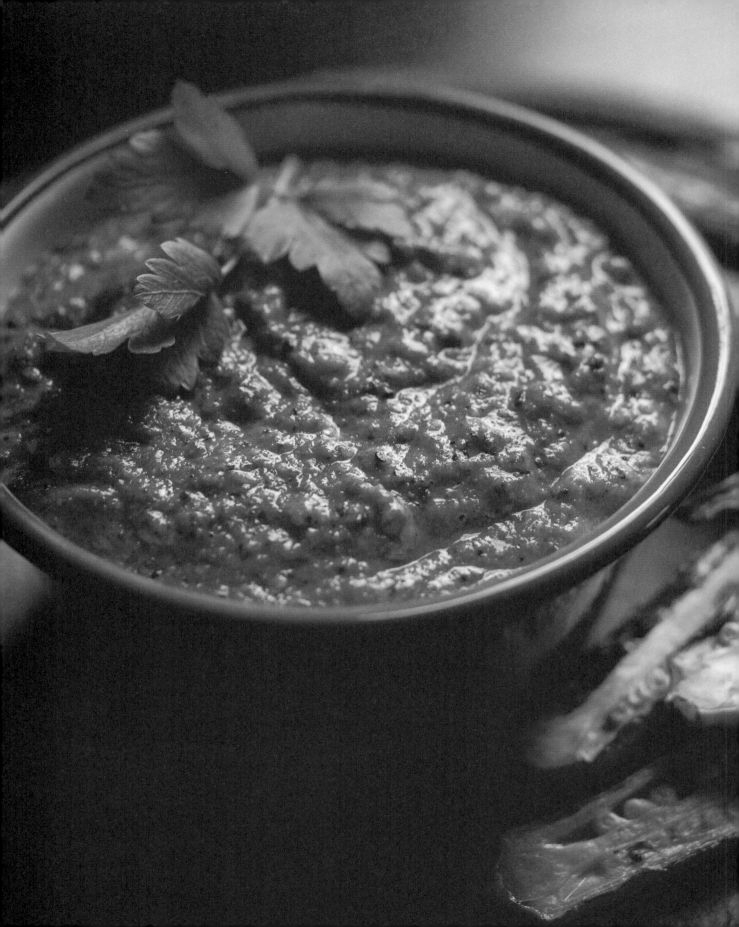

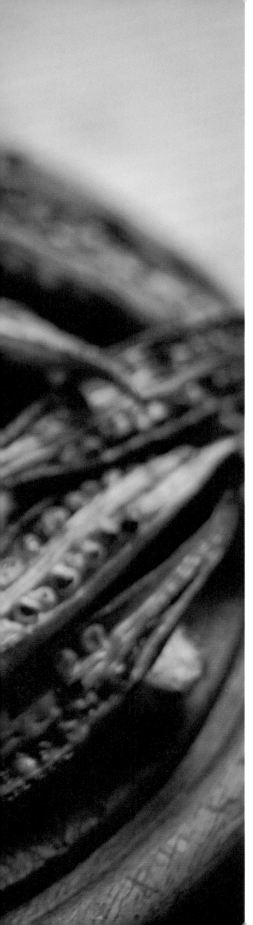

Muhammara
(Red Pepper Dip)

TOTAL COOK TIME: 50 MINUTES • SERVES 3

Chris DeBarr discovered this recipe back in the 1980s, when he first learned to cook Lebanese and Syrian cuisine and fell under the magic sway of pomegranate molasses. Muhammara remains one of Chris's all-time favorite dishes to make, and he's always thrilled to introduce the tart, sticky, sweet, crimson elixir known as pomegranate molasses to any cook. He considers it a life-changing ingredient and recommends the Cortas brand.

¾ cup toasted pecans or walnuts

4 red bell peppers, roasted and peeled

½ cup roasted garlic

2 tablespoons ground cumin

1 tablespoon ground Aleppo chili pepper

1 tablespoon Rumi Spice's Kabul Piquant Chicken seasoning blend

2 teaspoons kosher salt or 1½ teaspoons fine sea salt

1 teaspoon ground white pepper

¼ cup pomegranate molasses

½ cup extra-virgin olive oil

1 cup breadcrumbs, unseasoned

In a food processor, pulse the nuts until they are well chopped.

Add the remaining ingredients and pulse until smooth. Taste and adjust the seasonings, as needed.

Serve with pita bread or flatbread for dipping and scooping.

NOTES

• To toast the pecans or walnuts, preheat the oven to 400°F. Spread the nuts in a single layer on a baking sheet and toast in the oven for 7 to 8 minutes. Alternatively, you can toast the nuts in a skillet over medium heat until they become fragrant.

• You can substitute jarred roasted red peppers for the red bell pepper. Use one 25-ounce jar, drained.

• To roast the garlic, preheat the oven to 400°F. Slice the top ¼ or ½ inch off a head of garlic to expose the cloves. Place the garlic on a piece of foil and drizzle olive oil all over the garlic, rubbing it with your hands to coat it well. Wrap the garlic up loosely in the foil and roast it in the oven for 30 to 40 minutes, until the cloves are golden brown and very soft.

Frim Fram Sauce

TOTAL COOK TIME: 1 HOUR 45 MINUTES + OVERNIGHT COOLING • MAKES ABOUT 2 CUPS

"There's a silly song that I first heard Ella Fitzgerald sing about a secret sauce at a restaurant," said Chris DeBarr. "The secret stuff is called frim fram sauce, and I always believed that the secret signature had to have that New Orleans flavor." So he made his own version as a smoky roasted-tomato remoulade worthy of Ella's praises.

5 Roma tomatoes, cored and chopped

1 small or ½ large sweet onion, cut into fat half-moon slices

½ cup garlic cloves

1 tablespoon fine sea salt

4 tablespoons Spanish smoked paprika

3 tablespoons Chef Paul's Seafood Magic

2 teaspoons freshly ground black pepper

1 sprig fresh rosemary or 3 sprigs fresh thyme (optional)

¼ cup oil (use a neutral-flavored oil with a high smoke point, such as avocado or grapeseed oil)

¾ cup Creole mustard

2 heaping tablespoons prepared horseradish

1 tablespoon sweet paprika

1 tablespoon hot sauce (such as Crystal or Tabasco)

2 stalks celery, minced

8 scallions, minced

Preheat the oven to 400°F.

In a metal loaf pan, combine the tomatoes, onion, garlic, salt, 3 tablespoons of the smoked paprika, 2 tablespoons of the Seafood Magic, the pepper, and rosemary or thyme, if using, and toss to mix. Pour the oil over the top. Cover the pan with aluminum foil and roast in the oven for 1 hour.

Pull the pan out of the oven, give it a gentle stir, and return it to the oven for another 15 minutes.

Remove the pan from the oven and let it cool for 30 minutes to an hour, until it is still warm but no longer hot.

In a blender, combine the roasted tomato mixture with the remaining 1 tablespoon of smoked paprika, the remaining 1 tablespoon of Seafood Magic, the mustard, horseradish, sweet paprika, and hot sauce. Puree the mixture until smooth.

Let it cool completely, and then refrigerate overnight.

To finish, stir in the celery and scallions.

Black-Eyed Pea and Peanut Butter Hummus

TOTAL COOK TIME: 5 MINUTES • SERVES 6

Chef Chris DeBarr was one of the cooks who first introduced hummus to American dining guests back in the 1980s, before the chickpeas-and-tahini spread became ubiquitous across the country. Somehow it still took until the pandemic year of 2020 for him to imagine that the best Deep South version of hummus is to use black-eyed peas and peanut butter together!

Chris usually uses dried black-eyed peas in his cooking, giving them hearty doses of seasoning. For the hummus, though, he likes the plain meatiness of canned black-eyed peas. He makes up for the plainness of the peas with an extravagant multi-nut-and-seed "everything" crunchy nut butter from Fix & Fogg. You can use any peanut butter, but try to choose one without palm oil. If you can find a good roasted garlic olive oil, substitute that for the plain extra-virgin olive oil.

3 (14-ounce) cans black-eyed peas, drained

⅔ cup peanut butter

2 teaspoons ground cumin

½ teaspoon fine sea salt

½ teaspoon ground white pepper

2 teaspoons ground black urfa chili or 1 teaspoon ground Aleppo chili

2 tablespoons roasted garlic (see page 267)

⅓ cup extra-virgin olive oil

In a food processor, combine the black-eyed peas, peanut butter, cumin, salt, white pepper, ground chili, and garlic, and process until smooth.

With the processor running, slowly add the oil until the mixture is smooth and all the oil has been incorporated.

Grains, Beans, Nuts, and Moromiso Moringa Salad

TOTAL COOK TIME: 15 MINUTES • SERVES 4

The beauty of this salad is that you can add whatever your heart desires to this base. Moromiso is a product of the fermentation process used to make miso paste. It has much less sodium than soy sauce or table salt but adds umami to the dish. If you can't find moromiso, you can substitute miso paste mixed with a little bit of water to thin it out.

1 cup of packaged mixed grains (use a blend that combines rice, bulgur, barley, wheat berries, red rice, and/or quinoa)

2 cups water

2 tablespoons moromiso paste mixed with a little water

1 tablespoon sesame oil

2 tablespoons chickpeas

2 tablespoons black chickpeas

2 tablespoons pinto beans

1 tablespoon pumpkin seeds

1 tablespoon sunflower seeds

12 cherry tomatoes, halved

3 tablespoons cooked green beans, cut into 1-inch lengths

3 tablespoons fresh moringa leaves

6 fresh basil leaves, torn

2 tablespoons torn cilantro

1 tablespoon extra-virgin olive oil, for garnish

1 teaspoon nutritional yeast, for garnish

½ teaspoon bee pollen, for garnish

Add the grains to a medium saucepan with the water and bring to a boil. Reduce the heat to low and simmer for 10 minutes. Remove from the heat and let stand for 5 minutes. Fluff with a fork.

While the cooked grains are still warm, transfer them to a large bowl and stir in the moromiso and sesame oil.

Add the chickpeas, beans, pumpkin seeds, sunflower seeds, tomatoes, green beans, moringa, basil, and cilantro, and toss to mix.

Serve with a drizzle of olive oil and sprinkled with nutritional yeast and bee pollen.

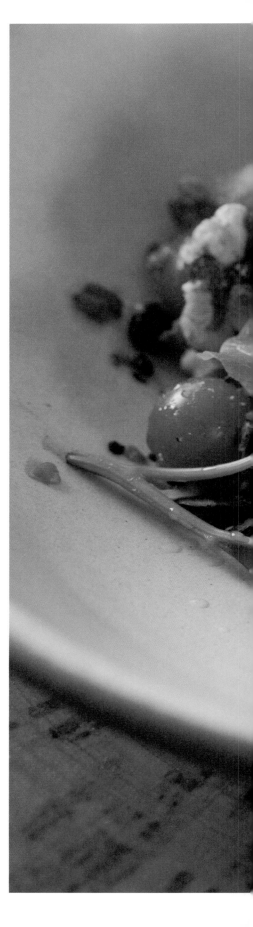

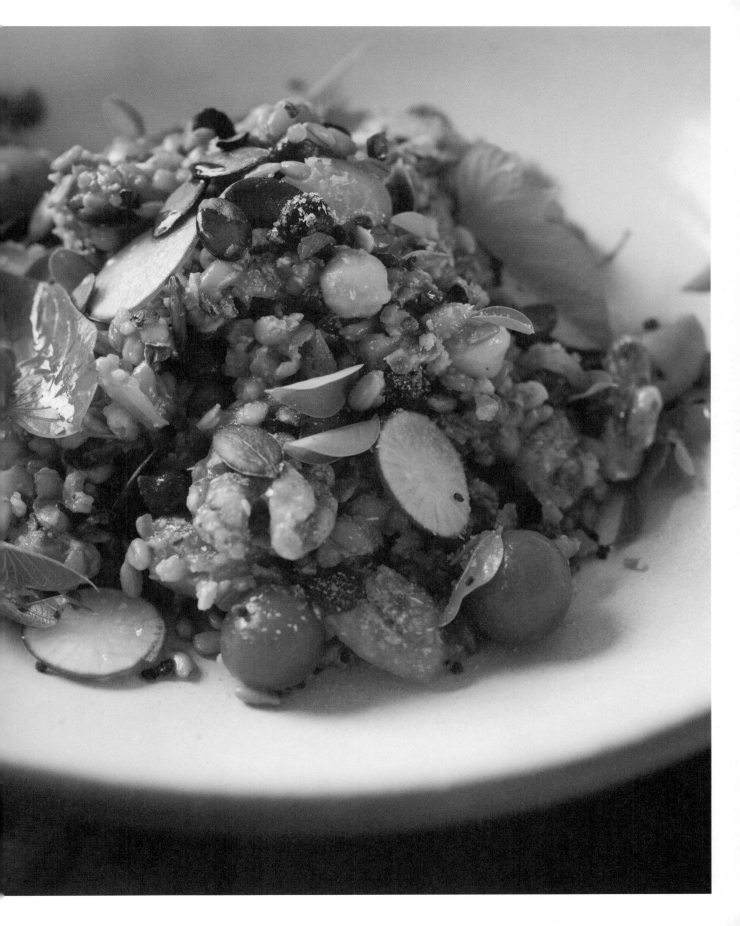

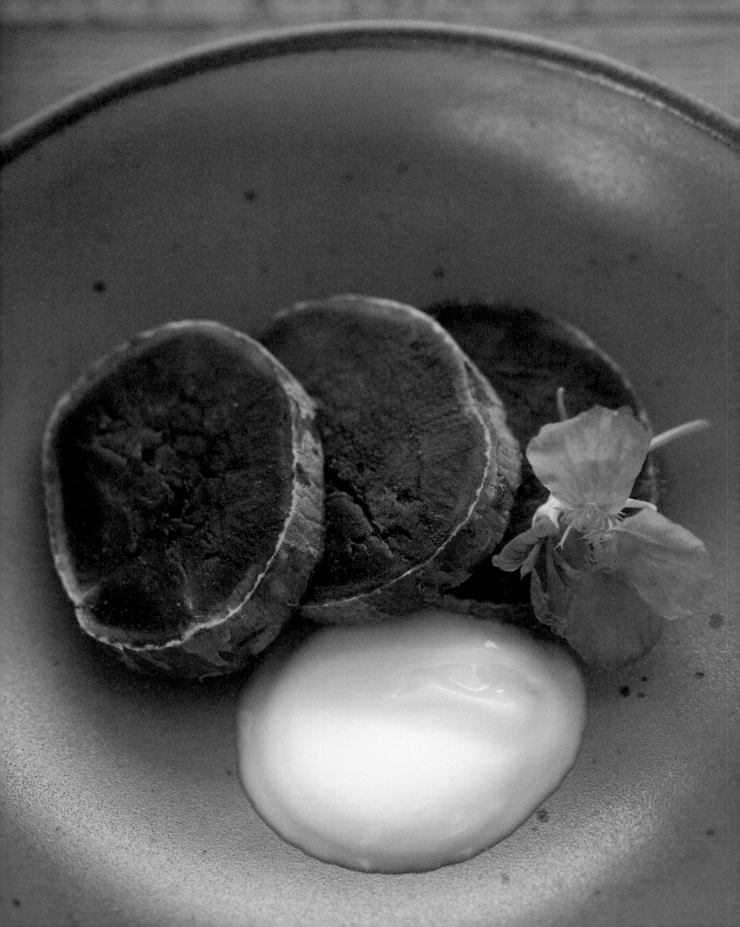

ALAN WONG CONTINUED

Roasted Okinawan Sweet Potato With Coconut Ginger Cream

TOTAL COOK TIME: 1 HOUR 10 MINUTES • SERVES 4

Okinawan sweet potatoes have been cultivated in Japan since the early 17th century and have long been a staple of Hawaiian cuisine. They usually have pale, tan skin and purple flesh. They become very sweet and creamy after cooking.

2 Okinawan sweet potatoes

1 (16-ounce) can coconut cream

6 to 8 thin slices peeled fresh ginger

2 tablespoons Wai Meli raw honey or your favorite honey

Preheat the oven to 350°F.

Sprinkle the sweet potatoes with a bit of olive oil and salt and wrap them in aluminum foil. Roast them in the oven for about 1 hour, or until a toothpick or skewer goes in nicely. The cooking time will depend on the size of the sweet potatoes.

Meanwhile, prepare the ginger cream. Combine the coconut cream and ginger slices in a medium saucepan over medium heat. Bring to a simmer and cook until the liquid is reduced by about 25 percent, 10 minutes or so.

Stir in the honey and then remove from the heat.

While the sweet potatoes are still warm, slice them into approximately ⅜-inch-thick round disks (with the skin left on).

Serve the sweet potato slices with the coconut ginger cream on the side for dipping.

NOTES
• Use a coconut cream that is thick and creamy.

• Look for a thick, creamy honey that won't thin out the coconut cream too much and will add lots of flavor.

Sweet Potato Gazpacho With Lomi Tomato Relish

TOTAL COOK TIME: 5 MINUTES • SERVES 3 TO 4

The word *lomi lomi* means "to massage" in the Hawaiian language. In pre-metal Hawaii, things were cut with a sharp rock or bones, or massaged by hand to soften or break them down.

A familiar dish at a luau today might be lomi lomi salmon, which uses salted salmon, an import from the Portuguese whalers who also brought bacalao (salted cod) and other salted meats to the islands in the early 1900s.

Chili pepper water was also from Portuguese sailors. The chili is high in vitamin C, which prevented scurvy during a long voyage at sea. Almost every household in Hawaii has a small bottle of their favorite chili pepper water to use as a condiment. In Alan Wong's restaurants, he keeps small cruets of soy sauce and chili pepper water on the table in lieu of salt and pepper.

FOR THE GAZPACHO:

1 medium or 2 small cooked sweet potatoes, peeled and diced into 1-inch pieces

2 ripe tomatoes, quartered

1½ cups water

2 teaspoons rice vinegar

¼ cup Hawaiian chili pepper water or hot sauce (such as Crystal or Tabasco), or to taste

Salt

FOR THE TOMATO RELISH:

¼ cup diced tomato

1 tablespoon finely diced onion

1 tablespoon thinly sliced scallion

Salt to taste

Chili pepper water or hot sauce

To make the gazpacho, in a blender or food processor, combine the cooked sweet potatoes and tomatoes. With the motor running, add the water slowly and then the vinegar, and puree until smooth. Add the chili pepper water and salt, and season to taste.

To make the tomato relish, in a stainless steel or glass bowl, combine all the ingredients.

To serve, ladle the gazpacho into bowls and top each with a dollop of the tomato relish.

NOTE
• Here's a quick way to make your potatoes ahead of time: Sprinkle the sweet potatoes with a bit of olive oil and salt and wrap them in aluminum foil. Roast them in a 350°F oven for about 1 hour, or until a toothpick or skewer goes in nicely. The cooking time will depend on the size of the sweet potatoes.

Mahaka Mango Cheeks
With Red Onion Shave Ice

TOTAL COOK TIME: OVERNIGHT • SERVES 4

FOR THE PICKLED RED JALAPEÑO:

4 teaspoons water

1 tablespoon raw, unprocessed
 Hawaiian Lehua honey or another
 honey

1 teaspoon rice vinegar

1 teaspoon white vinegar

½ teaspoon salt

1 red jalapeño, thinly sliced

FOR THE RED ONION SHAVE ICE:

½ red onion, diced large

1 cup water

1 red jalapeño pepper (seeded for a
 milder dish)

2 tablespoons freshly squeezed
 lime juice

Pinch of salt

FOR THE VEGAN NƯỚC CHẤM:

1½ tablespoons white soy sauce

1½ tablespoons powdered monk
 fruit sweetener

1½ tablespoons freshly squeezed
 lime juice

FOR THE MANGO CHEEKS:

4 mango cheeks (from 2 peeled
 mangos)

FOR THE GARNISHES:

Chopped basil

Chopped cilantro

Chopped mint

Chopped dill

Reserved pickled red jalapeño

To make the pickled red jalapeño, in a bowl, combine the water, honey, rice vinegar, white vinegar, and salt, and whisk to combine well, dissolving the honey and salt. Add the jalapeño slices and stir to coat. Cover and refrigerate for at least 24 hours.

To make the red onion shave ice, in a blender or food processor, combine all the ingredients and process until smooth. Pour the mixture into a stainless-steel bowl and freeze for a few hours.

When the mixture is frozen, scrape the ice with a spoon to create fine to medium-size ice granules. Keep frozen until ready to serve.

To make the vegan nước chấm, in a small bowl, stir together all the ingredients until the sweetener dissolves.

To serve, place the mango cheeks in a bowl, cut side down. Drizzle a tablespoon of the nước chấm mixture over the mango and let it drip into the bowl, slightly pooling around the fruit.

Garnish with the fresh herbs and pickled jalapeño, as desired, then top with about 2 tablespoons of the red onion shave ice.

NOTES
• White (shiro) soy sauce is made with more wheat and less soy than the regular soy sauce we're used to. The result is lighter in color and has a more delicate flavor. If you can't find it, you can substitute light soy sauce or a mixture of 2 parts regular soy sauce to one part water.

• A mango has two cheeks, one on either thick side of the pit.

Lentil and Mushroom Shepherd's Pie

TOTAL COOK TIME: 1 HOUR 40 MINUTES • SERVES 6

FOR THE MASHED POTATOES:

3 pounds russet potatoes, peeled and halved

4 to 5 tablespoons vegan butter

1 cup plant-based milk (such as oat milk)

3 tablespoons nutritional yeast

½ teaspoon nutmeg

1 teaspoon white pepper

Sea salt

FOR THE FILLING:

1½ cups dried brown or green lentils, soaked overnight and drained

4 cups filtered water

3 or 4 bay leaves

1 tablespoon olive oil

1 onion, diced

4 cloves garlic, minced

1 cup finely chopped cremini mushrooms

Pinch of sea salt

1 cup finely chopped carrots

1 cup finely chopped celery

2 teaspoons fresh thyme or 1 teaspoon dried thyme

2 teaspoons paprika

1 teaspoon smoked paprika

1 teaspoon ground cumin

½ teaspoon cayenne pepper

To make the mashed potatoes, in a large pot, cover the potatoes with water and bring to a low boil over medium-high heat. Season generously with salt, cover, and cook for 20 to 30 minutes, until the potatoes are very tender.

While the potatoes are cooking, preheat the oven to 425°F and lightly grease a 2-quart baking dish (or comparably sized dish, such as a 9-by-13-inch pan, or a cast-iron skillet).

Meanwhile, in a separate pot, start the filling: Combine the lentils with filtered water and bay leaves. Bring to a low boil. Cover and reduce the heat to a simmer. Cook until the lentils are tender, 35 to 40 minutes.

Drain the potatoes in a colander and then return them to the pot and let them stand for 5 minutes to give any remaining water a chance to evaporate.

Transfer the potatoes to a mixing bowl. Use a potato masher, pastry cutter, or large fork to mash the potatoes until smooth. Stir in the vegan butter, plant-based milk, nutritional yeast, nutmeg, white pepper, and salt. Cover loosely and set aside.

Once the lentils are tender, remove the lid and continue simmering, uncovered and stirring frequently, to evaporate any excess liquid.

To make the filling, in a large saucepan over medium heat, heat the olive oil until it shimmers. Add the onion and garlic, and cook, stirring occasionally, until they begin to brown, about 5 minutes. Add the mushrooms and a generous pinch of salt, and cook, stirring occasionally, until the mushrooms are caramelized, about 5 minutes more. Add the carrots and celery.

Add the lentils to the saucepan with the vegetables along with thyme, paprika, smoked paprika, cumin, and cayenne. Stir to mix and then taste and adjust the seasoning if needed.

Transfer the lentil mixture to the prepared baking dish and top with the mashed potatoes, smoothing the layer of potatoes with a spoon or fork. Place the baking dish on a baking sheet to catch any overflow. Bake for 10 to 15 minutes, until the potatoes are lightly browned on top. Remove from the oven and let cool briefly before serving.

Pasta-less Veggie Puttanesca Lasagna

TOTAL COOK TIME: 1 HOUR 30 MINUTES • SERVES 9

FOR THE VEGAN RICOTTA:

3 cups raw almonds, soaked in water for at least 6 hours or overnight, drained and peeled

2 tablespoons nutritional yeast

2 tablespoons freshly squeezed lemon juice

1 tablespoon olive oil (optional)

1 teaspoon salt

Pinch of freshly ground black pepper

½ cup water, plus additional as needed

FOR THE PUTTANESCA SAUCE:

1 tablespoon olive oil

3 cloves garlic, minced

2 tablespoons fresh rosemary

1 onion, diced

1 (15-ounce) can tomato sauce

2 tablespoons capers

½ cup water or as needed

FOR THE LASAGNA:

2 tablespoons olive oil

1 large onion, diced

2 cups cremini mushrooms

2 to 3 medium zucchini, thinly sliced with a mandolin

1 medium eggplant, thinly sliced with a mandolin

Preheat the oven to 375°F.

To make the vegan ricotta, in a food processor or blender, process the almonds to a fine meal, scraping down the sides as needed.

Add the nutritional yeast, lemon juice, olive oil, if using, salt, pepper, and water, and process to a smooth puree. Add more water a little at a time if the mixture is too dry.

Taste and adjust the seasonings as needed, adding more salt and pepper for flavor, nutritional yeast for cheesiness, and lemon juice for brightness.

To make the puttanesca sauce, in a skillet, heat the olive oil over medium-high heat. Add the garlic, rosemary, and onion, and cook, stirring occasionally, until the onion is caramelized, about 8 minutes. Add the tomato sauce and capers. Cook for a few minutes more, until everything is heated through. Add up to ½ cup of water, if needed, to achieve a saucy consistency.

To make the lasagna, in a skillet over medium-high heat, heat the olive oil. Add the onion and mushrooms and cook, stirring occasionally, until softened, about 5 minutes.

Pour about 1 cup of the puttanesca sauce into a 9-by-13-inch baking dish. Layer the zucchini slices, the eggplant slices, and the onion-mushroom mixture in the baking dish. Add small spoonfuls of the ricotta mixture on top of the vegetables and gently spread it into an even layer. Top with a layer of the puttanesca sauce. Repeat until all the ingredients have been used up, ending with a layer of zucchini slices and a layer of sauce.

Bake, covered, for 1 hour, until the zucchini and eggplant are very easily pierced with a knife.

Remove from the oven and let cool for 10 to 15 minutes before serving.

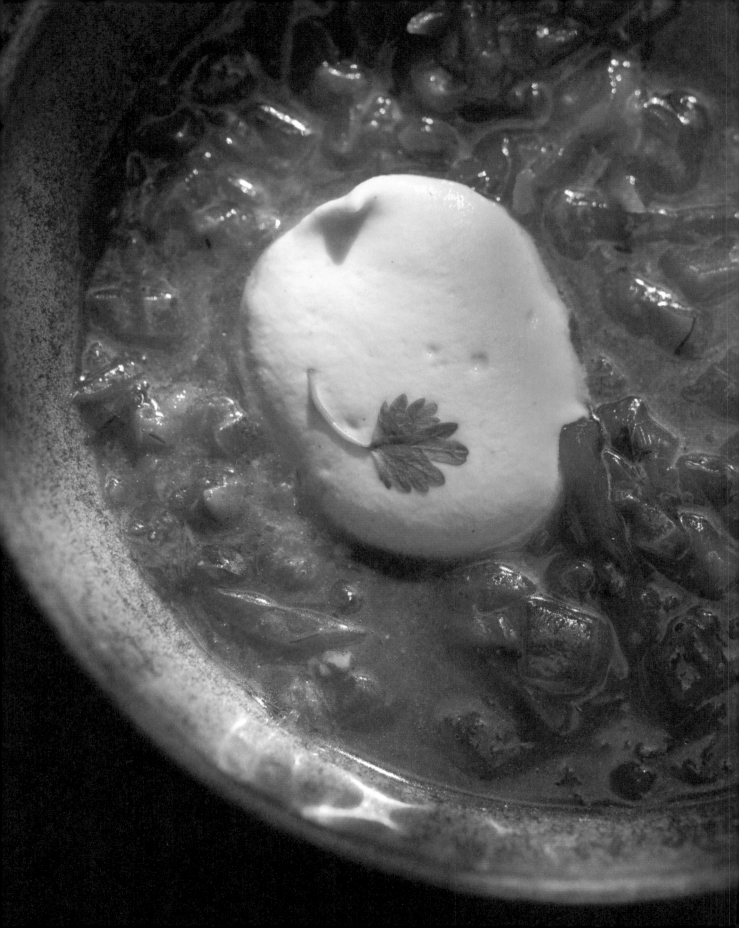

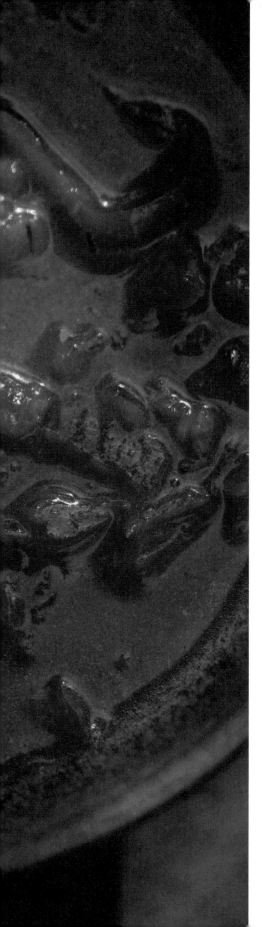

Modern Borscht

TOTAL COOK TIME: 1 HOUR 45 MINUTES + 10 HOURS SOAKING •
SERVES 4

½ cup beans of your choice, soaked
overnight and drained

6 cups vegetable broth

2 cups filtered water

½ small cabbage, chopped

1 large carrot, peeled and julienned

2 medium beets, peeled and
julienned

1 tablespoon lemon juice

1 medium sweet potato, diced into
medium cubes

2 to 3 bay leaves

½ large onion, diced large

1 teaspoon grapeseed oil

1 to 2 teaspoons tomato paste

3 cloves garlic, pressed

1 large red bell pepper, julienned

1 cup sauerkraut (optional)

¼ cup unsweetened coconut milk
(optional)

Salt

Freshly ground black pepper

1 cup cilantro, chopped

½ cup dill, chopped

Add the drained beans to a large
pot, cover with them water, and
bring to a boil. Lower to a simmer,
and cook for 45 minutes to 1 hour,
or until the desired tenderness.
Drain and set aside.

In a large soup pot, bring the
vegetable broth and filtered
water to a boil. Add the cabbage,
carrot, and beets to the broth.
Reduce to a simmer. Squeeze the
lemon in immediately to keep the
color of the broth.

Add the sweet potato and bay
leaves to the broth.

In a large sauté pan, sauté the
onion with the grapeseed oil.
Once the onion is softened, add it
to the pot of broth along with the
tomato paste, garlic, red bell pepper, and beans, as well as the sauerkraut and coconut milk, if using.
Bring to a simmer over medium-
high heat and cook until the vegetables are fork-tender. Add salt
and pepper to taste.

Turn off the heat and garnish with
the cilantro and dill.

Raw Okroshka Soup

TOTAL COOK TIME: 5 MINUTES + 30 MINUTES FOR SOAKING • SERVES 4

FOR THE BROTH:

1 cup cashews, soaked for at least 30 minutes

2 cups water, plus 1 cup of sparkling water (or 3 cups regular water)

2 tablespoons nutritional yeast

1 tablespoon champagne vinegar or wine vinegar

½ teaspoon lemon zest

1 clove fresh garlic

Salt to taste

Freshly ground black pepper to taste

FOR THE VEGETABLES:

2 to 3 cucumbers, cut into small dice

5 radishes, cut into small dice

2 avocados, cut into small dice

½ cup chopped dill

2 tablespoons chopped green onions

1 tablespoon radish sprouts

1 tablespoon onion sprouts

To make the broth, in a blender, blend the cashews, 2 cups of regular water (or 3 if you aren't using sparkling water), the yeast, vinegar, lemon zest, garlic, salt, and pepper, until smooth.

To assemble the soup, place all the vegetables into bowls for serving. Pour the broth over the vegetables and add the sparkling water, if using, to the broth right before serving.

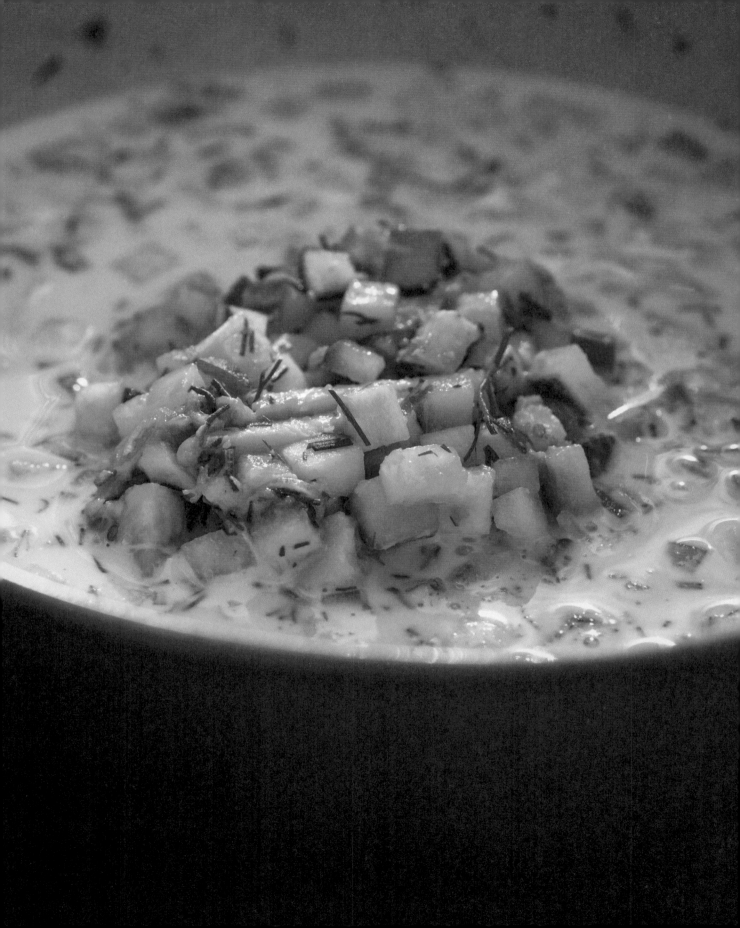

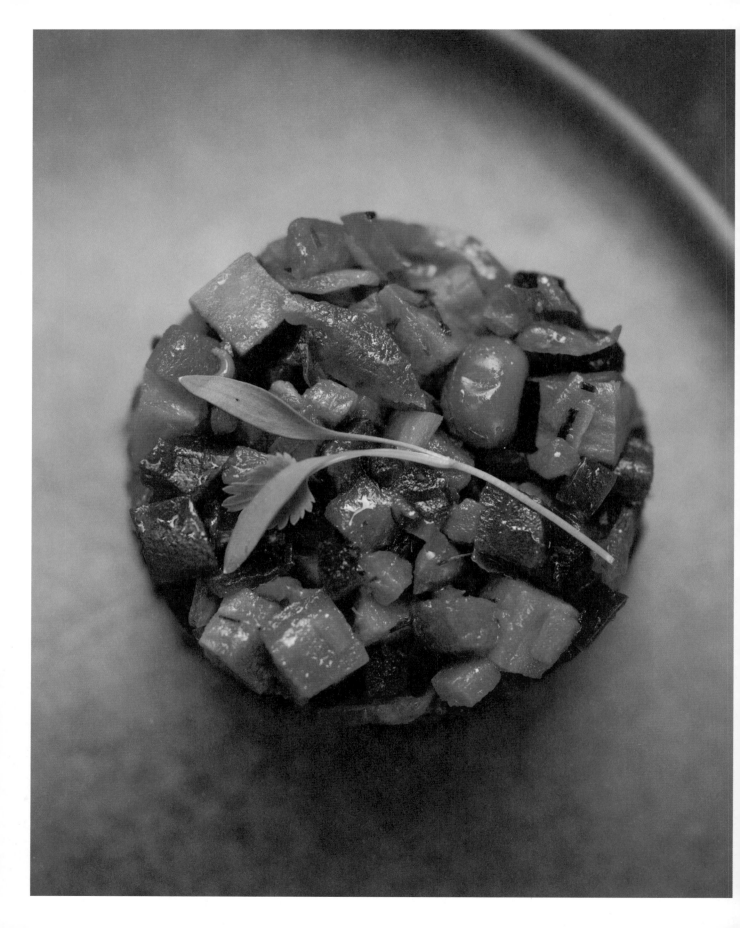

The Better Vinaigrette Salad

TOTAL COOK TIME: 6 HOURS • SERVES 4 TO 6

FOR THE SALAD:

½ cup navy beans, soaked overnight and drained

5 medium beets, scrubbed

3 medium sweet potatoes, scrubbed

2 carrots

½ cup frozen peas

½ cup diced pickled cucumbers

½ cup sauerkraut

½ cup diced raw Persian cucumbers

2 tablespoons olive oil

½ tablespoon apple vinegar

Salt

½ cup finely chopped green onion

Add the beans to a large pot. Cover with more than 3 inches of water, bring to a boil, and then reduce to a simmer. Simmer for 45 minutes to 1 hour, tasting after 45 minutes to get the desired tenderness.

Fill a separate large pot with enough water to cover the beets and bring to a boil. Add the beets and cook for 45 minutes to 1 hour, checking after 45 minutes to reach the desired tenderness.

In separate pots, boil the carrots and sweet potatoes for 30 minutes each until their skins easily come off with a fork or knife. Drain the vegetables and refrigerate them or let them sit in an ice bath until chilled.

Peel the skin from the beets, sweet potatoes, and carrots, and finely dice them into even cubes.

In a separate pot, boil the frozen peas for 6 to 8 minutes. Drain and cool to room temperature.

In a large mixing bowl, add all the vegetables, oil, vinegar, and salt to taste. Mix to combine.

Allow the ingredients to sit together for at least 2 to 3 hours (or overnight).

Serve topped with the green onion.

Blue Zones Food Guidelines

These 11 simple guidelines reflect how
the world's longest-lived people ate for most of their lives.

1 • ENSURE THAT YOUR DIET IS 90 TO 100 PERCENT PLANT-BASED

While people in four of the five blue zones consume meat, they do so sparingly, using it as a celebratory food, a small side, or as a way to flavor dishes. People in the blue zones eat an impressive variety of garden vegetables and leafy greens (especially spinach, kale, beet and turnip tops, chard, and collards) when they are in season; they pickle or dry the surplus to enjoy during the off-season. Beans, greens, sweet potatoes, whole grains, fruits, nuts, and seeds dominate blue zones meals all year long. Olive oil is also a staple in the blue zones. Evidence shows that olive oil consumption increases good cholesterol and lowers bad cholesterol. In Ikaria, for example, we found that for middle-aged people, about six tablespoons of olive oil daily seemed to cut the risk of premature mortality in half.

2 • RETREAT FROM MEAT

Averaging out consumption across the blue zones, we found that people ate about two ounces or less of meat about five times per month.

The Adventist Health Study 2, which has been following 96,000 Americans since 2002, has determined that the people who lived the longest were vegans or pesco-vegetarians who ate a small amount of fish. Vegetarian Adventists will likely outlive their meat-eating counterparts by as many as eight years.

While you may want to celebrate from time to time with meat, we don't recommend it as part of a Blue Zones diet. Okinawans probably offer the best meat substitute: extra-firm tofu, which is high in protein and cancer-fighting phytoestrogens.

3 • GO EASY ON FISH

If you must eat fish, consume fewer than three ounces up to three times weekly. In most blue zones, people eat small amounts of fish, up to three small servings a week. Usually, the fish that they eat are small, relatively inexpensive varieties like sardines, anchovies, and cod—middle-of-the-food-chain species that are not exposed to the high levels of mercury or other chemicals that pollute our gourmet fish supply today.

Again, fish is not a necessary part of a longevity diet, but if you must eat it, select varieties that are common and not threatened by overfishing.

4 • REDUCE DAIRY

Cow's milk doesn't figure significantly in any Blue Zones diet (except that of some Adventists). Goat and sheep milk products figure prominently into the Ikarian and Sardinian blue zones. We don't know if it's the goat's milk or sheep's milk that makes people healthier, or if it's the fact that they climb up and down the same hilly terrain as the goats. Interestingly, though, most goat's milk is consumed not as liquid, but as yogurt, sour milk, or cheese.

5 • CUT DOWN ON EGGS

People in all the blue zones eat eggs about two to four times per week. Usually they eat just one as a side: Nicoyans fold an egg and beans into corn tortillas; Okinawans boil an egg in soup; those in Mediterranean blue zones—Sardinia and Ikaria—fry an egg to eat with bread, almonds, and olives for breakfast. Blue zones eggs come from chickens that range freely and don't receive hormones or antibiotics.

People with diabetes and heart disease often limit their egg consumption for health reasons. Eggs aren't a key component for living a long life, so we don't recommend them—but if you must eat them, try to eat no more than three per week.

6 • EAT A DAILY DOSE OF BEANS

Beans reign supreme in the blue zones and are the cornerstone of every longevity diet in the world: black beans in Nicoya; lentils, garbanzo, and white beans in the Mediterranean; and soybeans in Okinawa. People in the blue zones eat at least four times as many beans as Americans do on average—at least a half cup per day—and so should you.

Why? Beans are packed with more nutrients per gram than any other food on Earth. On average, they are made up of 21 percent protein, 77 percent complex carbohydrates, and only a few percent fat. Because they are fiber-rich and satisfying, they'll likely help to push less-healthy foods out of your diet.

7 • SLASH SUGAR

Consume only 28 grams (7 teaspoons) of added sugar daily. People in the blue zones eat sugar intentionally, not by habit or accident. They consume about the same amount of naturally occurring sugars as North Americans do, but only about a fifth as much added sugar—no more than seven teaspoons a day. Between 1970 and 2000, the amount of added sugar in the American food supply rose by 25 percent (about 22 teaspoons of added sugar per day)—generally, the result of the insidious, hidden sugars mixed into soda, yogurt, and sauces.

If you must eat sweets, save cookies, candy, and bakery items for special occasions—ideally as part of a meal. Limit sugar added to coffee, tea, or other foods to no more than four teaspoons per day. Skip any product that lists sugar among its first five ingredients.

8 • SNACK ON NUTS
Eat two handfuls of nuts per day. A handful weighs about two ounces, the average amount that blue zones centenarians consume: almonds in Ikaria and Sardinia, pistachios in Nicoya, and all varieties of nuts with the Adventists. The Adventist Health Study 2 found that nut eaters outlive non-nut eaters by an average of two to three years. So try to snack on a couple handfuls of almonds, Brazil nuts, cashews, walnuts, and/or peanuts every day.

9 • SOUR ON BREAD
If you can, strive to eat only sourdough or 100 percent whole wheat bread. Most commercially available breads start with bleached white flour, which metabolizes quickly into sugar and spikes insulin levels. But blue zones bread is either whole grain or sourdough; in Ikaria and Sardinia, breads are made from a variety of whole grains such as wheat, rye, or barley, each of which offers a wide spectrum of nutrients.

Whole grains have higher levels of fiber than most commonly used bleached flours. Some traditional blue zones breads are made with naturally occurring bacteria called lactobacilli, which "digest" the starches and glutens while making the bread rise. The process also creates an acid—the "sour" in sourdough. The result is bread with less gluten than breads labeled "gluten free," with a longer shelf life and a pleasantly sour taste that most people like. Traditional sourdough breads actually lower the glycemic load of meals, making your entire meal healthier, slower burning, easier on your pancreas, and more likely to make calories available as energy than stored as fat.

10 • GO WHOLE
Strive to eat foods that are recognizable. People in the blue zones traditionally eat whole foods, which are made from a single ingredient—raw, cooked, ground, or fermented—and are not highly processed. Residents eat raw fruits and vegetables; they grind whole grains themselves and then cook them slowly. They use fermentation—an ancient way to make nutrients bioavailable—in the tofu, sourdough bread, wine, and pickled vegetables they eat.

And they rarely ingest artificial preservatives. Blue zones dishes typically contain a half dozen or so ingredients, simply blended together.

11 • DRINK MOSTLY WATER
If possible, strive to avoid soft drinks (including diet soda). With very few exceptions, people in blue zones drink only coffee, tea, water, and wine. (Soft drinks, which account for about half of Americans' sugar intake, were unknown to most blue zones centenarians until recently.) Here's why:

Water: Adventists recommend seven glasses of water daily. They point to studies showing that being hydrated facilitates blood flow and lessens the chance of a blood clot.

Coffee: Sardinians, Ikarians, and Nicoyans all drink coffee. Research associates coffee drinking with lower rates of dementia and Parkinson's disease.

Tea: People in every blue zone drink tea. Okinawans prefer green varieties, which have been shown to lower the risk of heart disease and several cancers. Ikarians drink brews of rosemary, wild sage, and dandelion—all herbs known to have anti-inflammatory properties.

Red wine: People who drink—in moderation—tend to outlive those who don't. (This doesn't mean you should start drinking if you don't drink now.) People in most blue zones drink one to three small glasses of red wine per day, often with a meal and with friends.

Contributors

I am grateful to the chefs, home cooks, and food historians who let us into their kitchens. We shared delicious plates of food, remarkable stories, and laughs along the way. For their contributions to my research and sharing their recipes in these pages, I give many thanks. They include the following:

NICO ALBERT, of the Cherokee Nation, is a self-taught chef, caterer, and student of Indigenous cuisine. Raised in California and Arizona, she returned to Tulsa, Oklahoma, the land of her mother's people, to reestablish a relationship with her Cherokee community. Her passion also drives her to improve the health and wellness of Native Americans. She is the owner of Burning Cedar Indigenous Foods, a catering, educational, and consulting service specializing in Native cuisine. *Pages 42–45*

MARIA ALEMANN learned to cook from her mother, aunts, and grandmother in their family kitchen. She was born in Argentina and grew up surrounded by meat, bread, and wine. Then, after working at a steakhouse in 2011, something clicked and she decided never to eat meat again. That's when her vegetarian journey began. Today, she is the chef behind The Plantisserie, an organic deli and market where she makes and sells artisanal, organic, and plant-based foods—all prepared from scratch—in Miami, Florida. *Pages 276–277*

TENAGNE BELACHEW is the chef behind Lalibela Ethiopian in Los Angeles, which she runs along with her six daughters and son. The restaurant's name comes from a town in Ethiopia that is known for its churches; Tenagne grew up nearby in Wole, where she learned to cook recipes passed down from her grandmother and mother. The family's restaurant embodies her native home's cultures and culinary traditions. *Pages 100–101*

ALAN BERGO, aka the Forager Chef, is a Minnesota native who loves to hunt for wild mushrooms. A 15-year veteran of the culinary industry, he worked for chefs in Italy and in James Beard Award–nominated restaurants in St. Paul. Now he is the leading authority on foraging and cooking wild mushrooms and plants, and he shares his knowledge and recipes at foragerchef.com. He is the author of *The Forager Chef's Book of Flora. Pages 242–245*

ROOSEVELT BROWNLEE is a Vietnam War veteran who spent years touring the European and Montreal jazz festival circuit, where he cooked for touring musicians. He's served food to the likes of Muddy Waters, Nina Simone, and Dizzy Gillespie. A Georgia native son, he continues to sell food at festivals closer to his home in Savannah.

ROGER BUETTNER is author Dan Buettner's father and the man who inspired him to seek adventure. He often took Dan canoeing and camping in the Boundary Waters and backpacking out west. At 85 years old, he's still going strong. A tried-and-true, meat-and-potatoes type of guy, he taste-tested every dish in these pages to make sure the average American, like him, would enjoy them. Consider this book Roger Buettner approved! *Pages 238–239*

SYLVIA CASARES is Houston's "Enchilada Queen." The chef and restaurateur is the owner of Sylvia's Enchilada Kitchen, where her flavorful menu includes 19 different enchilada varieties. She began her career as a food scientist for Uncle Ben's Rice, where she learned that flavor means always choosing the best ingredients and refusing shortcuts. With this wisdom, and her passion for the delicious flavors of authentic Mexican cuisine, she built her enchilada empire. She is also the author of *The Enchilada Queen Cookbook. Pages 129–131*

MARION "ROLLEN" CHALMERS grew up in Hardeeville, South Carolina, where he began growing Carolina Gold rice and Charleston Gold rice in 2010. He also grows the heritage crop on Daufuskie Island, which marks the first time Carolina Gold has been grown on the island in more than 100 years. A passionate woodsman who enjoys the outdoors, he credits his patience, humble spirit, and positive attitude for his successful harvests. *Pages 90–93*

RUTH CHANG will tell you that she made it to 94 years old with the help of a steady diet of tofu and cod liver oil, which she had a spoonful of every night as a child. Her sisters are 90 and 96. With a master's degree in social work, she learned to cook out of necessity after having children—learning from a Chinese friend and her church how to make the foods of her childhood. Her philosophy: Life starts at 60—enjoy it, your people, and your family. *Pages 160–163*

CAMRYN CLEMENTS is "just a person, not a chef" as she puts it. The home cook knows her stuff: After her husband discovered fatty liver disease runs in his family, they decided to shift to a plant-based diet for disease prevention and overall better health. With French ancestry, Camryn only knew how to cook Cajun cuisine, which she had picked up from her mother. She decided to take her favorite recipes—rice and gravy, étouffée, and cornbread, among others—and make them plant-based. That was three years ago. Today, she and her family continue to eat a plant-based diet, proof that you don't need a culinary education to change your lifestyle. *Pages 226–229*

CHRIS DEBARR is the executive chef behind a super-secret dinner club in New Orleans. He has been cooking and eating plant-based food since the 1980s and says plants have secret lives: "You open them up, and you get so many things." Born in Pensacola, Florida, he learned how to cook because it was cheaper than eating out. He spent time in restaurants in Dallas, Texas, and Athens, Georgia, before landing in New Orleans, where he has been for 25 years. *Pages 266–269*

BJ DENNIS is a chef and the leading expert on Gullah Geechee culture and cuisine. Based in Bluffton, South Carolina, he leads the food program at the International African American Museum (IAAM), where he creates a menu based on his Gullah Geechee heritage. Before joining the IAAM, he often hosted Gullah Geechee pop-up restaurants around Charleston. "Keeping the culture of the Low Country alive is important and necessary," he says. "Gullah Geechee is the heartbeat and soul of Low Country culture." *Pages 82–83*

NATALIE GOLBA was born in Russia, where her parents—both doctors—emphasized the importance of nutrition and farm-to-table foods. After a successful career in modeling in both Russia and the United States, she is now a trained personal chef based in Los Angeles. Along with sharing her knowledge of healthy cuisine with her clients, she shares her recipes and nutrition plans on her website, Naughty Delicious. *Pages 278–281*

BILL GREEN is the renowned "Gullah Chef." A farmer and huntsman, he is also the owner of the Gullah Grub Restaurant in the historic Low Country of St. Helena Island, South Carolina. At the restaurant, he and his family have been preparing authentic Gullah meals for more than 15 years. They follow the heritage traditions: Eat in season and eat locally. *Pages 84–87*

KATINA HANSEN is the chef and owner of Blue Ridge Bakery in Brevard, North Carolina, where the pies, cookies, pastries, and lunches are made fresh daily using only regional recipes and local ingredients. She's also an example of how the Blue Zones diet and lifestyle works: After making the decision to change her life, she followed the Blue Zones guidelines and lost 100 pounds by eating better and walking in the mountains. She now offers Blue Zones–inspired recipes on her bakery's lunch menu. *Pages 224–225*

JUAN HERNANDEZ is the executive chef of Gjelina in Los Angeles. He came to the United States at 15 years old from Oaxaca, Mexico, with an intimate knowledge of corn, tomatoes, and chickpeas. He worked his way up through kitchens in California until finding his place at his celebrated restaurant in Venice Beach. His love of fresh produce from local farms (he started helping his father on the family farm at seven years old) inspires the restaurant's dishes, but he also draws heavily from childhood memories of watching his mom in the kitchen. *Pages 250–253*

KIM HUYNH AND VIET PHAM are the chefs and co-owners of Good Vibes Cafe in Huntington Beach, California, where the motto is "From Soul to Bowl." Specializing in vegetarian and vegan cuisine, Kim, a Vietnam native, comes by her veganism naturally—her mother, a religious Buddhist, was vegan and raised her as such. She came to America in 1975 and has cooked for temple monks, hosted the Dalai Lama, and owned vegetarian restaurants for more than 30 years. *Pages 204–205, 246–249*

MATT JOHNSON is the sous chef at Thirty Nine Restaurant at the First Americans Museum in Oklahoma City, Oklahoma. A member of the Cherokee Nation, he contributes to a menu that brings awareness to the culinary distinctions between tribes and the cultural history behind Indigenous recipes. *Pages 46–47*

SOPHY KHUT escaped from Cambodia with her family in 1975. In 2000, she moved to Long Beach, California, home to the country's largest Cambodian community, where she opened Sophy's Restaurant, now called Sophy's: Cambodia Town Food and Music. The restaurant is a Long Beach institution, and Khut takes pleasure in introducing Americans to Cambodian cuisine, which she learned to make from her family's long line of chefs. *Page 153*

RACHEL KLEIN is the chef and owner of Miss Rachel's Pantry, a South Philadelphia restaurant and catering company that specializes in vegan and eco-friendly fare. An alum of Philly's renowned Vedge Restaurant, she turned lemons into lemonade during the pandemic, when catering wasn't so in demand, by creating and delivering meal kits of vegan comfort food to customers. *Pages 220–221*

RICH LANDAU is the chef and owner of Philadelphia's Vedge Restaurant and Fancy Radish. A pioneer of the modern plant-based dining experience, he aims to translate vegan cuisine to a broader audience. He and his wife and business partner, Kate Jacoby, cooked the first ever vegan meal served at the James Beard House in Manhattan. (Kate is a James Beard Award–nominated pastry chef and certified sommelier.) Rich has won many awards, including the James Beard Foundation's Best Chef: Mid-Atlantic and *Philadelphia Magazine*'s Best Chef in Philadelphia, and he won his episode of the Food Network's *Chopped*. *Page 234*

KEITH LIM learned his culinary techniques from his grandmother, who lived to 96, his mother (to 99), and his aunt (to 101). He learned his culinary techniques from them, and the lessons are straightforward: Eat your vegetables and avoid processed foods. He grew up on Chinese cabbage, beans, squash, and watercress, which are essential ingredients in the food he cooks today. His wife, Karen Dureg, is a registered nurse at Kaiser Permanente, where she helps doctors—and their patients—eat better, including teaching techniques to go vegan. They live in Honolulu, Hawaii. *Pages 164–165*

CLAUDIO LOBINA is the executive chef of the Patio at the Continuum in Miami, Florida. He was born and raised in Milan, Italy, and his family has a long tradition and passion for Italian cuisine. After meeting his Cuban wife, he moved to the United States in 2010 and started working at Puntino, an Italian restaurant in Key Biscayne, Florida. After establishing an authentic style of regional Italian cuisine, he joined the Patio in 2019, where he implements a unique menu of flavors with the highest-quality ingredients. *Pages 260–263*

CLAUDIA LOPEZ was born in El Salvador and moved to the United States when the country's civil war made life in her home country too dangerous. She graduated from the University of Southern California's Marshall School of Business in 2003 and spent nine years working for General Motors and AstraZeneca. Unhappy with her career, she decided to go after her dream of starting her own business. It began with selling artisanal candies and baked goods from El Salvador at Los Angeles farmers markets. Fast-forward to Claudia becoming chef and owner of the restaurant Mama's International Tamales,

where she specializes in plant-based dishes from Latin America. Her restaurant has won awards and was named one of PETA's top 10 Latinx-owned vegan restaurants. *Pages 126–128*

PAULA MARCOUX is a food historian who consults with museums, film producers, and publishers about the bygone pathways of food history and culture. She has worked professionally as an archaeologist, cook, and bread-oven builder and is the food editor of *Edible South Shore and South Coast* magazine, where she writes on food history. She also gives regular workshops on natural leavening, historic baking, and wood-fired cooking in her hometown of Plymouth, Massachusetts. *Pages 60–65*

NICOLE MARQUIS is the chef and owner of HipCityVeg in Philadelphia and Washington, D.C., and Philadelphia's Bar Bombón (a Latin-inspired restaurant reminiscent of those in Puerto Rico's Old San Juan) and Charlie Was a Sinner. A graduate of Temple University and the California Institute of the Arts in Los Angeles, she is part of the wave of health-conscious professionals leading a restaurant renaissance. Her award-winning HipCityVeg offers bold flavors with a 100 percent plant-based menu. The fast-food-inspired dishes are meant to be novel yet familiar, so diners can easily and happily discover a new way of healthy living and eating. *Pages 112–117*

SERIGNE MBAYE has worked at Michelin-starred restaurants around the country, most recently heading up New Orleans's Dakar Nola, named after his hometown in Senegal. The chef is inspired by the West African traditions that influenced many familiar New Orleans dishes (rice dishes cooked in one pot like jambalaya and a Senegalese gumbo made with okra). The fine-dining cuisine at Dakar Nola puts Senegalese food on the forefront in modern and innovative ways. *Pages 94–97*

DAVE SMOKE MCCLUSKEY is an Indigenous foods educator and member of the Mohawk Nation. He's also a chef and the founder of a movement he calls the Corn Mafia: In partnership with the Congaree Milling Company, he works alongside seed savers and growers to nixtamalize and coarsely grind hominy grits for chefs and specialty stores. His work with the Corn Mafia and the purpose of his cooking are part of his effort to make people think about the history of the ingredients in their meals. *Pages 38–41*

ADÁN MEDRANO is a chef, food writer, filmmaker, and the author of *Truly Texas Mexican: A Native Culinary Heritage in Recipes* and *"Don't Count the Tortillas": The Art of Texas Mexican Cooking*. After more than 23 years traveling and working throughout Latin America, he returned to the United States in 2010 to focus on the culinary traditions of the Mexican American community. A graduate of the Culinary Institute of America, he celebrates Indigenous traditions in his food and educational courses. He is also an award-winning filmmaker and the founder of the CineFestival San Antonio, the longest-running Latino film festival in the United States. *Pages 124–125*

ANNA NEEDHAM is the CEO of Mood Food Organic Catering and Tao Natural Foods. She has more than 15 years of practical experience and 20 years of work experience in natural health. Tao is a 50-year-old organic wellness shop that specializes in meals and herbal remedies for sustained health. *Pages 208–209*

VINH "KATHY" NGUYEN was born in Saigon and came to the United States in 1983 to find freedom. In the 1990s she hosted a cooking show on the radio in Vietnamese and was the host of *Cooking at My Kitchen* on Vietnamese TV. She is considered a "Rachael Ray of Vietnam," of sorts. Today, she hosts a YouTube cooking show, but mostly cooks for her family of 12. *Pages 166–171*

SUZAN LEE PAEK came to the United States from South Korea when she was two years old. Though she came to America at an early age, her diet was 70 percent Korean growing up—soybean-based soup for breakfast and grilled tofu or grilled fish for dinner. She raised her children on the same meals. Today, she works with the Fellowship, crafting dishes for the National Prayer Breakfast, which has been attended by every president since Eisenhower. She considers her food similar to her mother's but westernized. *Pages 192–193*

CHAD PHUONG is the chef behind Cambodian Cuisine and Battambong BBQ, a Texas-meets-Cambodia-style pop-up that serves Southern-style fare with Cambodian flair in Long Beach, California. Alongside his sandwiches are traditionally Cambodian eats, including Cambodian corn and a veggie "coleslaw," a medley of pickled cabbage, cucumber, and carrots. The pop-up is named after the countryside where he and his family would hunt and forage for food in Cambodia until they moved to Long Beach in the early 1980s. At 21, he moved to Hereford, Texas, where he became infatuated with barbecue and eventually melded these two traditions. *Pages 196–197*

HENRY PINEDA is the chef and owner of Modern Filipino Kitchen (MFK) by Aysee. The restaurant's origins began in the Philippines in 1986, with a restaurant called Aysee that inspired his own endeavors. Half Guatemalan and half Filipino, Henry modernizes traditional dishes, including

the *kamayan* feast, to reflect the rich history of his family's home country in every bite. *Pages 188–191*

MATTHEW RAIFORD is the James Beard Award–nominated chef behind Gilliard Farms, just west of Brunswick, Georgia. The farm was first purchased by his great-great-grandfather more than 150 years ago. Today, Matthew honors his Gullah Geechee roots tending the farm and creating authentic farm-to-fork experiences. He received his certification as an ecological horticulturalist from the Center for Agroecology at the University of California, Santa Cruz. In 2015, he and his partner, Jovan Sage, a food alchemist, opened the Farmer and the Larder to help jump-start the revival of Brunswick's historic downtown. *Pages 78–81*

JUAN RODRIGUEZ from a young age traveled between his home in Chicago to Monterrey, Mexico, where he spent time with his grandmother Magdalena in her kitchen. After obtaining a degree in the culinary arts from the Art Institute of Dallas and spending 15 years working his way up in kitchens, he is now the chef and owner of Magdalena's Catering and Events, created to honor his grandmother's legacy and follow her culinary traditions. Once a month, he and his wife, Paige, host a supper club for their Fort Worth, Texas, community. *Pages 118–121*

STEPHEN ROUELLE is the chef and owner of Under the Bodhi Tree in Pahoa on the Big Island in Hawaii. The restaurant serves vegan dishes, with vegetables and fruits sourced from local farms. Stephen's personal journey from the standard American diet to raw veganism inspires his menu. He seeks to share the physical and mental benefits he gained from a plant-forward diet while also showcasing the quality of Hawaii's organic produce with vibrant and flavorful dishes. *Pages 240–241*

NARINTR "NAT" RUENGSAMUTR was born in Bangkok, Thailand, and moved to the United States at 29 years old. She learned to cook from her mom, who cooked both in restaurants and at home. Her mother's specialty was curry, which Nat has learned to perfect (the secret, she says, is fresh chili paste). At her restaurant, Bulan Thai Vegetarian Kitchen in Los Angeles, 90 percent of her customers aren't vegetarian, but they enjoy her food because it's made with quality ingredients and robust flavors. *Pages 182–183*

SHERRY SAKATA was born in Japan's Hyogo Prefecture and raised in Osaka. She learned to cook from her father after her mother left the family when Sherry was six years old. After a career in computer animation and web design and founding her own company in Tokyo, she moved to the United States to raise her family after having triplets. Wanting to make better food, she studied at Le Cordon Bleu in Los Angeles for a year. She practices her kitchen skills at home, as well as cooking for 200 people at her Methodist church every month. *Pages 184–187*

SEAN SHERMAN, born in Pine Ridge, South Dakota, and better known as the Sioux Chef, is a member of the Oglala Lakota Sioux tribe. His culinary focus has been on the revitalization and awareness of Indigenous food systems in modern cuisine. He has shared his knowledge with crowds at Yale University, the Culinary Institute of America, and the United Nations, among other institutions. A recipient of the 2019 James Beard Leadership Award, he also won the James Beard Award for Best American Cookbook for *The Sioux Chef's Indigenous Kitchen.* His team at his nonprofit North American Traditional Indigenous Food Systems is working to make Indigenous foods more accessible to as many communities as possible. *Pages 48–51*

JASMINE SILVERSTEIN developed a passion for food during her personal journey of healing through diet and plant-based medicine. A certified master food preserver, chef, and caterer, she believes cooking is a way to connect more closely with her community in Hilo, Hawaii. When she's not working at her family's business, Sweet Cane Café, she tends to their organic garden or experiments with new recipes—ones without wheat, soy, GMOs, or refined ingredients. *Pages 56–59*

TAMMY MAHEALANI SMITH is the dietary manager of Lunalilo Home. She traces her lineage back 10 generations in Hakipu'u, a small *ahupua'a* on the island of Oahu. This is where the navigator Kaha'i is credited with bringing one of the first *ulu* trees to Hawaii from Samoa. Tammy honors this tradition as a keeper of ulu recipes and is introducing the food to a new generation. *Pages 52–53*

LAURA RHATMENY SOM is the executive director and founder of the MAYE Center, a wellness destination in Long Beach, California, that focuses on physical, spiritual, and community growth. Born in Cambodia, she was kidnapped and dropped off in an orphanage, where she learned to cook and farm. A refugee of the Cambodian genocide that lasted from 1975 to 1979, she opened the MAYE Center to help others find the tools for healing. At the center, they practice meditation, agriculture, yoga, and education. The urban farming she teaches allows the center's members to grow their own food and control their health and well-being. *Pages 198–199*

KRISSY SONG is the president and executive chef of Zip Banchan catering in Gardena, California. Her aim is to share Korean *banchan,* traditional small plates that are often very healthful. Though she is familiar with westernized fusion, she is committed to studying and cooking authentic and traditional Korean cuisine—and delivering it to American dinner tables. *Pages 200–203*

LYNETTE LO TOM is an enthusiastic home chef who has been cooking for more than 50 years—since her mother first asked her to prepare dinner for her five younger siblings. She grew up eating mainly Chinese food made by her mother in Hawaii, though she cooks cuisines from around the world and is often inspired by Japanese, Korean, and Vietnamese dishes. She shares her recipes on her website, lynettecooks.com, and is the author of three cookbooks: *A Chinese Kitchen: Traditional Recipes With an Island Twist, Back in the Day: Enjoy Hawai'i's Comfort Foods From Family and Friends,* and *Yum Yum Cha: Let's Eat Dim Sum in Hawai'i. Pages 154–155*

DIEGO TOSONI and his wife, Veronica Menin, not only share a love for each other but also for cycling, plant-based foods, and animals. So it was no surprise that they teamed up to start Love Life Café, a delicious and conscious food spot in Miami, Florida. A graduate of the T. Colin Campbell Center for Nutrition Studies, Diego is a self-trained cook who understands the relationship between the food on our plate and our health. He uses beautiful natural ingredients to achieve incredible flavors that make plant-based eating delicious. *Pages 134–137*

HAO TRAN is a culinary adventurer and one of four co-founders of The Table, a combined retail market and culinary studio in Fort Worth, Texas. She grew up in the Vietnamese community in South Arlington, Texas. As the daughter of immigrants, she spent her early years in her parents' home kitchen learning Southern Vietnamese cooking from her mother and the spicier Hue-style cooking from her father. She spent summers at her aunt's French Vietnamese restaurant in Montreal and developed a repertoire of classic and colonial dishes. A high school chemistry teacher, she juggles school with pop-up events, collaborative dinners, and cooking classes. *Pages 150–152*

YIA VANG was born in a Thai refugee camp, where he lived until his mother, Pang, and his family resettled in central Wisconsin. A trained chef, he uses his food at Union Hmong Kitchen in Minneapolis to tell a story. Sourced from what's in season and combining local traditions from his family, his cooking brings Hmong flavors to American palates and invites people to change how they think about food with every bite. He was named Chef of the Year by *MSP Magazine* in 2019 and Best Chef 2020 in *City Pages,* has appeared on nationalgeographic.com and CNN's *United Shades of America,* and is the host of the Twin Cities Public Television series *Relish. Pages 148–149*

ASHWIN VILKHU is the head chef, general manager, and beverage director of Saffron Nola. The James Beard Award–nominated family restaurant has garnered numerous accolades after creating its first brick-and-mortar location following 26 years as a catering business and six as a pop-up restaurant. The restaurant was born from his parents, Avinder and Pardeep, who immigrated to New Orleans from India and fell in love with the city's traditions and ingredients. Saffron Nola's menu is Indian at its core but inspired by flavors from around the globe. *Pages 174–181*

TESS VILLEGAS-RUMLEY is the chef and owner of Barefoot Zone in Kona, Hawaii. She aims to transform lives through food by teaching others to eat healthy, all in the aloha spirit. Her dishes are 100 percent plant-based, and she offers a weekly Facebook and Instagram Live cooking show, which is as full of energy as it is good flavors. *Pages 256–259*

JAMES WAYMAN is the executive chef of Oyster Club in Mystic, Connecticut, executive chef and partner of Nana's Bakery and Pizza and the Grass and Bone butcher shop and restaurant, and a founding member of Moromi Shoyu, an artisanal shoyu shop. He was born and raised on a farm just outside Greensboro, North Carolina, and his passion for nurturing the culinary community in southeastern Connecticut has made a significant impact on the local food economy. His restaurants have contributed to a rise in demand for hyperlocal, sustainable, and seasonal products and a more thoughtful approach to everyday eating. His mission is to continue to make a lasting impact on the broad food system. *Pages 230–233*

WILLIAM WOYS WEAVER is an internationally known food ethnographer and the author of 20 books, including *Flavors From the Garden: Heirloom Vegetable Recipes From Roughwood.* He is the founder of the Roughwood Table, a nonprofit organization devoted to heritage foods and heritage seeds. His grandfather H. Ralph Weaver established the Roughwood Seed Collection in 1932, the oldest private seed collection in the eastern United States, which houses the largest collection of Native American seeds in the country. William received his Ph.D. in ethnography from University College Dublin. *Pages 222–223*

BRAD WILLCOX is a professor and director of research in the Department of Geriatric Medicine at the John A. Burns School of Medicine, University of Hawaii at Manoa.

He trained in internal medicine at the Mayo Clinic and received his medical degree from the Division on Aging at Harvard Medical School. He is also a co-investigator of the Okinawa Centenarian Study and co-author of *The Okinawa Program. Pages 158–159*

ALAN WONG is a critically acclaimed chef known for his creative flair. A renowned master of Hawaii Regional Cuisine, he marries elements of different ethnic cooking styles using the finest island-grown ingredients. Born in Japan, he opened his first restaurant in Hawaii in 1989, where he started integrating cuisine from his home country with his French culinary background and Western cuisine. In 2015, his two Honolulu restaurants were inducted into the Hawaii Restaurant Association's Hall of Fame. *Pages 270–275*

CAROL WYNNE is a Mashpee Wampanoag culture keeper and Otter Clan mother. A tribal Elder, she shares her tribe's traditions and history through food, dance, and song. She celebrates traditional Wampanoag ingredients, including squash, hazelnuts, and dried blueberries, which she often cooks over an open fire. *Pages 36–37*

ANDREW ZIMMERN is an Emmy Award–winning and four-time James Beard Award–winning TV personality, chef, writer, and social justice advocate. Known for the Travel Channel's Bizarre Foods franchise, he is also the host of *Andrew Zimmern's Driven by Food, The Zimmern List, What's Eating America,* and *Wild Game Kitchen.* He has devoted his life to promoting cultural acceptance, tolerance, and understanding through food. He serves on City Harvest's Food Council and is a goodwill ambassador for the United Nations World Food Programme. A founding member of the Independent Restaurant Coalition, he resides in Minneapolis, Minnesota. *Page 235*

RECIPE INDEX

Boldface indicates illustrations

Acknowledgments

To Angelo and Irene Palermo and Henry and Madeline Buettner,
my grandparents, whose Blue Zones values imbue my life to this day.

This book required a shockingly enormous two-year effort by a multidisciplinary team of experts, many of whom put just as much time and effort into this as I did.

Our editor in chief, Naomi Imatome-Yun, oversaw the entire project, from shaping the recipes to the cover shoot. She somehow managed to shepherd this book to fruition while still holding down a full-time job with Blue Zones, LLC.

Producer Karen Foshay helped us track down America's best plant-based chefs in every city we visited. Her blend of fearlessness and resourcefulness got us into 65 kitchens, despite my ever shifting requests as the book evolved.

My chief of staff, Sam Skemp, managed the storm of details, from travel itineraries to archiving the recipes to conducting social media polls. Speaking of social media, I want to shout out my Instagram followers, who selected this cover for us. I consider you all collaborators.

At National Geographic, director of photography Adrian Coakley worked with David McLain to wade through more than 20,000 frames to choose the images for this book. Creative director Elisa Gibson created the stunning look and feel, and senior editor Allyson Johnson oversaw the entire process. I thank them, and my longtime friend, editorial director Lisa Thomas, for their painstaking collaboration on every facet of *The Blue Zones American Kitchen.*

I want to thank Remar Sutton and Mary Abbott Waite, who have been shaping my writing and encouraging me for four decades. Thanks for carving the roast, as it were.

When the idea for this book occurred to me, my first call was to former *Esquire* food editor Jeff Gordinier, who opened his Rolodex of America's best chefs and got me properly introduced. And to Marion Nestle, who helped connect me to food researcher James Malin. James spent more than 100 hours in the archives to underpin the book's premise with data.

At the Blue Zones office, I'd like to thank April Lunde, Aislinn Kotifani, Nick Buettner, Amelia Clabots, Danny Buettner-Salido, and especially CEO Ben Leedle for their support and logistical help.

Few get far in life without support from close friends. I want to thank Kevin Moore, Pilar Gerasimo, Tom Boesen, Varda Nauen, Rudy Maxa, Rob Perez, Ellie Andersen, and especially Stephanie Blanda for supporting me during the writing of this book.

At NBC, special thanks go to Cynthia McFadden and the enormously talented Jake Whitman for producing the Blue Zones Kitchen series for the *Today Show.*

David McLain would like to thank Raymond McLain for instilling a love of food and travel in me. Anne, Finn, and Myla McLain for being the best family I could ever wish for. Susan Welchman and José Azel for teaching me so much about photography over the decades. And Neal Manowitz, Matt Parnell, and Kayla Lindquist at Sony, the innovative company that built the cameras and lenses used to bring this book to life visually.

About the Blue Zones

Blue Zones employs evidence-based ways to help people live longer, better. Beginning in 2004, Dan Buettner teamed with National Geographic and the National Institute on Aging to identify pockets around the world where people lived measurably better, longer lives. After locating the world's blue zones, Buettner took teams of scientists to each location to pinpoint lifestyle characteristics that might explain the unusual longevity. The original researching and findings were released in Buettner's best-selling books *The Blue Zones, The Blue Zones Solution, Thrive,* and *The Blue Zones of Happiness.*

In 2009, Buettner and Blue Zones worked in partnerships with AARP and the United Health Foundation to apply the Blue Zones principles to Albert Lea, Minnesota. It was a "stunning success" and formed the blueprint for the Blue Zones Project, which has since expanded to 70 communities across the United States, impacting millions of people. This groundbreaking initiative has occasioned double-digit drops in obesity, smoking, and body mass index (BMI).

Learn more about the Blue Zones on Facebook (facebook.com/BlueZones) and Twitter and Instagram (@BlueZones), and at bluezones.com.

About the Author

DAN BUETTNER is the founder of Blue Zones, an organization that helps Americans live longer, healthier, happier lives. His groundbreaking work on longevity led to his 2005 *National Geographic* cover story "The Secrets of Long Life" and four national best-sellers: *The Blue Zones, Thrive, The Blue Zones Solution,* and the number one *New York Times* best-seller *The Blue Zones Kitchen.* He is also the author of *The Blue Zones of Happiness.* He lives in Miami, Florida. Find him on Instagram (@danbuettner) and at danbuettner.com.

About the Photographer

DAVID McLAIN is a Maine-based photographer and filmmaker whose work explores big questions through intimate stories. Over his career, he has shot seven feature-length assignments for *National Geographic,* co-produced and shot *Bounce,* a feature documentary that premiered at SXSW, and worked around the world for commercial clients including Sony and Apple. McLain has been collaborating with Dan Buettner for the past 20 years, including photographing the number one *New York Times* best-selling *The Blue Zones Kitchen.* He is a founding member of the Sony Artisan Program and lives with his wife and two children in a 220-year-old farmhouse in Maine.

Blue Zones American Kitchen

Since 1888, the National Geographic Society has funded more than 14,000 research, conservation, education, and storytelling projects around the world. National Geographic Partners distributes a portion of the funds it receives from your purchase to National Geographic Society to support programs including the conservation of animals and their habitats.

Get closer to National Geographic Explorers and photographers, and connect with our global community. Join us today at nationalgeographic.org/joinus

For rights or permissions inquiries, please contact National Geographic Books Subsidiary Rights: bookrights@natgeo.com

ISBN: 978-1-4262-2247-4

Printed in South Korea

22/SPSK/2